AF443162

Lameness
In Cattle

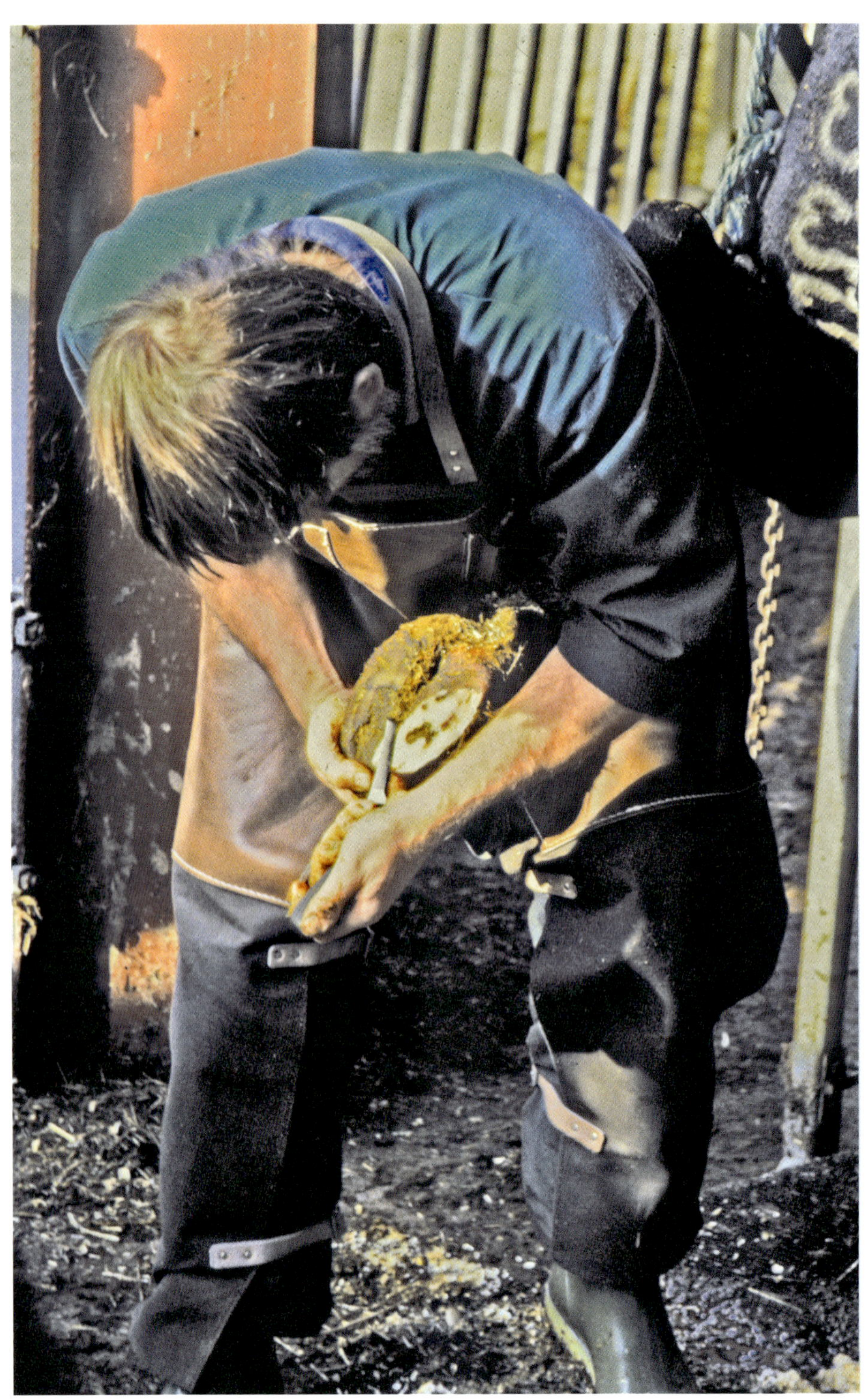

Lameness In Cattle

Chris Watson

Foreword by David Logue

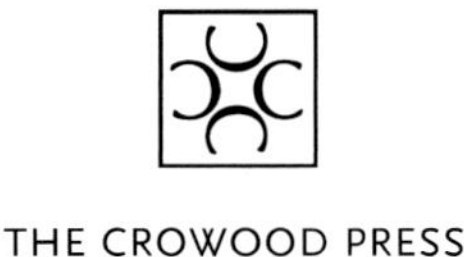

THE CROWOOD PRESS

First published in 2007 by
The Crowood Press Ltd
Ramsbury, Marlborough
Wiltshire SN8 2HR

www.crowood.com

British Library Cataloguing-in-Publication Data
A catalogue record for this book is available from the British Library.

ISBN 978 1 86126 905 8

Acknowledgements
I am very grateful to all my colleagues in the practice who have spent many hours with me discussing lameness and the best ways to deal with it. My clients have been more than patient whilst I took photographs instead of getting on with the job, and my wife has been extremely patient whilst I have been writing this book. She has put in a lot of hard work correcting my use of the English language. I am also very grateful to Keith Cutler who, despite being quite capable of writing the text himself, instead offered to do the more difficult task of commenting and correcting someone else's approach to the subject.

Disclaimer
The author and the publisher do not accept any responsibility in any manner whatsoever for any error or omission, nor any loss, damage, injury or liability of any kind incurred as a result of the use of any of the information contained in this book, or reliance upon it.

Typeset in Century Schoolbook by Bookcraft Ltd, Stroud, Gloucestershire

Printed and bound in Singapore by Craft Print International Ltd

Contents

Foreword

Chris Watson has a wealth of experience in farm animal practice in Gloucestershire and in this readable yet comprehensive book he shares this with all those who are interested in lameness in cattle. The book has been written with herdsmen and veterinary students in mind, but others more experienced in lameness would benefit from reading it. Lameness, especially in dairy cattle, is rightly considered a welfare problem and, as detailed in Chapter 2, it has a considerable economic impact. I particularly liked the pragmatic approach to lesion management; it is clear that this is based on first-hand experience. Readers must remember that the use of antibiotic foot-baths for the treatment of digital dermatitis is generally frowned upon and even banned by some countries. In the UK the statutory interpretation is that where the antibiotic is used 'off label', the milk from treated animals should be withheld from human consumption for 7 days – a requirement that astonishes most farmers. I enjoyed reading the section on the environment in Chapter 9 and the emphasis on the importance of thinking holistically about the herd. The author returns to this theme in the final chapter, which offers sound advice on how to approach a herd problem. In my opinion he identifies the main areas of approach, although I have to confess I have not tried vinegar on cows newly introduced to the milking herd to prevent 'bullying'. Since I have just heard and read how concentrated chilli extract can stop marauding elephants, it's probably worth a try.

David Logue

Introduction

Lameness in cattle is an ongoing struggle for most producers, who are forced to confine cattle on concrete either to meet the demands of modern agricultural production or during the winter period simply to protect grazing from poaching. The problem is most acute for the dairy producer where the demands of milk production put a significant strain on the animal along with the effects of housing and management, which are unfortunately a consequence of modern milk production. For this reason most of this book is targeted at the dairy cow, although the principles are the same for all other cattle. Beef producers who are reliant on suckled calf production are starting to see many lameness problems appear in breeding stock as units become larger and more intensive. Diseases such as digital dermatitis are now a significant part of the suckled cow's health issues and many producers are now looking at control measures that have until recently been the remit of the dairy herd.

Lameness is the third most important disease of the dairy cow after infertility and mastitis. It is both a significant economic disease and a welfare issue, especially for the dairy cow. In 1997 the Farm Animal Welfare Council identified lameness as the most important welfare problem facing the dairy industry. Lameness is very painful for the cow, causing reduced milk yield, loss of body weight, poor fertility, significant treatment costs, and the risk of premature culling from the herd. Many surveys looking at the problem have shown a lameness incidence of around 25 per cent of cows in the herd affected annually. However, more thorough surveys have shown that the true annual incidence of lameness in dairy herds is around 50 per cent, or 50 cases of lameness per 100 cows in the herd. The Reading University team, in their report on the economics of lameness, showed that the direct cost of lameness is, at 1998 prices, £50 per case with a further cost of £86 for all the indirect costs that occur (fertility and culling etc.), which means that each average lame foot is costing £136. On a herd basis this amounts to £40 for every cow being lost due to the effects of lameness. An affected dairy cow will lose around 400ltr of milk production due to the disease and this works out at around 0.7 pence per litre off the milk price, which is more than most farms spend on their total veterinary and health care for the herd. This is only the average figure; the range of lameness incidence seen on farms shows that potential losses are enormous for some units. The best herds manage to achieve lameness incidence levels of less than 10 per cent compared with some herds that have incidence levels of over 100 per cent.

A recent survey of manpower in the dairy industry showed that in the six years up to 2003 labour input has dropped from 4.3 hours per 1000ltr produced to 3.2 hours. This means that the opportunity costs on a herdsperson's time are very high and dealing with lame cows is a significant burden for the stockperson, taking valuable time away from other tasks.

I have spent over thirty years dealing with lame cows in cattle practice. Dealing with the individual lame cow is rewarding when you can apply the right skills and treatment to produce satisfactory results. However, it is easy to become absorbed in individuals and lose sight of the overall herd. Herd problems can be significantly reduced by the use of inexpensive prevention regimes along with sensible cattle husbandry and good environmental management and design.

This book aims to help both the stockperson and the professional address the immediate need for individual treatment and how to develop and apply future herd control strategies. Many of the skills are common to both groups of people and even though some techniques such as surgery are going to be professional tasks, the herdsperson should appreciate what treatment options are available and what action is required.

Good recording is an essential management tool in reducing lameness by targeting resources and effort. Also important is a thorough understanding of what produces lameness and what principles can be applied sensibly to prevent the disease or significantly reduce it.

If we are to create a credible health programme for cattle lameness, we need to have a commitment to 'completing the circle'. We initially need to use good records and accurate diagnosis along with methodical investigations to be able to promote 'best practice' for the foot care of a herd. We then need to use ongoing monitoring to make sure that the protocols adopted actually produce results, which brings us back full circle to the assessment stage again. This is the difference between active *health initiatives* and what we are often faced with in practice – *health assurance*. We need to promote the former and not simply settle for the latter.

Chris Watson
May 2006

CHAPTER ONE

Form and Function –
How and Why the Foot Works

INTRODUCTION

To successfully treat and prevent lameness requires a thorough understanding of the structure of the bovine foot and how it works. Normal and abnormal changes arising within the foot affect the way it functions, often producing lameness. Appreciating the details of the 'form and function' of the bovine foot will give an insight into why lesions occur, as well as providing us with the expertise necessary to treat and, more importantly, prevent them.

EVOLUTION OF THE BOVINE FOOT

Cattle are ungulates (hoofed animals) that originally evolved to graze on large open grasslands or plains. The structure of the bovine foot has developed to meet the basic requirements of this original environment. This lifestyle required that an ungulate had to carry a large abdomen to cope with digesting plant material (the rumen in the bovine) and had to be fast on its feet to escape predators on the open plains. Therefore the ungulate foot had to adapt to support this large abdominal weight and yet ensure the animal could make a rapid escape if predators were present – the 'flight' response.

There is a physical advantage in taking weight on a small area at the extreme tip of the foot. A human athlete, when sprinting,

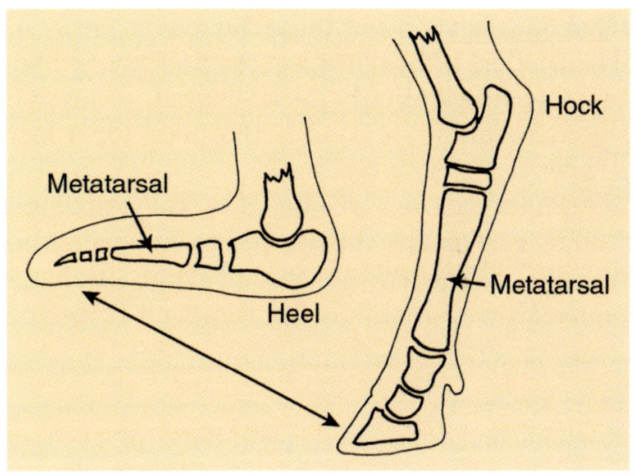

The arrangement of bones in a human and a bovine hindlimb to show the bovine taking weight on the toe and creating a longer stride for speed.

will rise up onto the tips of the toes and run with little or no contact with the back of the foot. This stance creates more leverage and enables the athlete to extend the length of the limb, which increases the stride length and gives the speed required. This principle has been adopted by ungulates such as the bovine to give them speed, but this must be balanced with the necessity to carry a large abdominal weight. The foot has adapted to meet these requirements by first reducing the number of digits and then changing the shape of the foot to bring the animal's weight up onto the toes. Combining some bones into a single, larger structure, therefore losing digits, gives strength, whilst rising up onto the toes extends the limb and produces the speed required.

This evolutionary process started with the loss of the large first digit or 'thumb' altogether and progressively the outer two digits started to reduce in size and no longer played a role in weight bearing. These digits are clearly seen today in bovines as vestigial accessory digits above the fetlock area. The centre two digits became enlarged and formed the typical cloven hoof of the bovine group so that the whole weight is taken down through the leg on a single bone column and ends up at the tips of the two remaining digits. These digits have become covered in horn to protect them from damage and to enable the foot to perform its function of bearing weight and being able to move the animal quickly, what is known as 'cursorial adaptation' – the need for a fast getaway!

Adaptation has produced a very specialized foot to enable the animal to function and become successful in its original environment. However, this is far removed from the present-day surroundings in which we keep the majority of our cattle, especially during the winter. The present bovine has a foot that is not adapted to the current demands we place on the animal, and this is almost certainly why lameness is such a major disease issue.

SKIN STRUCTURE

The end of each foot is covered with a piece of specialized skin – the hoof – that consists primarily of a protein called keratin, arranged into a specific pattern to form horn. To understand how the hoof is constructed we need to look at skin, as hoof is simply a specialized piece of skin that has been modified to do a specific job.

Skin is made up of two basic layers:

1. The outer epidermis. This is normally a thin structure that is mostly dead or dying cells that are constantly being worn away at the surface and being replaced from below. It is this layer that becomes modified to create the many specific structures that are associated with the outer layer of the skin – hairs, feathers, glands and, most important in this case, the horn that comprises the hoof of the cow. The lower layers of the epidermis (the stratum germinativum) are responsible for the continuous supply of cells that move outwards to form the outer layer as the epidermis loses surface cells. As cells move outwards they die, become flattened and are cornified or keratinized, which means they have keratin laid down in them to make them hard and resistant to wear. The degree of keratinization varies according to where the skin is found and what function it has to perform.

2. The inner dermis (or corium as it is referred to in the hoof). This is the 'support' structure that looks after the nerves and blood vessels that allow the epidermis to form and survive. It is an insulating layer between

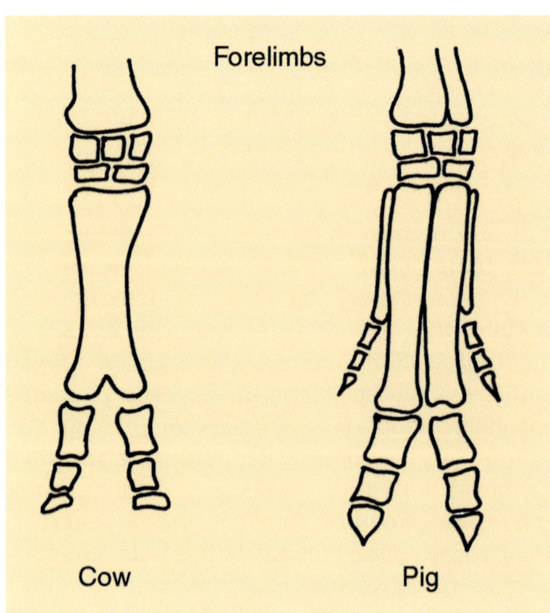

A comparison of the forelimbs of a cow and a pig to show the adaptation of the limb towards an ungulate way of life – less digits and single leg bones.

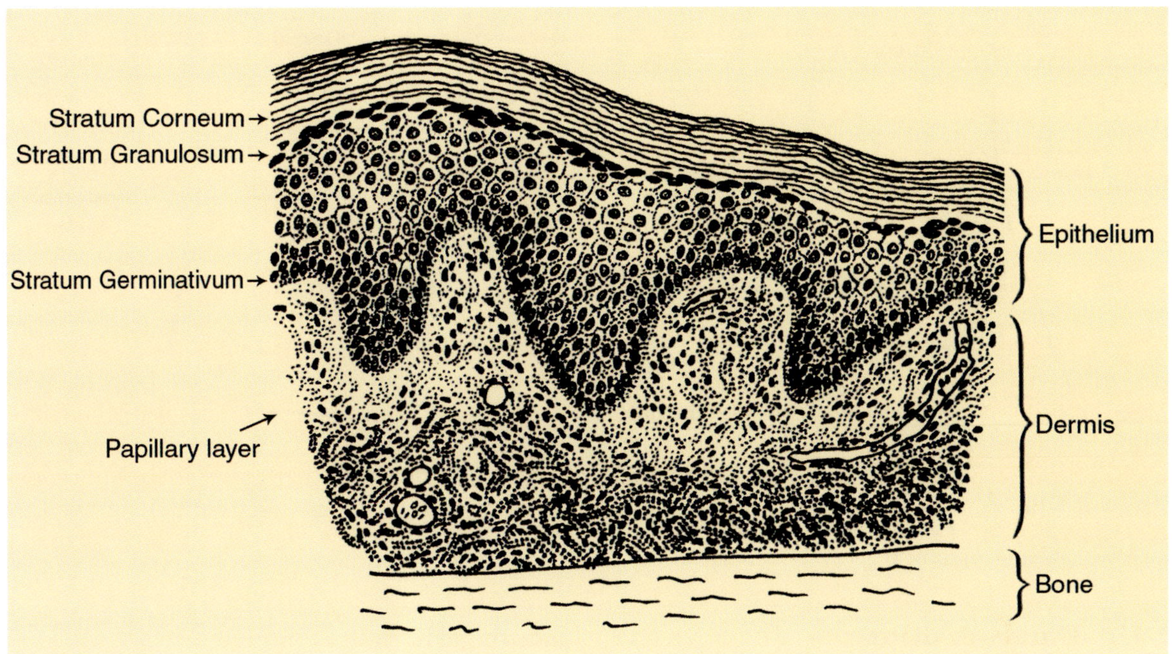

A section through a piece of skin to show the different cell layers. Note the large undulating surface that joins the two layers together.

the epidermis and the bone. When it is present in thick sections such as in the foot it forms a deeply indented pattern called dermal papillae ('fingers'), enabling blood vessels to come into closer contact with the outer epidermis, thereby forming a much closer union between the two layers. This principle is used extensively in the foot to support horn production.

In simple terms the horn of the hoof is skin that has been specially keratinized. This process is not random but occurs in an organized way to allow horn to wear and ensure it fulfils its function of being strong and protective, yet allowing some movement.

Horn preserves many features that we see in skin. Not only is it continually wearing away and being formed, but it allows water movement through from the surface, causing the horn to become harder when it dries out and softer and more supple when water is retained. It also has nerves closely associated with it that induce pain and hence lameness. Pigment cells are present so that the horn is coloured randomly with dark areas.

STRUCTURE OF THE FOOT

General

We need to be precise when using terms to describe the various structures and areas of the foot. This necessitates looking at the anatomy of the foot in detail and the language used to describe it.

There are basically four parts to the structure of the foot:

1. The hoof, which is made of a horn casing.
2. The corium underneath.
3. The bones of the leg in this area – the pedal bone and navicular bone.
4. The joints, ligaments and synovial structures (sheaths and bursae).

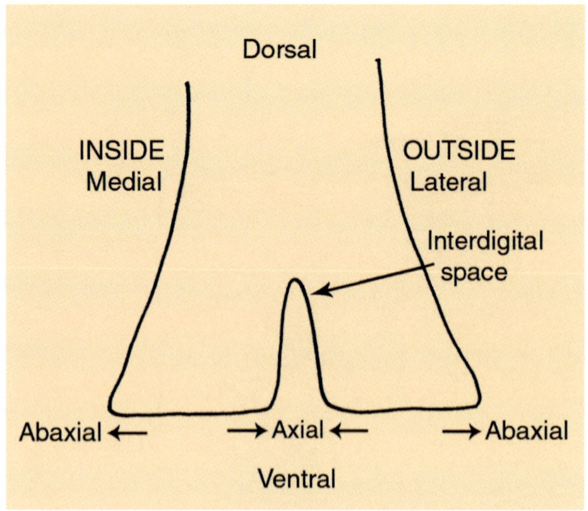

A hind view of a foot showing the various terms used to describe areas of it.

A side view of a foot to show the various terms used to describe it.

Skin–Horn Junction

The skin of the leg joins with horn at the coronary band and the bulbs of the heel. Both are covered with a soft waxy type of horn (periople) that is pliable and forms a functional transition between mobile skin and more rigid horn. Its function is to allow movement between the skin and the horn as the animal walks and also to secrete a waxy coat over the horn that helps to regulate water content of the horn. If this wax coat is intact and covers the horn surface, water is retained

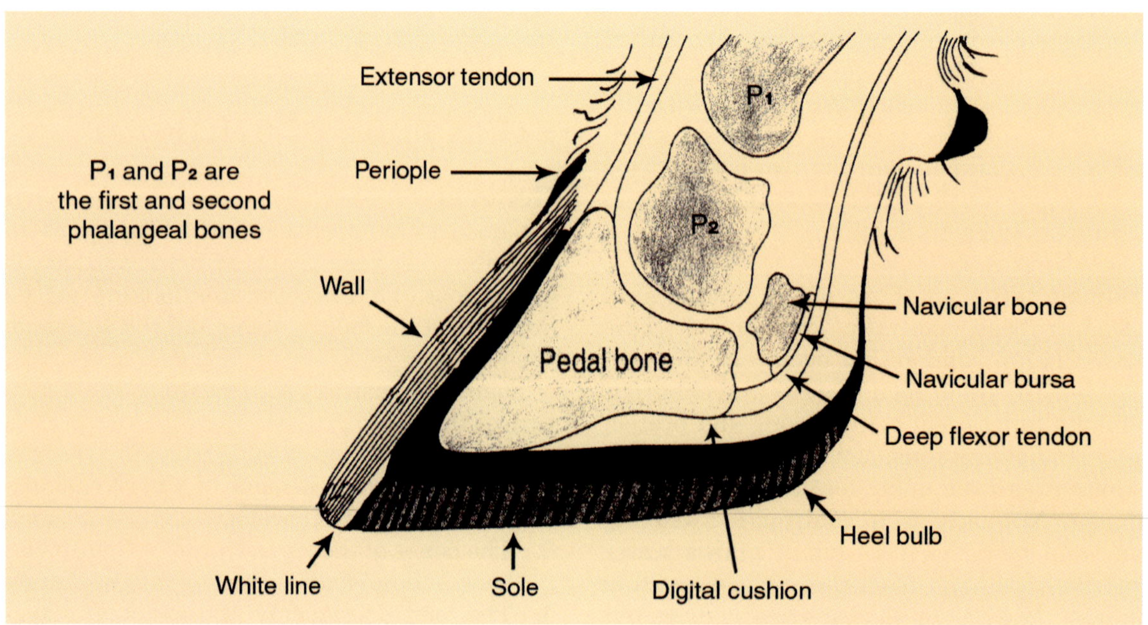

A section through the foot to show the main structures.

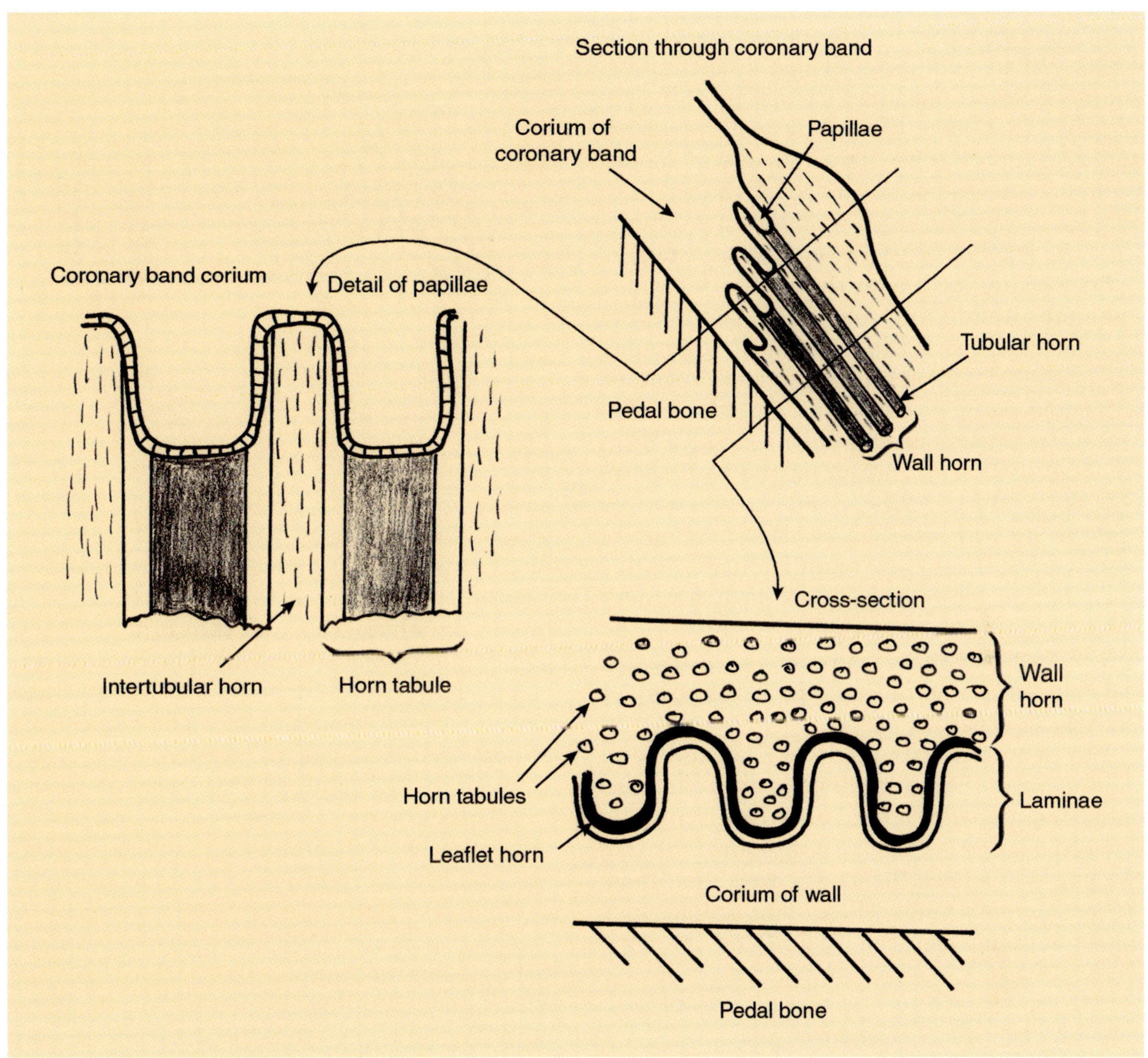

(Left) A cross-section across the papillae of the corium showing how horn tubules are formed. (Top right) A detailed longitudinal section through the coronary band to show how the wall horn is formed. (Bottom right) A cross-section of the hoof wall to show how the horn structure fits onto the laminae.

and the horn becomes more supple and soft. If the wax is thin or is removed by wear, water loss increases and the horn becomes hard and brittle. Both of these conditions can be problematic and it is essential to try to manipulate the water content of the horn to get the right balance.

Wall

Horn is not simply a layer of epidermal cells that have been keratinized to harden them, as would be the case with a footpad in, for instance, a dog or cat. To gain strength and perform well the horn is formed into distinct structures to form a hard layer that can support the foot and cope with constant wear from contact with the ground as the animal walks. When building a bridge a mechanical engineer would use steel formed into girders or tubes that have inherently more strength and are lighter than simple sheets of metal. In much the same way horn is shaped into tubules to give strength with lightness, along with the efficient use of essential materials.

The corium just below the coronary band is distinctly undulating and forms pronounced papillae or 'fingers' that manufacture tubular horn. These tubules are then 'glued' together with non-specific horn (intertubular horn) and grow outwards and downwards to form the hoof wall. The corium on the wall of the hoof below the coronary band is also strongly undulating with papillae, as described above. However, it does not manufacture tubular horn but forms a large area of attachment bonding the horn very tightly to the corium. The more tissue there is in contact the greater the grip, so an undulating junction is stronger than a flat sheet.

The undulating structure of the papillae in the corium of the hoof wall is arranged in folds called laminae. The laminae run longitudinally down the length of the horn wall and look like the pages of a book, hence the word 'laminae' – the leaves of a book. These regular folds give added grip between the corium and the horn

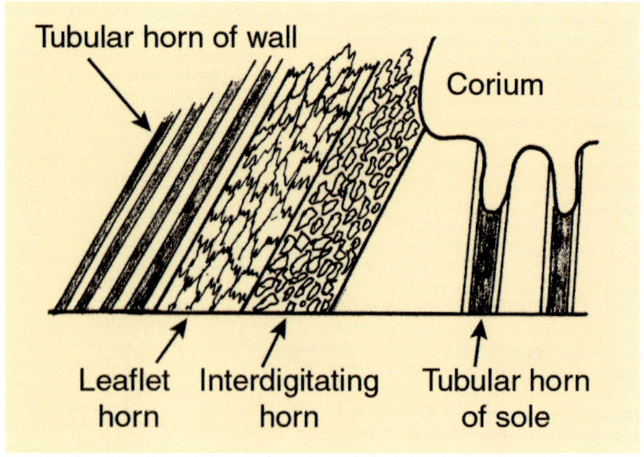

A more detailed section of the white line area.

by forming a tight joint – almost like a dovetail joint in a piece of furniture. This longitudinal pattern also allows horn to slip slowly downhill as it wears at the floor surface and is replaced with new horn at the coronary band, pushing horn down the wall. The growth rate of horn is around 5mm per month and the total length covered means that a complete change of hoof wall horn occurs approximately every 15 months. The laminae of the corium form a small quantity of loose horn that is designed to lubricate the horn tubules as they move down the wall over the laminae. This horn is known as the leaflet horn.

If you look at a human fingernail, you can see the laminae under the surface as faint white lines running down the length of the nail. There is the same progression of horn from the pale bed of the nail cuticle (equivalent to the coronary band) down to the nail edge where it wears away or is regularly trimmed off.

Sole

The horn of the sole is fashioned in the same way as the horn of the wall, by the papillae of the solar corium, and like the horn of the wall it is formed as clusters of tubules. However, these tubules grow directly outwards towards the solar surface and thus do not need to pass over laminae, as does the horn wall. The horn of the sole is around 10–15mm thick and as it wears away it is replaced at the same rate as

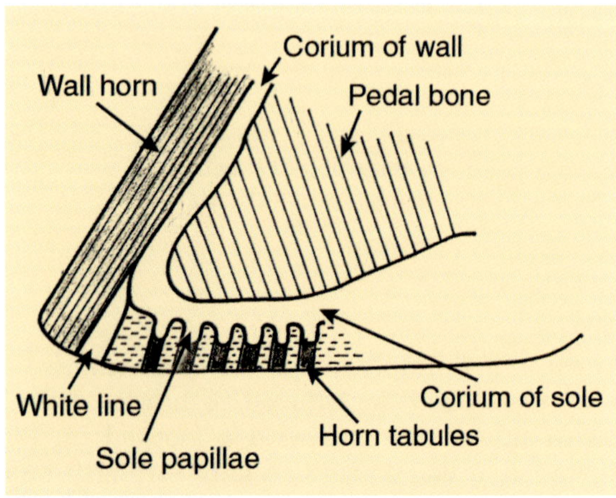

A section through the sole area showing the formation of horn from the solar papillae.

the wall horn (5mm per month), but because it passes out vertically the complete change occurs approximately every 100 days.

The white line is the distinct pale horn that is seen around the edge of the sole where it meets the horn of the wall. The white line extends right round the foot as far as the wall limits, as shown in the diagram on page 18. The area of weight bearing occurs where the tough tubular horn of the wall comes into contact with the ground surface at the white line area. The white line itself is composed of both leaflet horn that has been 'sliding' down the laminae, lubricating the horn of the wall, and a small area of horn produced between the wall and the sole that is known as interdigitating horn. The white line has evolved to allow some 'give' at this junction and permit movement of the pedal bone up and down within the casing of the wall horn. However, this 'give' can also be a weak point in the design of the foot because, if the white line is damaged, foreign material may enter the foot. White line horn is the softest horn produced in the hoof and as such it is more prone to fissures.

The heel or bulbs of the heel are found at the posterior aspect of the sole. They are composed of softer horn that forms the boundary between skin proper and the horn of the sole. The heels have sacks of fat and elastic tissue under them, which is an adaptation of the corium in this area. This forms a shock-absorbing mechanism that works like a damper being squashed and released as the foot comes into contact with the ground. It is known as the digital cushion. This compression area may also have a role to play in blood circulation in the foot, preventing it from pooling and damaging tissues. Blood that pools contains less oxygen and nutrients and this could damage tissues in the area that are relying on a fresh supply of nutrients for normal growth and horn production.

Bones and Joints

The bones of the foot are the mechanism by which weight is ultimately transferred from the animal's body to the floor to allow it to stand and move normally. These bones are arranged in such a way as to give strength and yet allow movement through the joints. This is necessary not only to allow bending of the limb but also to absorb the shock of taking weight on a solid surface. The main bone in the foot is the pedal bone (or third phalangeal bone), which is the final point of contact with the ground and is fully encased in the horn.

Each foot of the cow has to take the entire animal's body weight on just two digits, and only at the end of each digit (in a standing human the weight is taken on several bones as a flat-shaped foot). The pedal bone fits snugly into the hoof where it rests tightly at the tip of the hoof. It is suspended within the horn case of the foot by the corium of the wall – through the connective tissues and the laminae joints along the length of the wall. There is also a 'hammock' arrangement of ligaments from

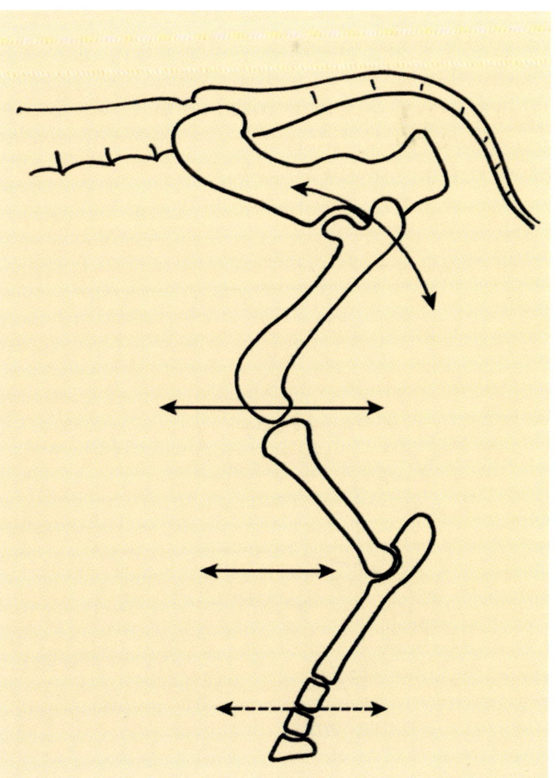

A diagram of the bones of the hindlimb and how they flex to take the animals weight. Part of the 'shock absorption' system.

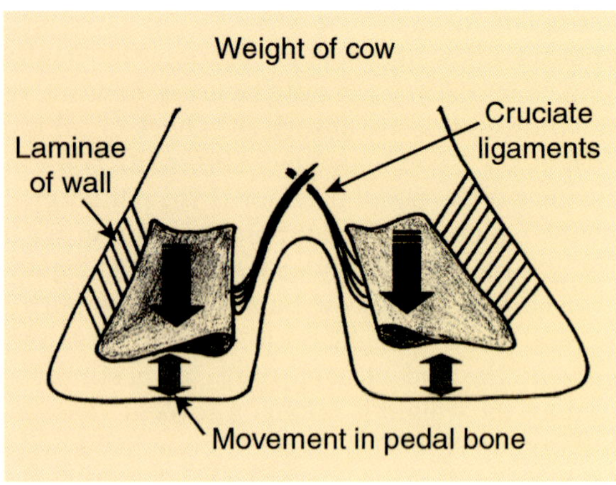

The hammock arrangement of ligaments supports the pedal bone but allows some up and down movement.

the interdigital space (the cruciate ligaments). This attachment of the pedal bone is designed to shift slightly when the foot takes weight, so preventing damage to the bones and the joints above. The pedal bone will move down somewhat as weight is taken. The shape of the pedal bone and its position in the hoof means that if this downward shift is too great then

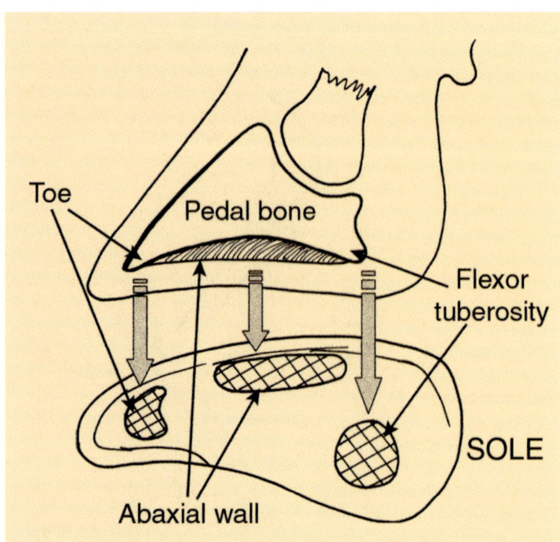

The pedal bone movement can be enough to press on the corium of the sole at specific points.

there is the potential for damage to occur.

The key impact points for the pedal bone are:

- the flexor process at the rear edge of the bone,
- where the toe arches down and comes close to the sole at the front and
- where it is cupped so that the outside (abaxial) edge takes most of the weight down on to the sole.

Tendons

Movement of the foot is achieved by a flexing of the joints that is controlled through the muscle mass higher in the leg. This force is transmitted down to the foot via a series of

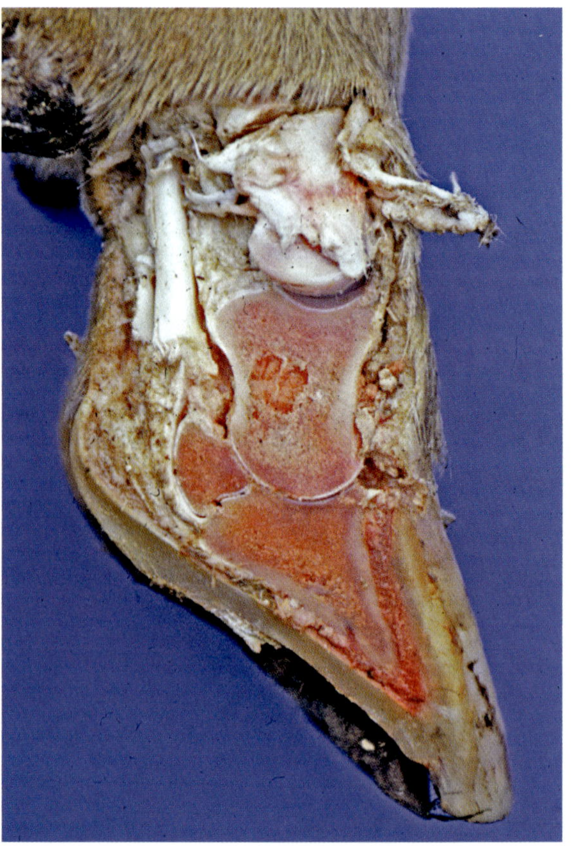

A section through a cow's leg shows the structures of the foot. The deep digital flexor tendon is obvious as a large white band at the back of the foot.

tendons extending down to the hoof. These tendons fall into two groups:

1. The extensor tendons extend down the anterior aspect of the leg and foot and connect onto the pedal bone at its uppermost edge.
2. The flexor tendons extend down the back of the leg and join, via the navicular bone, to the bottom of the pedal bone at the back. They attach at a distinct point called the flexor tuberosity. The navicular bone acts like a pulley to allow the tendon to bend round a corner as it passes from the straight leg round the curve of the pedal joint to the pedal bone itself.

These tendons pass through a series of sheaths and run over sacs of fluid called bursae, which lubricate them and allow them to act without damaging themselves or the bones and tissue they run over.

HOW THE COW WALKS

We have now covered the basics of how the foot is constructed and how the individual elements of it function. The ability of the cow to use all these elements in moving around is the final stage in combining form and function of the leg. Looking at the way a cow actually uses all these elements should enable us

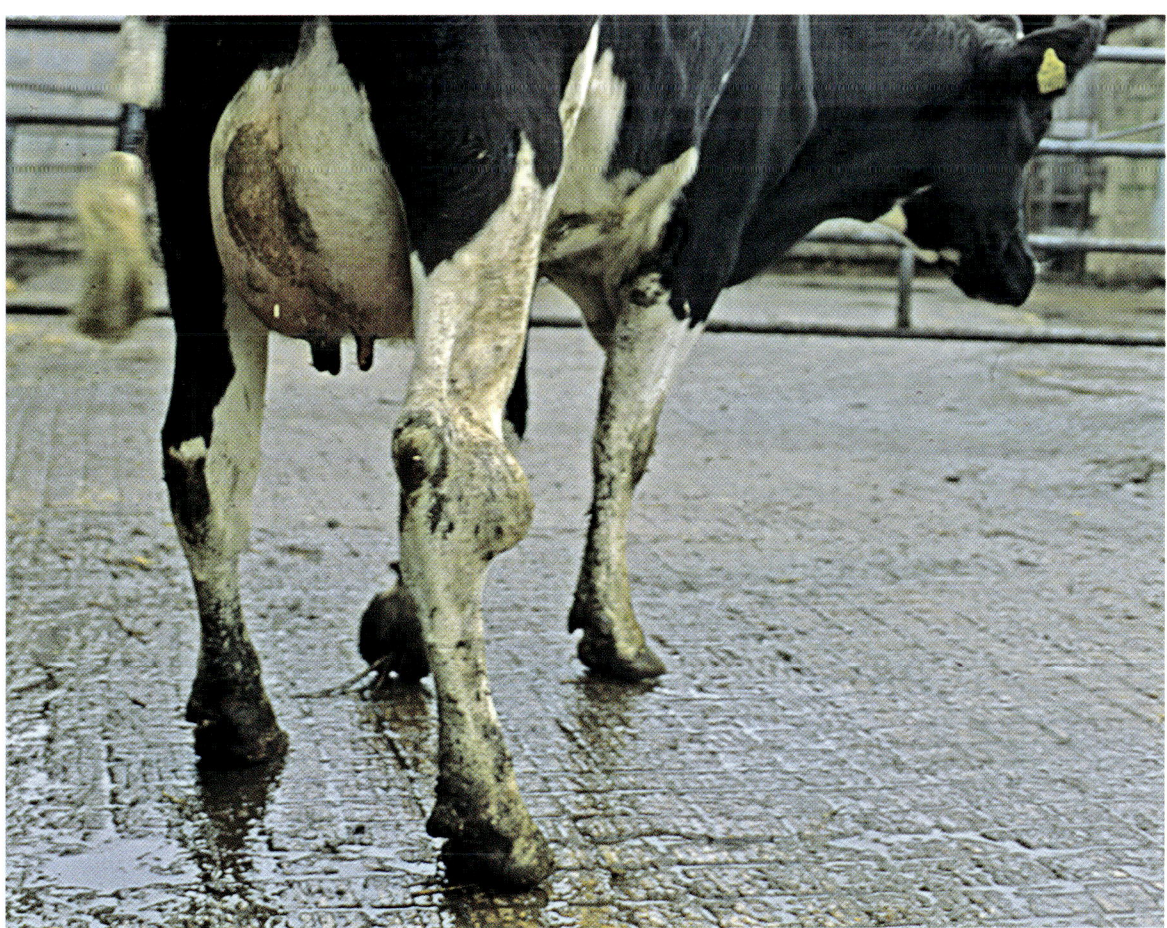

How is weight distributed when a cow walks?

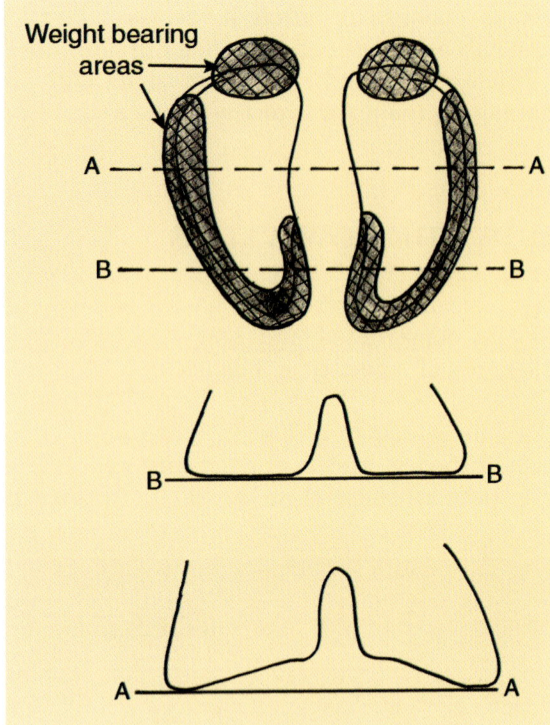

A view of the sole shows where weight is taken during normal movement. The sections A and B indicate the cross-section shape of the sole at these points. Note that the toe area is flat.

to understand why things go wrong and why a cow shows lameness when various parts of the process fail. First, it is worth going through the cycle of movement to understand the normal actions involved before starting to look at disease processes.

The act of walking begins when the heel of the foot contacts the ground. The heel horn is softer and elastic so it stretches and distorts to absorb the animal's weight on initial impact with the ground. The fat pad in the heel (digital cushion) then distorts under pressure to take up more of the weight, much like the shock absorbers of a vehicle. The weight then reaches the hoof wall around the abaxial edge of the hoof and part of the axial surface.

The sole should be concave and therefore non- weight bearing. This means that most weight is taken on the wall of the hoof and is transmitted through the laminae supporting the horn to the pedal bone. Although the laminae are the primary attachment of the corium to the horn, ultimately weight is eventually taken through the various connective tissues of the corium that join the laminae to the bone structure. Once weight is taken onto the hoof wall the pedal bone 'sinks' in its hammock arrangement as it transfers the weight directly up the bones of the leg via the various joints involved. These joints and tendons complete the process by moving, bending and 'giving' to take up the weight without producing too much impact shock that could damage the leg.

DISEASE PROCESSES

Now that we have considered the normal form and function of the foot, we need to relate this to the types of disease and injury we see in lame cows. How is the structure affected by disease? We will deal with the specific diseases in later chapters, but here we consider the common set of circumstances involved in the way foot lesions are formed.

General

One of the main issues with the bovine foot is that most of the damage and horn lesions we see externally are derived from weaknesses that occur within the foot itself.

The pedal bone moves up and down inside the horn casing of the claw as part of the normal process of supporting and transferring weight. If the pedal bone attachment is disrupted in any way, it becomes loosened and there will be excessive movement of the bone downwards onto the delicate structures in the corium below. This loosening normally occurs at calving to some degree, and it predisposes the foot to damage from other factors. These factors usually involve the environment and management of the cow, and it is this combination of events that may go on to produce lameness. The process can be split up into three clear stages:

Stage 1. Disruption in the tissues of the claw.
Stage 2. The pedal bone sinks.
Stage 3. Lesions are formed.

Stage 1.
The 'Disruption' Theory – Coriosis

There have been arguments over the nature of this disruption for many years and the answer is still far from clear. Originally the theory was that the primary lesion was due to 'laminitis'. Laminitis is specifically an inflammation of the laminae of the horn wall that causes the pedal bone to loosen from the wall and sink in the foot. There are many descriptions of this disease in the literature on horses, where it can be a severe and common disease. True laminitis in cattle is very rare. Occasionally beef cattle on very high concentrate diets (barley beef systems) present with a severe tenderness of all four feet and this laminitis is due to the effects of grain fermentation in the rumen. In dairy cows laminitis is extremely rare. It can be seen after a bout of severe illness such as mastitis, where it often induces an effect in all four feet with a severe disruption to horn growth. This creates a fault line in the wall (horizontal fissure) that is often seen growing out some months later (*see* Chapter 5).

If true laminitis is very rare, and not the clinical picture we see in most cases of lameness, the next suggestion is that the effect could be a 'subclinical laminitis'. The assumption is that there are subtle changes occurring to the laminae that could cause less obvious clinical signs of laminitis but still predispose the foot to other damage that could cause lameness. Again the actual effect seen in the bovine foot does not involve the laminae of the horn wall, so the anatomical use of this term is incorrect.

The primary tissue to be affected is the corium. There appears to be a breakdown in the connective tissues in the corium, hence the best technical term for it may be coriosis – a dysfunction of the corium.

Possible Causes of Coriosis

It is not clear exactly what is happening and why, so we must wait for further research to address what and where the weakest link is in the disruption of claw horn. There are, however, two general theories:

1. The endotoxins theory. During the period around calving there are major changes to the feeding of the dairy cow. These changes cause the release of metabolites and possibly endotoxins as the rumen adapts to lactation. It is proposed that these products induce changes in the blood circulation to the foot and damage the tissues of the foot in a process similar to 'laminitis'. There is no evidence to support this theory and attempts to reproduce it have been largely unsuccessful.
2. The collagen theory. Collagen is an important tissue in the corium. It is ultimately responsible for connecting the hoof to the pedal bone. It is proposed that the hormones of parturition could weaken the matrix of suspensory collagen in the corium, especially in hoof wall, and cause the disruption necessary to allow the pedal bone to loosen and move. It has been suggested that there may be a biochemical change due to an enzyme mediator, 'hoofase', that breaks down the collagen between the corium and the pedal bone.

At present it is perhaps more useful to talk in terms of a 'disruption' to the basic tissues and structures that suspend the pedal bone within the horn capsule and avoid too much scientific debate.

Stage 2.
The Effects of Disruption

Disruption of the support mechanism of the pedal bone will allow it to loosen from its position and 'sink' inside the horn casing. It will then press onto the corium of the sole and may put some side pressure onto the walls, causing the white line to become weaker. This means that the potential impact sites we described above for the pedal bone may become badly damaged by pressure on the corium at these points. The attachment of the pedal bone is much stronger on the abaxial wall horn (through the laminae) than it is on the axial wall because there are not as many laminae. This causes the pedal bone to rotate as well as sink, especially in the axial area (adjacent to the interdigital space), and compresses the corium axially (*see* Chapter 5).

Stage 3.
The Formation of Lesions

A cascade effect is initiated, with other factors (environmental, management etc.) adding pressure to the sole area. These effects control how much damage is done to the hoof and whether lameness occurs. The circumstances the cow finds itself in dictate whether damage to the claw becomes severe enough to cause lameness. The most important issues are the effects of the environment, management and nutrition, which we will address in more detail in Chapter 9.

What happens when the corium becomes damaged? First, the damage is usually to the germinal layer of the solar corium and it may be many weeks before it shows, as it takes time for the effects of this to grow out and cause changes in the surface horn. The basic lesions are due to compression of the corium and this shows primarily as haemorrhage and the formation of poorer quality horn. The horn cells being laid down start to show degenerative changes:

- Damaged cell walls. This will result in a lot of debris in the area, with various bits and pieces of cells.
- Poorer keratinization. The horn will be softer.
- Large spaces between cells – loosely packed. Cellular disruption means that cells are not laid down in a tightly ordered fashion, which is what gives the horn its strength.
- Blood and debris between cells. This will move the cells apart as blood and serum are released from damaged blood vessels.
- Bacteria are sometimes seen invading the spaces.

The horn created from the germinal layer of the corium will be weaker and therefore more structural damage may occur. The overall effect is to allow specific lesions to occur in the horn of the claw and so cause lameness. These effects are seen clinically as:

- Yellow soft horn. The horn is friable and damaged easily; the yellow colour is caused by serum leaking out from between the horn cells after damage to the blood vessels.
- Haemorrhage. The blood vessels are damaged enough to leak blood that clots and becomes incorporated into the horn.
- Double sole. There is enough cellular debris from the damaged corium to separate the sole into layers as it grows towards the surface. These separations can under-run to the heel or axial surface and allow infection in.
- Fissures can form at the white line due to poor-quality horn, which then opens up

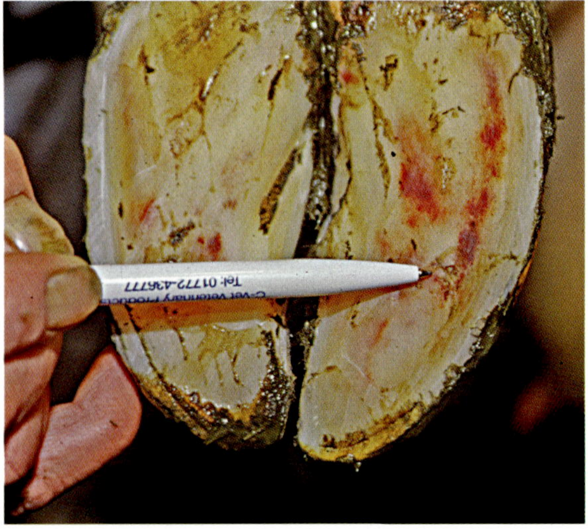

A view of the sole showing haemorrhages in the key areas associated with the pedal bone moving (see page 16).

and allows infection and foreign material in.

- Ulcerations of the solar horn. If the horn is of poor quality, the whole thickness of the sole in that area is lost and the underlying corium is exposed.
- Deformed horn. Horn production at the coronary band is also affected and shows the typical stress lines or hardship grooves. These can cause abnormal horn growth (*see* page 22).

The above lesions give rise to a list of potential claw diseases that produce lameness.

- Solar haemorrhage and bruising.
- White line disease.
- Solar ulcer.
- Heel ulcer.
- Toe ulcer.
- Solar penetration.

Lesions occurring in the first lactation are also likely to incur changes in the foot that predispose the animal to the risk of further lameness in subsequent lactations. Once a pedal bone has loosened and sunk, compressing the corium, it never regains its original position. This not only creates abnormal horn growth for the rest of the cow's life but also predisposes it to further bouts of lameness. A lameness incident in the first lactation makes the cow three times as likely to have lameness in later lactations. For example, cows with solar ulcers in one lactation will more frequently suffer from them in future lactations.

HORN GROWTH

Horn is being constantly laid down and worn away in a natural cycle aimed at always providing support and protection for the hoof. The rate of growth is approximately 5mm per month, enabling us to calculate when new horn growth reaches the wearing surface of the wall (15 months) or the sole (100 days). We need to understand the difference between normal and abnormal processes of the horn growth cycle because these growth patterns will, and often do, affect lameness incidence.

Normal Horn Growth

Horn growth shows consistent seasonal variations in both proliferation and keratinization – higher activity in summer and lower activity in winter. This most likely relates to the original need of the bovine in the wild when, during the summer, it was more likely to be on hard, dry surfaces and subject to increased wear and surface damage, so needing extra growth and keratinization. However, in winter, horn growth is reduced. When housing cattle on concrete, especially during the winter months, this causes difficulties because the need for new horn is increased.

There is also a change in horn growth rate in response to challenges such as lameness. It has been shown that after an incident of lameness, keratinization is increased in an attempt by the cow to repair the damage quickly.

Calving has an effect on horn growth as well. After calving, horn growth rate is found to be higher in the cows calving in winter than those calving in summer. This is perhaps a response to the demands placed on the foot. In winter an increase occurs after calving because it is needed to try to combat the increased prospect of lameness, damage, or wear on the foot. This is not the case in summer when the calving cow is able to reduce the rates of horn growth because there is no demand for the same damage repair or increased horn wear on modern grazing. The cow calving in summer has good horn growth before she calves so she can afford to down-regulate horn growth as nutrients go into milk production.

In summary, cattle calving in winter have lower horn growth rates but are exposed to more environmental stresses and trauma. They try to produce more horn after calving but this is too late. Their horn growth is unable to cope with winter housing stresses and calving so they are more likely to become lame.

Abnormal Horn Growth

Abnormal hoof growth is involved in many lameness diseases and can exacerbate any of the issues outlined above. Horn structure is mostly determined at birth and the process of ageing means that the foot becomes larger and the quality of the horn being formed starts to decline. There are also some specific issues, such as biotin in the diet, which can seriously affect the quality of horn being produced. Conformation of the leg and the way the animal walks – its gait – can alter horn growth and is closely related to the incidence of lameness. The type of environment the animal is kept in will also affect the way horn grows, which may lead to overgrowth or abnormal ledges of horn that can create pressure from outside on the sole.

Horn is affected by the quantity of water in its structure. If water is retained in the hoof, for example in slurry conditions or a wet environment such as spring grazing, the horn will become softer and more easily damaged. It will also be unable to support the pedal bone. In dry weather or on well-drained grazing the foot will lose water through the horn and it will become harder and more brittle; this can also damage horn, with more likelihood that the horn will break or crack.

Horn growth will be affected by the pedal bone pressing on the solar corium and also more generally by the disruption that occurs at calving. These disease processes and normal physiological changes will affect horn growth. 'Stress lines' – sudden defects in horn structure originating at the coronary band – arise as the horn is formed. These lines are common and will grow down the foot with time. They can cause difficulties if they are severe by altering the growth pattern of the horn or becoming horizontal fissures. Occasionally these stress lines occur after a severe mastitis or a true case of laminitis.

It is possible that abnormal horn growth will form pressure points in key areas of the foot such as the sole. We often see horn overgrowth of the lateral wall forming an 'overhang'. This creates a thick wad of extra horn over the sole, and frequently solar horn becomes damaged or ulcerated underneath. This wad of horn produces external pressure on the sole and will augment any pedal bone disruption, thus becoming yet another risk factor for the cow who may form claw lesions after calving.

SUMMARY

Research has shown that defects or weaknesses will occur at or around calving regardless of environmental pressures; they are an inherent consequence of parturition and due to basic physiological changes occurring at this time. This disruption, however, becomes magnified in response to adverse conditions at or around calving.

At present we can conclude that the most probable underlying cause for most lameness affecting the claw and horn is based on an underlying weakness, which is then amplified by outside influences to produce lameness.

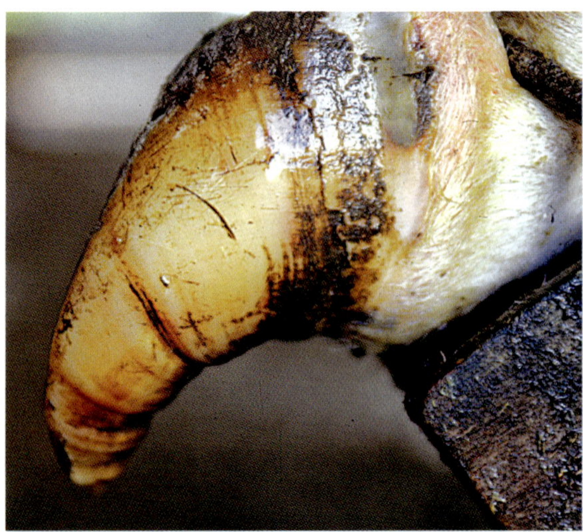

The hoof shows clear hardship lines due to the growth of the horn being 'disrupted', and is now starting to grow out of shape – 'corkscrew claw'.

CHAPTER TWO

Incidence and Recording of Lameness

To understand what is happening with lameness and to create accurate benchmarks for comparison of herds we need accurate records of the level of lameness and what is producing it. This will require definitions of incidents of lameness and an exact diagnosis of the problem concerned. The chosen system can be used to assess the herd against a benchmark and to monitor what action, if any, is needed for improvement.

Without good records it is difficult to obtain information about the level of lameness in a dairy herd. Lameness is a subjective disease and people's definitions may vary about whether a cow is lame or not and also as to the type of lesion involved. It is important that we consider the definitions associated with recording lameness in order to decide what these definitions mean in practice and how they can be used to investigate a herd problem.

DEFINITIONS FOR THE LEVEL OF LAMENESS IN A HERD

Individual Parameters

We need to decide the length of time it is reasonable to allow one incident of lameness to last before we record it again as being a 'new' case of lameness. This is slightly pedantic, but over-enthusiastic recording may make a cow appear to be repeatedly lame when it is still the same incident. We need to set a limit as to when an ongoing case becomes another lameness problem and not the same case. It is usual to accept a period of about 28 days for a single case of lameness to occur and heal fully, which should be reasonable unless there are complications.

- A 'limb case' is one foot or leg of the animal affected with lameness for a maximum period of time – say for a maximum of 28 days. If the cow has two limbs affected during this period, this will count as two limb cases.
- A 'cow case' is one individual cow in the herd affected with lameness once during a period of 28 days. If there is more than one leg affected, this still counts as only one cow case during the same period of time.

Herd Parameters

When comparing herd parameters we need to find a common denominator that allows herds of different sizes to compare their herd incidence of lameness. Usually the best measure is the percentage of cows in the herd that have been affected, or the number of cases of lameness per 100 cows. Again we need to specify what period of time this is being measured over, but the most common time span is over a year – the annual incidence. Figures for herd incidence are based on the average herd size over the period in question. This is usually not difficult to calculate as a best guess from the farm records, but it is possible to be very accurate by using NMR (National Milk Records) data where they count the number of cows in the herd for every day in the year (cow-days) and then divide this by 365 to give an accurate figure of the average number of cows in the herd (see the NMR web-based programme 'Herd Companion').

Herd measures of lameness would be:

- Percentage of cows affected with lameness. This is the number of cows affected in a period of time expressed as a percentage of the herd. The figure can also be expressed as the number of cases of lameness per 100 cows.

$$\frac{\text{No. of cows affected in 12 months}}{\text{Average herd size over 12 months}} \times 100 = \begin{array}{l}\text{Annual cow}\\\text{case incidence}\\(\% \text{ of herd})\end{array}$$

- Number of limb cases. This is the number of limbs (feet) affected in a period of time expressed as a percentage of the herd. This is more precise than the cows affected figure above as it takes into account when more than one foot is affected at the same time, which is not uncommon.

$$\frac{\text{Total no. of limb cases in 12 months}}{\text{Average herd size over 12 months}} \times 100 = \begin{array}{l}\text{Annual limb}\\\text{case incidence}\\(\% \text{ of herd})\end{array}$$

- Number of limb cases per affected cow. This gives some idea of either the repeat case incidence of lameness in the same cow or the fact that more than one leg is affected at once. It is not accurate enough to distinguish between these two options, but it does give some idea of continuing risk factors or ongoing disease problems that may produce either of these options, for example digital dermatitis (DD) will produce a high recurrence rate.

$$\frac{\text{Total no. of limb cases affected over 12 months}}{\begin{array}{l}\text{Total no. of}\\\text{cow cases over}\\12 \text{ months}\end{array}} = \begin{array}{l}\text{Annual incidences}\\\text{of limb cases}\\\text{per cow}\end{array}$$

- Percentage of cows affected more than once. The total number of cows affected more than once as a percentage of the total number of cows affected. This will give some idea of continuing risk factors that are producing repeated lameness in some cows, similar to the above limb cases per affected cow.

$$\frac{\begin{array}{l}\text{No. of cows}\\\text{affected more}\\\text{than once}\end{array}}{\begin{array}{l}\text{Total no. of}\\\text{cows affected}\\\text{with lameness}\end{array}} = \begin{array}{l}\text{Annual repeat}\\\text{case incidence}\end{array}$$

INCIDENCE OR PREVALENCE?

Once we have a system for recording the incidence of lameness we need to distinguish the difference and the relationship between what we call incidence and what is known as prevalence.

- Incidence is an occurrence happening once in a set period of time, for instance if, over the last year, we have had 100 cases of lameness, the incidence is 100.
- Prevalence is the level of lameness in the herd that is observed on any one single occasion during a period under observation. For instance, if, on a single day, locomotion scoring found 14 cows to be lame,

Incidence and Prevalence

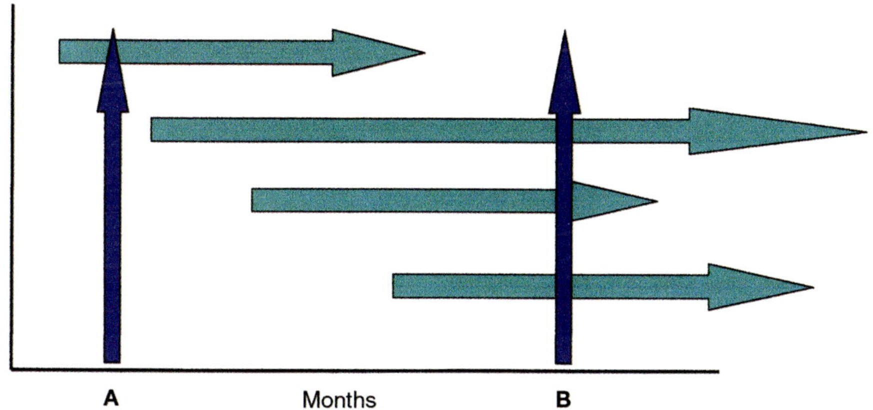

Each horizontal arrow indicates a case of lameness and extends for the period of time that the cow is actually lame. The longer the arrow the longer the cow is lame.

the prevalence within the herd on that day was 14.

The difference between the two can be shown in the diagram above.

If we visited a herd every 4 months and observed cows for lameness, at a point in time 'A' the prevalence of lameness is 1, i.e. one cow was observed to be lame. However, at time point 'B', 4 months later, the prevalence is three lame cows. The incidence over the whole period of time is constant at one case per month. The difference is that the separate incidents of lameness will last for dissimilar lengths of time, so although the actual incidence appears to be constant the observed prevalence changes. This raises the important point that the length of time over which any lameness incident occurs is affecting the cow's health, welfare, and also their production.

Prevalence can be measured by assessing lameness in the herd with what is known as a locomotion scoring system.

Locomotion Scoring

The principle is that cows are examined for lameness by visually assessing their gait and posture as they individually move past the

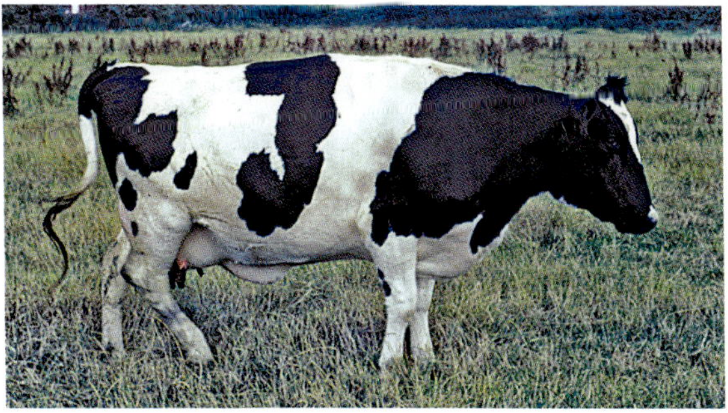

Watch for the pelvis moving and the head coming up.

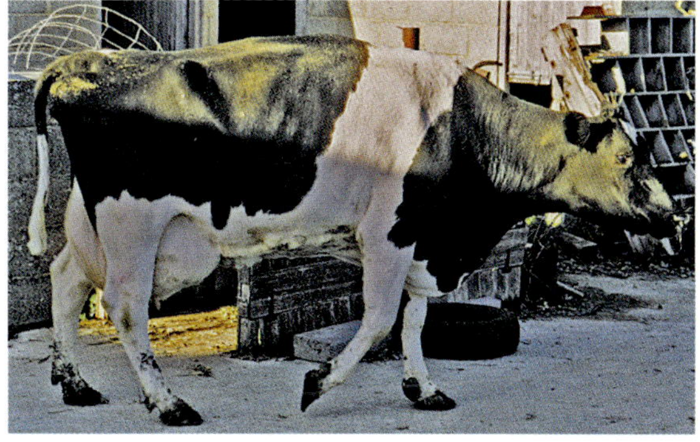

Lame cows soon start to arch their backs when walking.

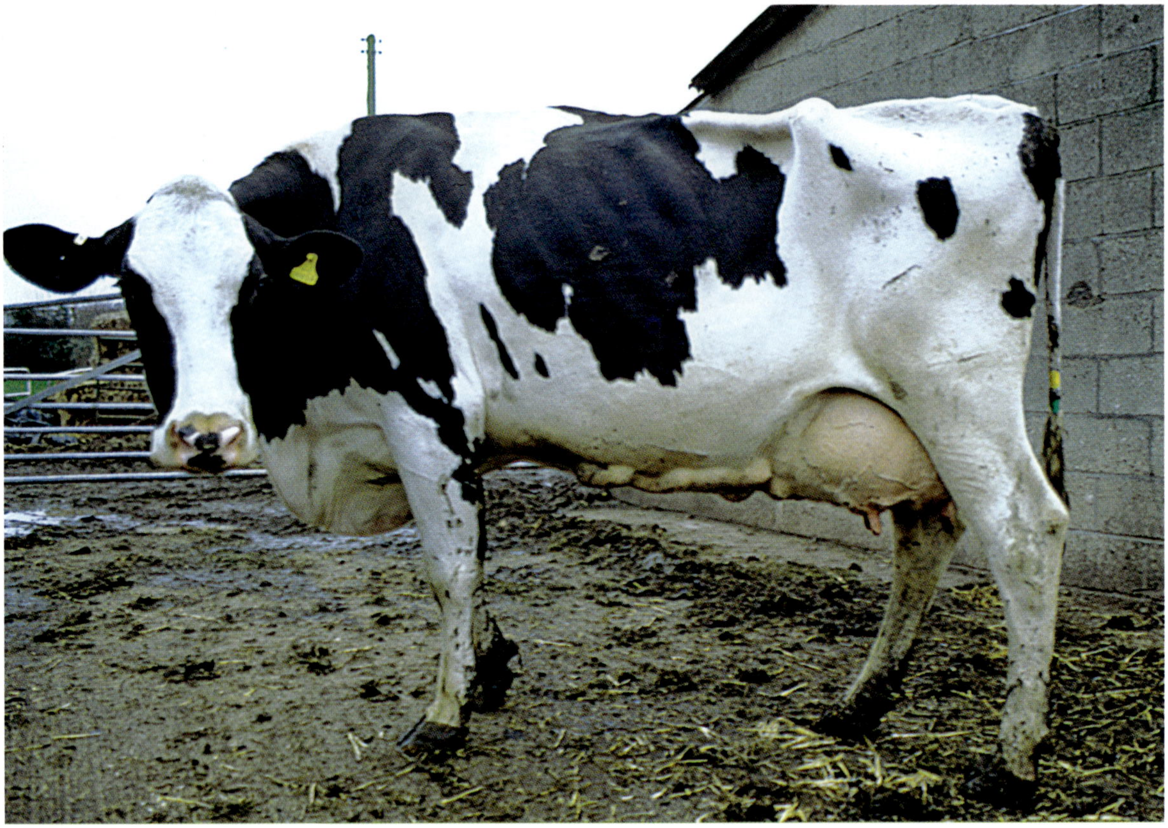

Weight loss is often apparent with lame cows.

observer. Most scoring systems are carried out by checking the cows as they walk back from the milking parlour after milking.

Lame cows walk with varying signs of lameness in the affected limb. Signs are usually associated with an attempt to take the weight off the lame foot and they do this by lifting their bodies or head.

Look for head lifting or pelvis tilting to show which leg is affected. Always check a cow from the front first as it is easy to miss forelimb lameness because a cow will always tilt the pelvis in lameness even if it is the front foot that is affected. Looking at the head first will tell the observer if the head lift is the dominant feature, indicating that the front leg is affected.

Lame cows arch their backs when walking, but if lameness is severe enough they will start arching their backs when standing as well.

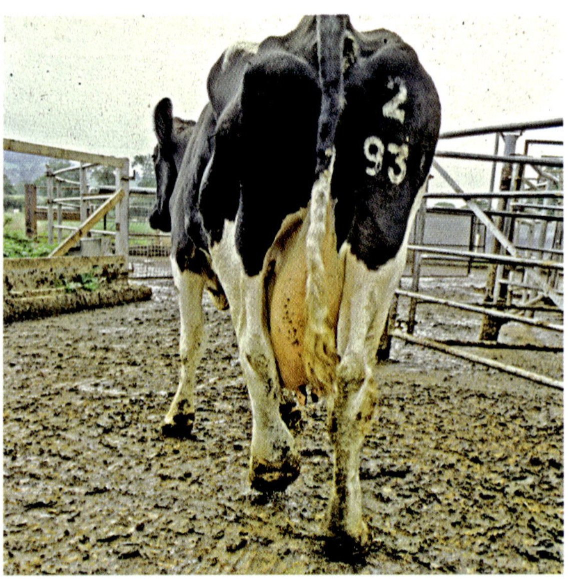

Eventually the foot is lifted from the ground and the cow is reluctant to walk.

Score	Definition	Criteria
1	Normal movement	No observed gait abnormality – long strides and no arching of the back.
2	Slightly lame	Walks slowly, shorter stride length and arches back on moving only. Stands normally. Normal weight transfer with no obvious leg affected.
3	Moderately lame	A short step taken with arched back and often stops when walking. Definite head or hip movement shows distinctly which leg is affected.
4	Severely lame	Very short steps, often resting the affected limb. Only partially weight bearing on affected leg, which is now very obvious. Seen to stand and walk with arched back. Weight loss.

Table 1 Locomotion scoring. Only scores 3 and 4 are indicators of lameness. Score 2 may indicate either a healing lesion or the early signs of a new case

The stride length is often shorter if the limb is causing pain. This is because the cow can take weight for a shorter period of time if it moves quickly through the painful foot with a short stride. Also look for other characteristic features such as weight loss.

In severe lameness other features start to become apparent, such as resting the lame foot off the floor or tilting the body to one side to take less weight on it. Severely lame cows also walk slowly and stop frequently.

Locomotion scoring can be very complicated, with many levels of scoring, but in practice a simple three- or four-point method is sufficient and more likely to be used. An example is shown in Table 1 above.

The herd locomotion scoring system can be made even simpler by carrying out what

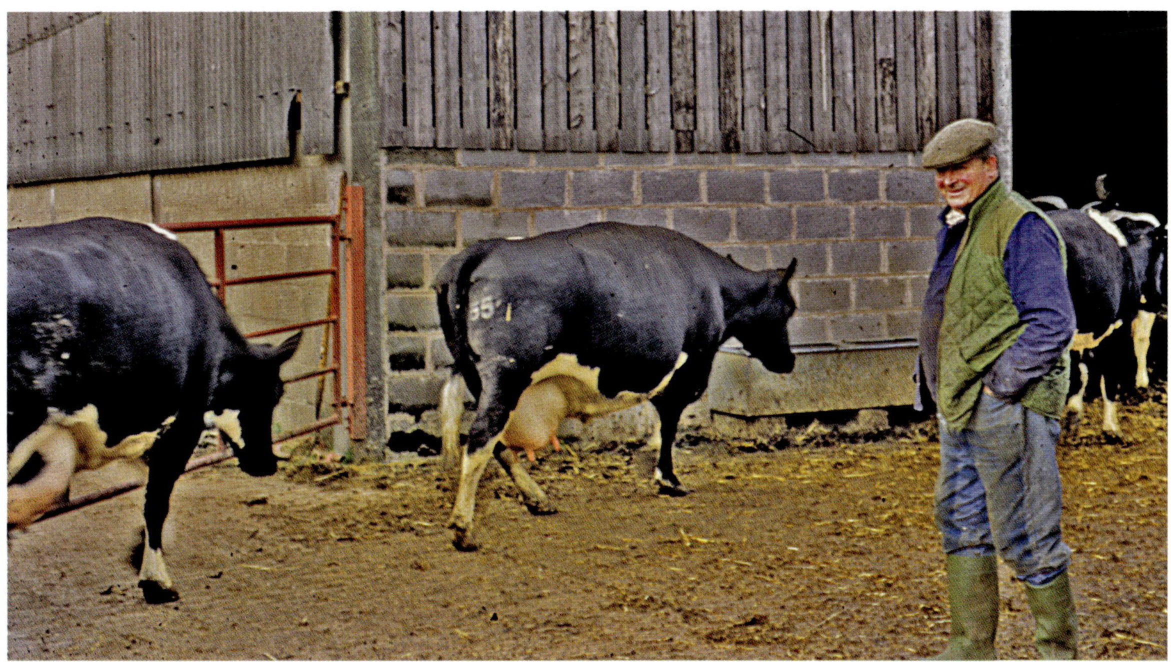

A 'walk past' locomotion score is a useful and quick method of assessing lameness.

is known as a 'walk-past' – observing the cows as they walk through a set opening and recording which cows are visibly lame. The actual mechanics of doing this take some practice, but it is very quick and remarkably effective at assessing lameness prevalence. Consideration must be given to how wide the gap is that the cows walk through for observation. It needs to be restricted so that the cows walk through in single file. The distance the observer stands away from the cows is also critical; too close and the cows will not walk through or will go past too quickly. A lame cow that is hurried or frightened may not show a lameness that is present. If the observer stands too far away, the cows will bunch up and make observation of individuals difficult. If you are careful and think about the cow's 'comfort zone' the walk-past will work well and give a good evaluation of the prevalence of lameness in the herd quickly and without a lot of fuss.

Many research workers have found that recording the prevalence of lameness in a herd on as few as two occasions per year can give a good estimation of the actual incidence of lameness in the herd during that period. For instance, a measurement of lameness prevalence in the herd in December is a good indicator of the level of lameness in the herd during the winter housing period. In June a single assessment would indicate the background level of lameness for the summer grazing season. This can be used as a simple, practical way to reflect the overall lameness prevalence over the 12-month period as it correlates well with observations taken more frequently. It is recommended that at least one of the observations be during the winter housing period.

The measurement of herd prevalence can be used to indicate the overall incidence. It has been observed by several workers that the incidence of lameness (individual cases) is between 2.5 and 3 times the average prevalence (lameness seen at the scoring visits). This is useful when investigating lameness in a herd where there are no records, or very poor ones, as

you can simply carry out a prevalence scoring visit and calculate the approximate incidence. In a few herds, however, where the length of time the cow is lame is very short, this sort of relationship breaks down. For instance, if there is a high incidence of digital dermatitis or where cows are treated promptly, each incident of lameness will last for a shorter period of time and looking purely at prevalence may underestimate the incidence because cases have resolved quickly. Prevalence works well when the lameness damage lasts for a reasonable period of time, which is usually the case with horn disease.

All herds should undergo some sort of locomotion scoring twice a year as part of their overall health initiative. The feedback will help to determine the level of lameness present in the herd and the effects of any protocols put in place to treat and prevent the disease.

DEFINITIONS FOR THE TYPE OF LAMENESS

Proper investigation and diagnosis of the type of lameness lesion or disease is very subjective; even amongst professionals who are familiar with dealing with lame cows there is often disagreement about what type of lesion is present. Therefore, obtaining accurate lameness records at farm level is difficult. However, we should restrict our definitions to distinct problems, as it is essential that we recognize and distinguish between the different causes of lameness. Both stockperson and veterinarian can then investigate the underlying causes to choose the best treatment and long-term preventative measures for the herd.

In general, it is best to restrict recording to specific diseases that are easily defined and recognized. Terms that describe effects rather than the primary problem are of little use. For instance, to say a foot has an 'under-run sole' is a valid description, but it does not indicate why the foot has an under-run sole. Was it due to white line disease, an ulcer, or a foreign body? These terms will be defined clearly in subsequent chapters, but the terms that should be used for recording lameness diagnoses are shown in the box below.

Suggested list of diagnoses to be used in recording lameness

Horn disease
Sole ulcer
White line abscess
Foreign body penetration
Slurry heel
Solar haemorrhages or bruising
Vertical fissures
Horizontal fissures

Skin disease
Interdigital necrobacillosis – 'foul'
Digital dermatitis
Peracute interdigital necrobacillosis – 'super foul'
Interdigital fibroma

Leg injuries
Joint disease
Leg injuries
NAD, no abnormality detected
Other

HOW MUCH OF A PROBLEM IS LAMENESS?

Several workers have looked at the level of lameness in the dairy herd (Table 2).

Three surveys record between 25 and 30 per cent cow incidence and two record 55 per cent. The difference here is due to the method of recording. When working only from farm-based recordings, the lameness incidence is around 25–30 per cent. If, however, lameness is investigated by going on farm and actively inspecting cows (Clarkson and Wood Vet Group studies), more lameness is seen to be present. Stockpersons have a different perception about lameness, especially when they are working with the cows all the time, and this difference is often highlighted when someone else visits to assess the herd.

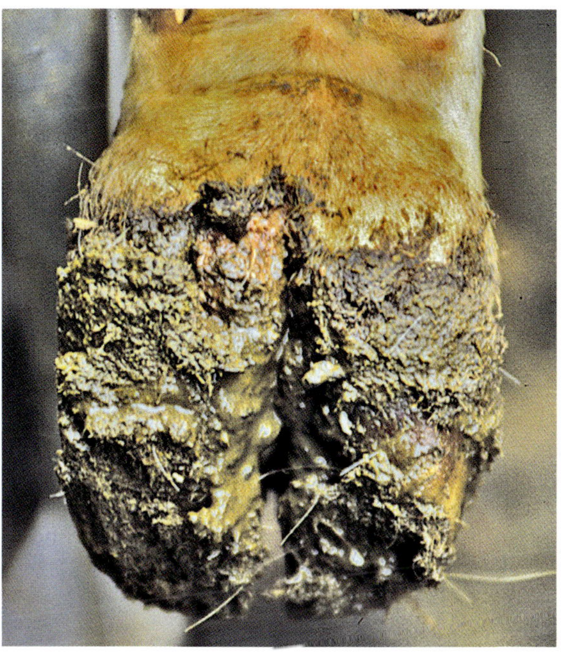

Make sure that recording lameness lesions is consistent. This cow shows digital dermatitis affecting the heel - bulbar digital dermatitis.

Table 3 (on the following page) shows one of the lameness surveys in more detail (DAISY, University of Reading).

The survey is based on farm records collected with the University of Reading DAISY herd health programme. The records are in line with other similar studies and probably reflect

Source	Cow incidence (%)
Whitaker (1980)[1]	25
Clarkson (1996)[2]	55
DAISY (1996)[3]	26
Weaver (1998)[4]	30
Wood Veterinary Group (1999)[5]	55

Table 2 Cow incidence expressed as per cent of cows. *The dates refer to the year the study was carried out.*
DAISY is the 'Dairy Information System' computer programme produced by the University of Reading

	Total average	Lowest quarter	2nd quarter	3rd quarter	Highest quarter
No. of herds	50	12	13	13	12
Herd size	150	133	149	148	170
% Cows affected	25.6	9.4	18.7	27.4	43.2
% Cows affected more than once	26.5	8.6	14.3	25	36.3
No. of cow cases per 100 cows in herd	35.2	10.4	22.5	35.7	66
No. of limb cases per 100 cows in herd	38.2	11.4	23.7	38.5	72.6
No. of limb cases per cow	1.5	1.2	1.3	1.5	1.7

Table 3 DAISY data 1995–96[3]. *The data is sorted by limb cases per 100 cows in the herd*

a true incidence of lameness based on farm recordings. The survey shows that 26 cows per year in an average 100-cow herd are affected with lameness; this consists of 38 individual limb cases. Over one-quarter of cows were affected with lameness more than once. This could be due to them being exposed to the same repeated environmental factors. Also, once a cow has been lame, its chances of a repeat incident are increased, probably due to changes occurring within the foot after the first lameness incident.

The survey also shows the range of lameness that existed in different herds. The difference between the best and the worst is over five-fold. The best herds managed an incidence rate of less than 10 per cent of the herd or only 10 cows per 100. The survey also showed that:

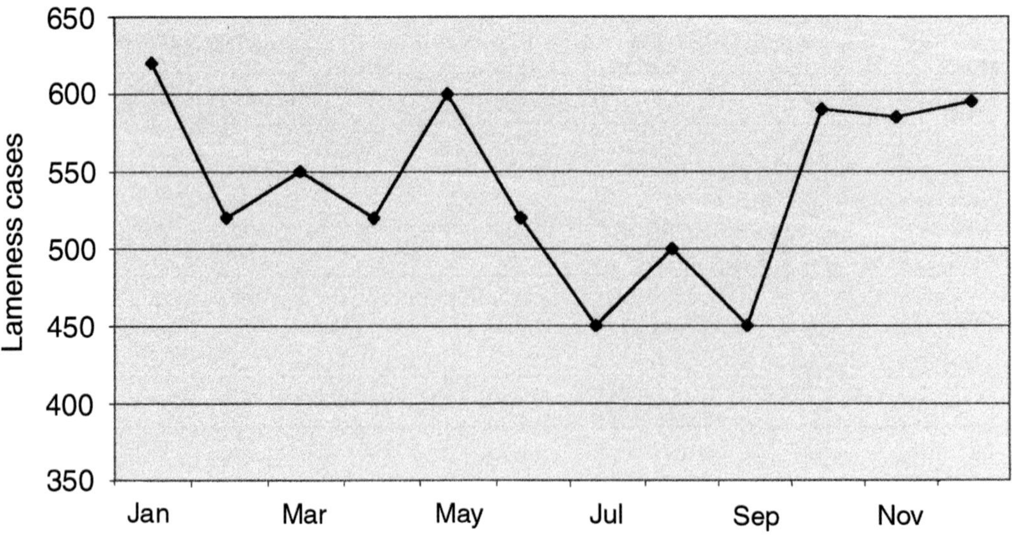

Graph of seasonal lameness incidence. Source: NADIS 2004 – based on 40 veterinary practices reporting. The trend is more important than the overall figures.

- Older cows were more prone to lameness – nearly twice as many cases in their fifth lactation and over.
- The peak incidence was during the winter, associated with the housing period, with a further increase in April and May associated with turnout. This is probably due to feet being in a poor condition after the winter and wet conditions on tracks and in gateways in spring. The lowest incidence is during the summer at grazing (*see* graph opposite).
- Sixty-five per cent of all foot lesions will be in the hindlimbs.
- The outer claw of the hindlimb is four times as likely to be involved in lameness lesions compared to the inner claw. The reverse is true for the forelimb; the inner claws are more likely to be affected.

The results of the most common causes of lameness recorded vary depending on whether they are based on veterinary records or the stockperson's records. Table 4 shows the distributions seen in three lameness surveys. If we look at two of these surveys in detail:

- Wood Veterinary Group, Gloucester[5] – only five commercial herds, but all cases of lameness were examined by a veterinarian and therefore recording should be more

consistent. The figures are based on the cows present during the trial and are not corrected for length of stay in the herd.
- Kossaibati *et al.* (DAISY, 1996)[3] – based on records from 50 farms. Note the high level of 'foreign body' diagnosed, which is probably confusion on the part of the stockperson between white line disease and a true foreign body.

Although there are some differences due to the person recording and diagnosing the type of lameness, the proportions of each condition are similar. Less than 2 per cent of all lameness is due to injuries or disease affecting the leg. The vast majority of cases are due to lesions in the foot itself. Of these, horn lesions (solar ulcers, white line disease and foreign bodies) account for approximately 60 per cent of lameness cases, and skin lesions (digital dermatitis and foul) account for about 38 per cent. Solar ulceration remains the most commonly diagnosed condition, but recent surveys indicate that digital dermatitis is rapidly overtaking this and becoming the main cause of lameness in the national dairy herd. For comparison, figures from some states in the USA, where cows are housed constantly, show that over 50 per cent of all lameness is due to digital dermatitis.

One interesting feature of these figures is that although the incidence of lameness has remained remarkably consistent over the years that surveys have been carried out (nearly 20 years in the examples quoted in Table 2: 1980–99), the type of lameness has changed enormously. In 1980 there would have been no records of digital dermatitis because the disease was not known in the UK until 1988. In fact the Clarkson work (Table 4) shows a very low incidence of digital dermatitis (only 8 per cent) as this study was done during 1989. As digital dermatitis is now one of the most common causes of lameness in dairy cows, the incidence of other causes of lameness must be declining. To maintain the overall herd incidence at the levels shown in Table 4 there must have been some reduction in the actual

Lesions	Clarkson (1996)[2]	DAISY (1996)[3]	WVG (1999)[5]
Ulcers	36	20	25
DD	8	20	22
White line	22	9	23
Foul	5	13	13
Foreign body	5	18	6

Table 4 Lameness surveys. *The figures refer to the lesion seen as a percentage of total cases recorded (only the main lesions are listed)*
DD = digital dermatitis
WVG = Wood Veterinary Group

numbers of other lameness conditions. We now know a lot more about lameness and are steadily improving the health of cow's feet. If it were not for the introduction and enormous spread of digital dermatitis, the level of lameness in the national dairy herd would probably be dropping.

THE COST OF LAMENESS

Before leaving the subject of incidence and occurrence it is worthwhile looking at the costs involved with lameness. The costs for any lame cow depend on the type of lesion involved, the severity of it, and the stage of lactation when the cow is affected. The economic consequences of lameness can be divided into direct and indirect costs. Direct costs are those that are specifically attributed to dealing with the lameness. Indirect costs are the consequential effects of the lameness that cause loss in another area of the animal's production, for example weight gain, fertility and so on.

Direct Costs

Veterinary Treatment
Professional fees, drugs and treatments have a cost related to the amount of work involved and the specific therapy needed for the type of lameness presented. For instance, a solar ulcer will, on average, require more time and more treatments than a case of digital dermatitis.

Herdsperson's Time Dealing with the Cow
The stockperson's costs involve time handling the cow for treatment or in helping the veterinarian treat the cow. There are also time costs for any ongoing treatment and also the extra time often involved in getting these cows in from the field or from a hospital pen at milking. Again the time spent on the cow depends on severity and type of lameness.

Milk Withdrawal from Medicines Used
Nearly all drug treatments have a drug withdrawal time, which means that milk has to be discarded. All types of lameness carry the risk of drug use and therefore a withdrawal time. For horn lesions this may be 10 per cent of all cases, but for skin lesions (e.g. 'foul') it will be 25 per cent or more of cases treated.

Reduced Milk Yield
Lame cows spend longer lying down and less time feeding. This will have a direct effect on milk production. The pain of the lameness will also affect the cow's ability to let milk down and this will have an effect on yield. Once the lactation curve has dropped off it does not normally recover, so lost milk production extends over the rest of the lactation period.

Indirect Costs

Reduced Fertility
Depending on the stage of lactation, lameness can affect fertility. As lameness is more common in the early part of lactation, at the time when we want to start serving the cow again, it is likely that it will have an effect on breeding. A lame cow may lose body weight through reduced feeding time. This will accentuate the negative energy balance of the cow, which can have a profound effect on the cow's ability to carry out reproductive functions such as proper maturation of ova, ovulation and survival of the early embryo. The behaviour of the cow will also be affected; she will not spend as long socializing with the rest of the herd and is more likely to be missed when in oestrus. This results in the cow being served more often and therefore taking longer to get back in calf. Again we can grade the effects on fertility according to the type of lesion and the severity of the lameness.

Increased Culling
Chronic lameness is one of the most common reasons for a cow being culled from the dairy herd. The costs of any lameness must bear in mind the increased chance that the disease episode may result in the cow being culled. A solar ulcer will increase the chances of

an infected cow being culled by 18 per cent, whereas skin disease lameness will probably have no effect on culling as it is less likely to become chronic and produce ongoing secondary problems. Culling cows is very expensive.

From the above list we can put costs on each of the various types of lameness seen in the dairy herd (based on 1998 costs).

1. The type of lesion dictates the costs likely to be incurred. For instance:

   - Solar ulcers have a direct cost of £72 but also have an effect on fertility and probable culling, which adds another £174. The total cost of a single case is likely to be about £246.
   - Horn disease (white line and foreign body penetrations) has a lower direct cost of about £50 and the knock-on losses from fertility and culling will be less as treatment is likely to be more effective. If we put indirect costs at £102, the total cost for horn disease lameness is £152.
   - Skin disease (digital dermatitis or foul) has a direct cost of about £37 with much reduced risks of indirect costs (£22), so the overall cost of a skin disease lameness incident is £59.

2. Allow for recurrence of cases, as lameness tends to make the animal more prone to further lameness. On average, a repeat limb case will be 0.5 incidence, i.e. each case of lameness will have a repeat 'half case'. We need to allocate repeated costs for this repeat lameness but not for all the elements we listed for the initial case. It can be reasonably assumed that there will be no further milk loss and no extra risks of indirect costs, so the recurrence simply entails time, drugs and milk withdrawal. A half cost for a repeat limb case can be calculated by adding half the extra direct costs of lameness apart from reduced yield. For instance, for a sole ulcer the veterinary costs, the herdsman's time and milk withdrawal total £45.60, so an extra

half case will be about £23. The calculation is:

- Solar ulcer = £23, add this to the costs in 1. above (£246) = £269.
- Horn disease = £16 + £152 = £168.
- Skin disease = £14 + £59 = £73.

3. Applying an incidence to the type of lameness in the herd will show the likely herd costs for each of these diseases. If, for instance, the incidence is 21 per cent for solar ulcers, 41 per cent for white line and other horn disease and 38 per cent for skin infection, and we allocate a typical 100-cow herd with a lameness incidence of 26 per cent overall, the following costs can be accumulated:

   - Solar ulcers – 26 × 0.21 = 5.5 cases @ £269 = £1470.
   - Horn disease – 26 × 0.41 = 10.7 cases @ £167 = £1787.
   - Skin disease – 26 × 0.38 = 9.9 cases @ £73 = £722.

4. The herd costs will be £1470 + £1787 + £722 = £3979 for an average herd with a 26 per cent cow case incidence. An average cost will be £153 (£3979 divided by the incidence of 26 per cent).

We can draw up a balance sheet to summarize the costs of lameness and work out a figure for an average case of lameness (*see* Table 5 on the following page).

The end result of these calculations is the key message to get across. The cost of lameness for a typical 100-cow herd with an average level of lameness is:

- Average cost of lameness per cow = £153.
- Average cow incidence of lameness = 26 cow cases per 100 cows.
- Costs for 100-cow herd = £4000.

If we look at the range of herd incidence results that were reported by Kossaibati (Table 3), the

	Sole ulcer	Horn disease	Skin disease	Average case
Proportion of lesions (%)	21	41	38	
Direct costs (£)				
Veterinary treatment – time, blocks and drugs	33.3	24.8	21.8	25.4
Herdsperson's time	10	5	5	6.1
Milk withdrawal	2	1.6	1.6	1.7
Reduced yield	27	18	9	16.5
Total	72.3	49.4	37.4	49.6
Indirect costs (£)				
Increased culling	104.9	64.1	0	48.3
Extended calving interval (fertility)	55	30	17.5	30.5
Extra services (fertility)	14	8	4	7.8
Total	173.9	102.1	21.5	86.6
Allow 0.5 cases of repeat limb lameness per cow per year	22.7	15.7	14.2	16.6
Total cost of a single limb case (direct and indirect costs)	246.7	151.5	58.9	136.3
Total cost for a lame cow per year single limb case plus 0.5 recurrence	269.3	167.2	73.1	152.9

Table 5 *Summary of costs of lameness.* *Calculations are based on 1998 prices*
Source: Kossaibati et al. 1999[3]
Note that the allowance for the extra recurrence of 0.5 limb cases per cow only takes into account direct costs of veterinary treatment, herdsperson's time and drug withdrawals. It is assumed that the recurrence will not further damage the milk production curve.

losses range from £1300 for the top quartile of herds down to £6800 for the lowest quartile. In an average herd the cost per cow is £40 and this equates to milk production costs of around 0.7 pence per litre of milk sold.

As mentioned at the beginning of this chapter, the incidence of lameness in a dairy herd depends on how the information is recorded. Locomotion scores carried out on a farm will give a true incidence of probably nearer 50 per cent than the 26 per cent we have used in the costing example above. This brings the cost up to nearer £80 per cow in a 100-cow herd or 1.4 pence per litre of milk sold. Substantial amounts of money are being lost on lameness and there are profound welfare issues for the cows concerned.

Lameness is an expensive disease for the dairy herd. Costs of between 0.7 and 1.4 pence per litre are substantial amounts of money, and recording and costing lameness is an essential part of any herd health initiative.

CHAPTER THREE

General Techniques for the Examination and Treatment of Feet

Handling a cow's foot need not be difficult. It should not be a daunting physical task as, with the right equipment and the right technique, you can examine a cow's foot safely, and should be able to reach the correct diagnosis. Good technique is vital to treat the cow effectively at the outset. Most treatments described in the following chapters are targeted at specific foot conditions. However, there are several basic supportive treatments that are common to many foot conditions and it is useful to look at them first and be sure you can use them effectively.

A basic approach for any lame cow must be:

1. The ability to restrain the cow simply and safely.
2. To examine the foot fully and reach a diagnosis – find out what is wrong.
3. To apply general supportive treatment.
4. To apply any specific treatment.

The last item in the list above will be dealt with in subsequent chapters that describe the specific defects we see in lame cows.

RESTRAINT

The cow needs to be restrained adequately before any attempt is made to lift the foot. To examine the foot properly you will need a stall or cattle crush that meets certain minimum requirements. There are various options available, but there are certain common requirements for almost any stall or crush.

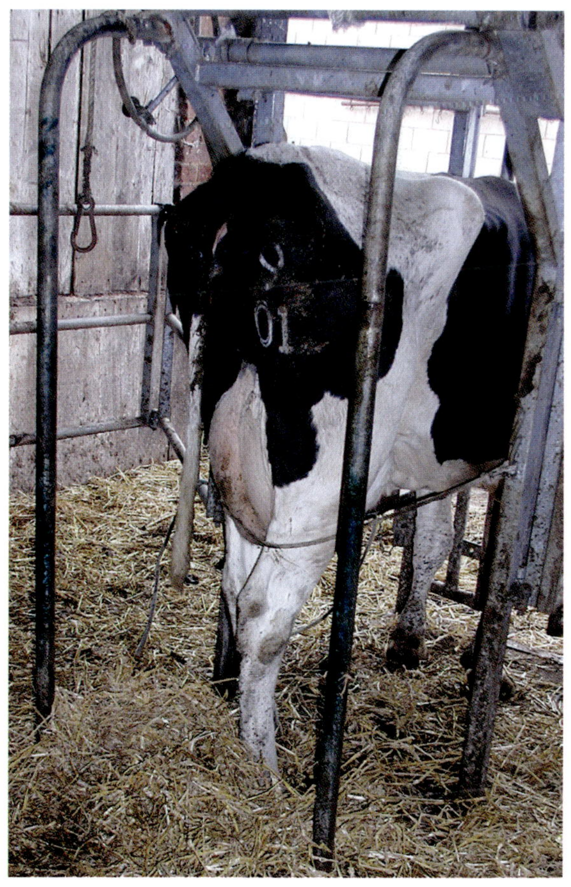

A simple stall made on the farm for foot work.

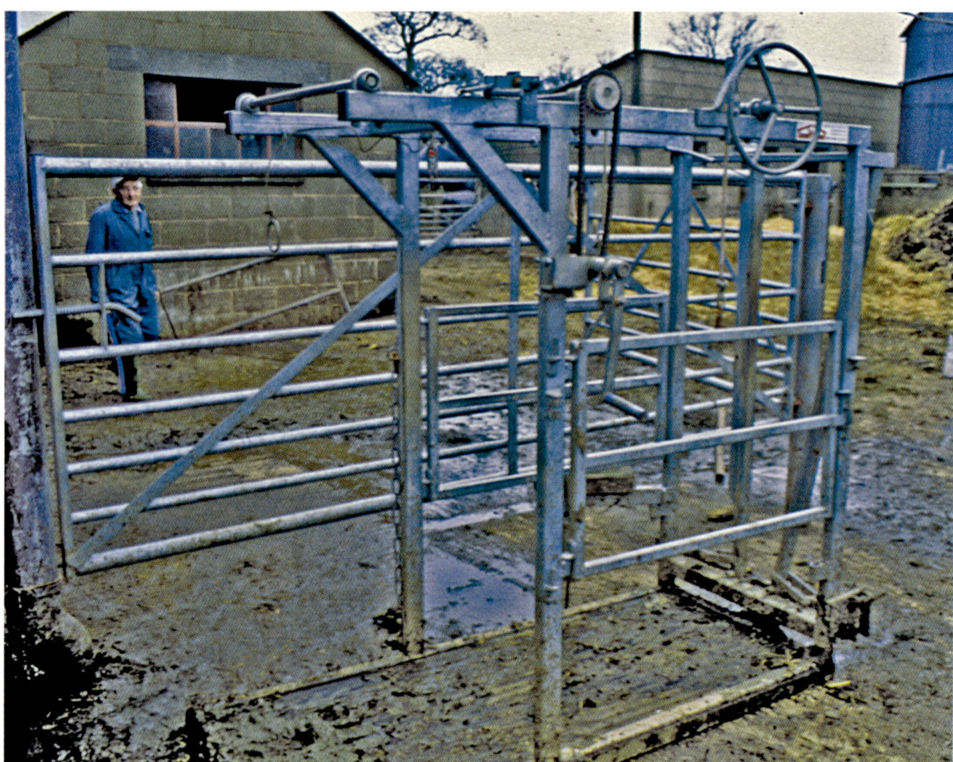

A purpose-made trimming crush. It is very open with few anchorage points to strap the foot to.

- Both side-to-side and forwards and back-wards movements should be restricted enough to comfortably lift and handle the foot. It is important that the cow fits the stall and is restrained far enough forward to allow the foot to be lifted and extended behind it. This will require a head-locking system and possibly a rear rump chain.
- A non-slip floor is essential. If a cow goes down in the crush or stall, it is very time consuming and dangerous to remove.
- There needs to be a cross member joining the two sides of the stall or crush, prefer-ably just above head height at the rear of the crush or stall. This will enable a lifting mechanism to be used.
- A method of restraining the foot once it is lifted.
- There should be no hinges or catches on the crush to injure the foot when lifting and working on it.

There are basically two design options avail-able – one is the traditional crush with a head restraint and the other is a purpose-built stall with some form of headlock yoke. Both can meet the requirements successfully if they are well constructed.

The cattle crush is the most common restraint device used. They come in different shapes and sizes and with a variety of adap-tations to handle feet. Some may need simple modifications to make them easier to use, whilst others are purpose made for dealing with feet. Crushes used for routine foot trim-ming have different design requirements to those intended for treating lame cows. For instance, lame cows are usually suffering some pain and discomfort (which is why the cow is lame). When handling a lame foot a secure fastening is needed to stop the foot moving around too much. The foot trimming crush often has the foot suspended freely, allowing the operator to work closely with the foot to

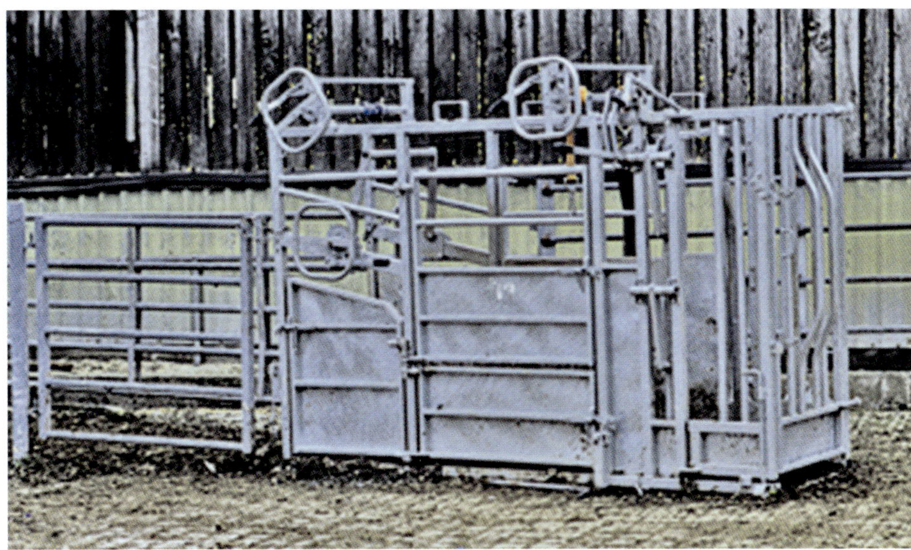

A robust general-purpose crush, usually used on the farm for both trimming and lame cows.

create the best angles for forming the shape of the foot. It is important to realize the difference between the two types of crush when deciding on a farm design. Most farms will only have the option of one type of crush and it is best that this is a more substantial crush rather than the trimming version.

Most crushes are perfectly adequate and it is personal taste as to what you choose as your favourite to work with. If the crush is not designed specifically for the task, it can be adapted easily to make handling feet easier.

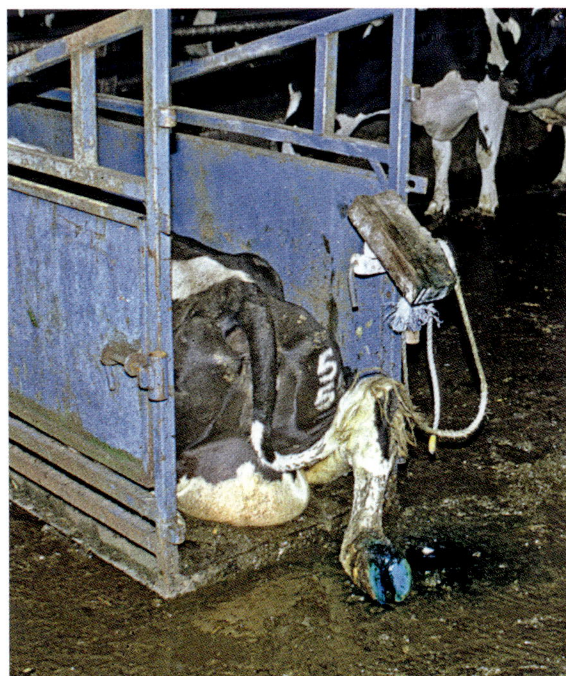

Cows that go down in the crush whilst being examined are difficult to handle.

- The front side panels can be removed to give access to the front feet.
- An extension can be added to the rear of the crush to angle the sole of the foot upwards and so allow better viewing and access to the foot. Dedicated crushes have an extension block to allow the foot to be restrained beyond the back of the crush, but a simple 'D'-shaped piece of metal can be welded to the back stanchion to produce a good fixing for the foot.
- A winch mechanism makes work easier; some sort of lifting aid is essential if the operator is working single-handed.
- Belly straps are useful to prevent the animal going down in the crush and they make lifting the front feet much easier because the animal allows the limb to come up without a struggle.

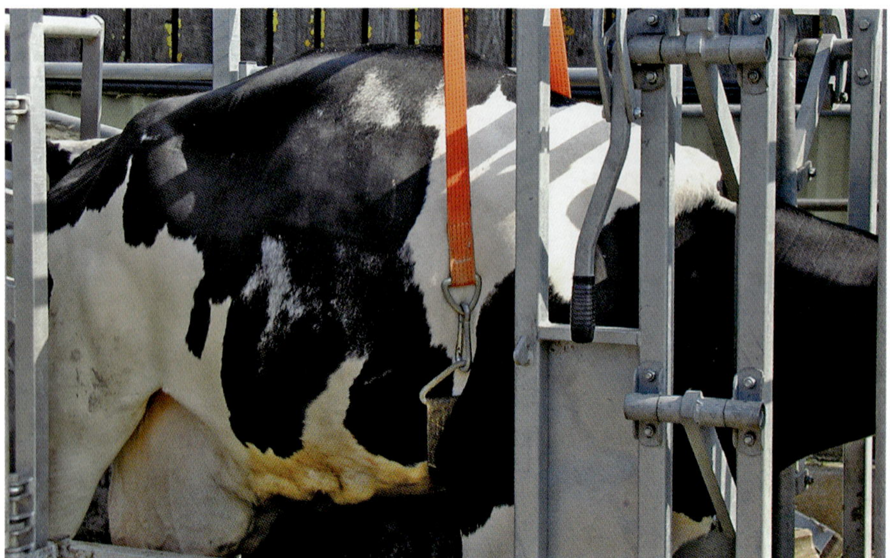

Always try and use the belly strap to support cows – especially if working alone.

HANDLING THE FOOT

After locking the cow in the stall or crush and applying the belly support, lift the foot with a wide strap or non-tightening rope. The foot can be lifted with a good winch system on the back of the crush or using a rope as in the diagrams below. If the lame foot is a hindlimb, the strap should be placed above the hock. With front feet the lift should be from the mid metacarpal area – between the fetlock and the knee. If you are using a manual system, a heavy gauge (18mm minimum) rope is important so as not to damage the leg or produce

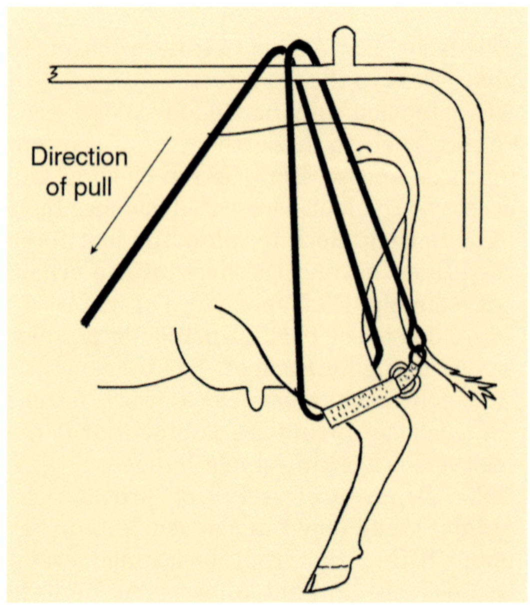

Side view of a cow being roped up for lifting.

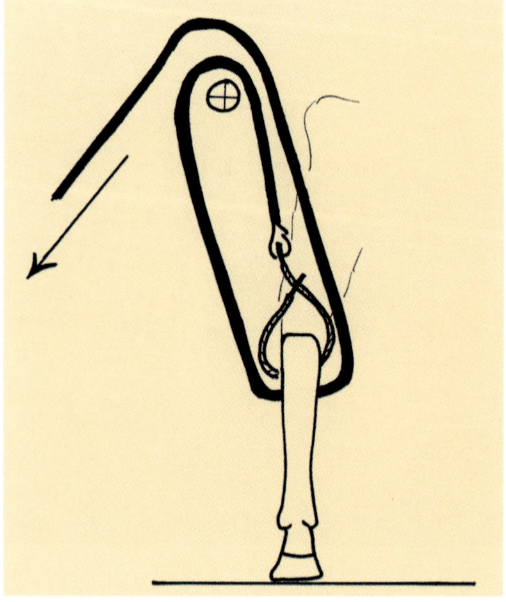

Rear view to show the layout of the ropes – they form a pulley system with the crush and the leg.

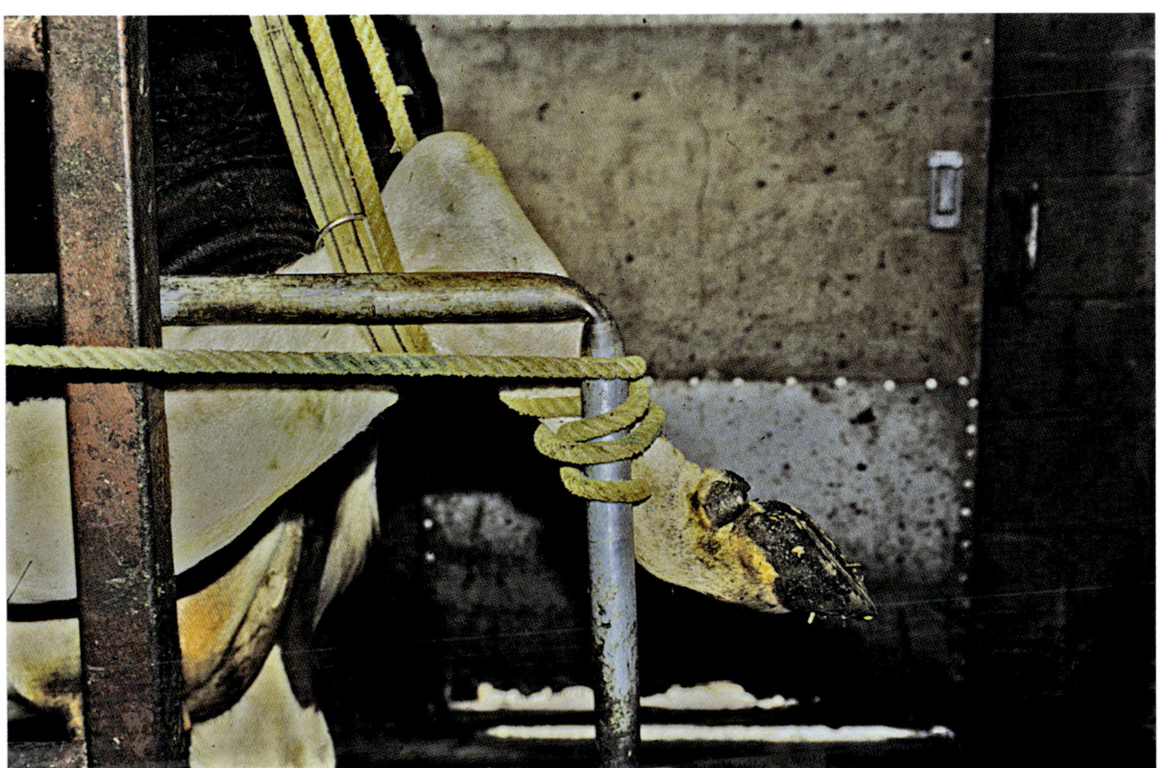

A simple piece of bent tube has been welded to the back of the crush in a 'D' shape to extend the foot back.

discomfort before you deal with the foot itself. Ropes of this size are much easier to handle and less likely to slip out of the operator's hands. Raise the foot to a comfortable working height and fix it to a solid structure low down at the fetlock area and preferably a distance of about 300mm behind the back of the crush. This extension of the foot backwards 'opens' the face of the foot by rotating the sole of the foot backwards and upwards into a better working position. A separate rope is usually applied for this final fixing if a winch is used.

The forelimb should be fixed to a convenient cross member or a specially designed cradle that attaches to the stall or crush. These cradles usually angle the front limb slightly outwards away from the body of the cow and outside the main crush area. This is very important because it not only makes the foot easier to work on but it stops the oper-ator getting kicked by the hindlimb coming forward, which commonly occurs.

Bulls are particularly difficult to handle because of their weight and the fact that they will not fit into most crushes. It is worthwhile using some light sedation with a bull to make sure the 'odds' of completing the job success-fully are in your favour.

Equipment

Complicated equipment is unnecessary for examining and treating lame cows. A sharp knife and a pair of hoof clippers are all that is required. Most people choose dedicated left- and right-handed knives. The author has a preference for a single, good-quality steel knife with a full double edge that allows the direction of trimming to be reversed without having to change knives. It is worthwhile getting a good steel knife because they last longer, remain sharper and do not rust. Hoof

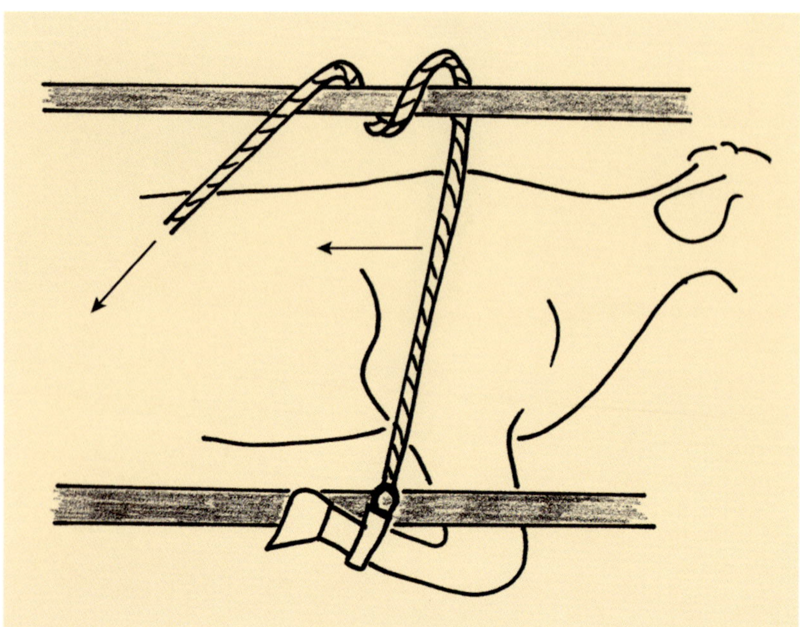

A front foot can usually be brought up with this method of roping up.

clippers, like knifes, are personal choice, but there is a huge advantage in having small, easily managed clippers rather than the large, cumbersome ratchet or double-action types. One of the best choices on the market are the 'Diamond'- type clippers – especially the 18in long model.

Although rarely used, a pair of hoof testers is a useful backup.

Good lighting is essential. Crushes are often sited in covered areas and bending over the foot creates shadows and prevents a good view of the foot. A halogen light, or preferably two to prevent shadows, situated high up behind the cow will make it easier to work on and to view lesions and abnormalities.

Softwood sawdust is a better cleaning agent on the feet than water because it prevents the whole area from getting sodden and dirty. Rubbing sawdust over the foot removes faeces easily and soaks up moisture. Keep a bucket of it by the foot crush.

Approach

Always note which foot the animal is lame on before putting it in the crush. This will save time, as it can be difficult to decide which foot needs examining when the animal is restrained.

Be careful to progress reasonably rapidly when examining the foot as, if the cow is lame, it may be painful for it to be restrained and left standing on three legs for any period of time.

There are a definite series of steps to work through when examining a lame foot:

- Clean the foot off and check for visible differences between the claws, such as swelling

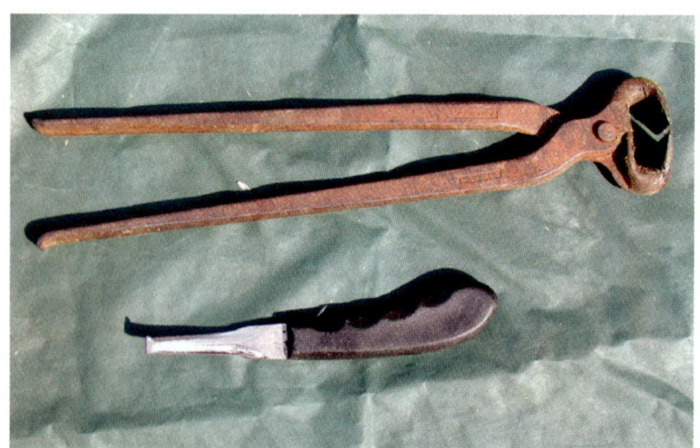

Equipment for trimming or lame cows. A double-bladed knife and a 'Diamond' set of clippers.

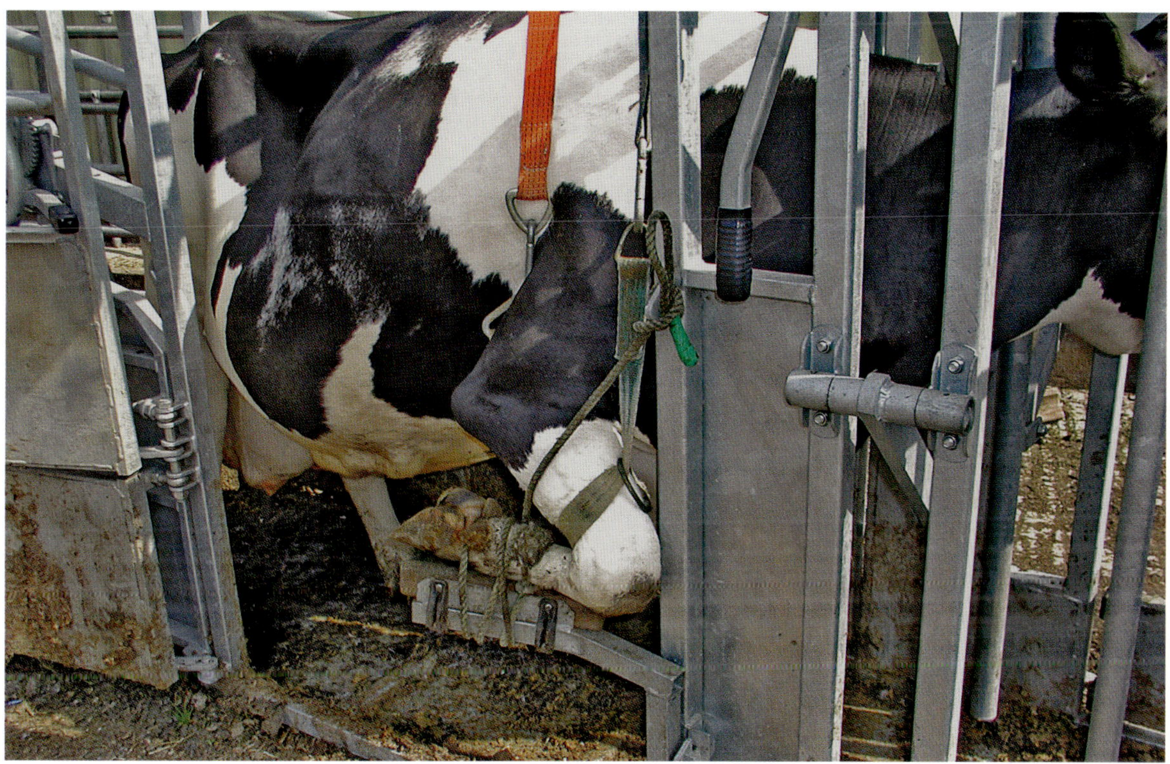

A purpose-made block is used to attach the foot rigidly to the crush.

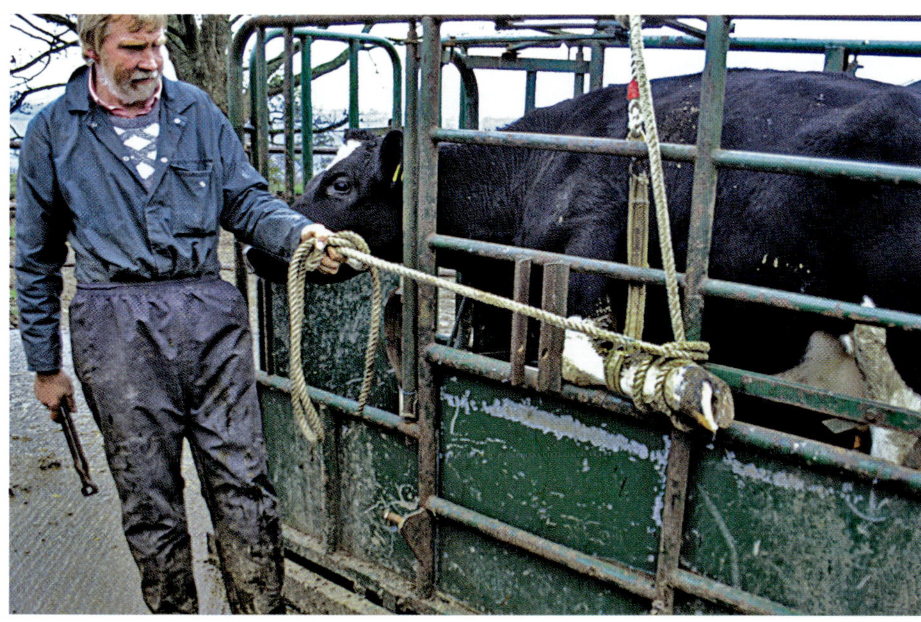

An ordinary crush successfully used for a front foot – it is a bit of a fiddle but it works.

and any obvious horn abnormalities. Look at the foot from above to see if there is any abnormal horn growth producing different weight bearing between the claws. Look between the claws and check for breaks in the skin or foreign bodies. Compare the conformation of the two claws, one against the other.

- Scrape the skin around the bulbs of the heels and around the coronary band to check for lesions. Gently scrape the skin in the interdigital space to check for cracks or swellings in the skin.
- Scrape the sole and the walls to make sure there are no cracks or fissures.
- Start paring the soles with the aim of finding the problem and also restoring any misshapen claw to normal (see the chapter on foot trimming). Start at the heels and trim off an area over the white line region while looking for defects. Work round the full length of the white line, making sure all discoloured areas are followed through to clean horn. Remember that the white line runs all the way from the heel on the outside (abaxial) wall round to one-third of the way up the interdigital (axial) wall.
- Use a knife to trim the sole. It may at first look normal, but, if defects are present, they may only start to appear when successive layers are removed – especially with solar ulceration.
- Look for flaps of horn at the bulbs of the heel or the coronary band that indicate where pus has escaped. These can then be followed back to find the original lesion.
- Always watch the animal's response to your actions. The cow will show pain when the causal area is examined and pared. Often a cow that shows no response whilst you are paring the foot is lame elsewhere in the leg rather than the foot.
- Although rarely required with cattle, a pair of hoof testers may be used to ascertain, by applying localized pressure, which area of the foot is causing problems.

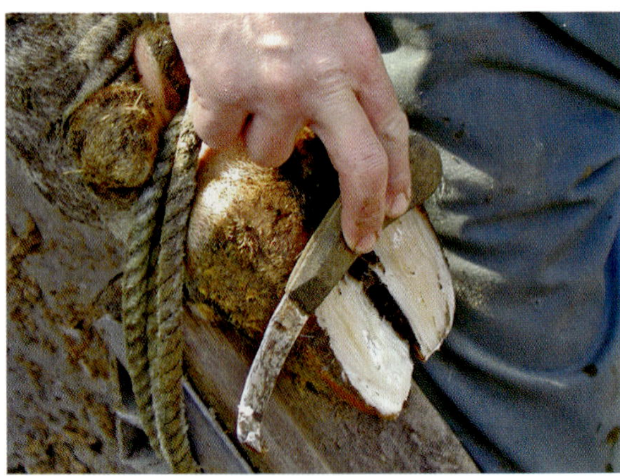

Visually judge whether the soles are even – 'balance' the foot.

- Examine joints higher up the limb – fetlock, hock etc. – if nothing is found in the foot.

This approach will, with care, find most causes of lameness. However, do not be afraid to let the cow out of the crush and check that you have examined the correct leg if nothing obvious is found.

Removing too much horn is risky and likely to do more harm than good. It is important to know when to stop trimming horn and not to remove more horn in a second attempt to find out what is wrong.

In many cases of lameness the defects seen in one foot may be present in the other 'unaffected' foot even though it is not apparently lame. Many claw horn diseases are due to processes that are likely to affect both feet, so it is worth examining the unaffected foot. Be careful not to produce damage that may cause the cow to become lame on both feet.

Try to balance the need to investigate for lameness with the requirement to preserve or create proper foot conformation; do not damage the foot and thus produce more problems. Always use foot trimming techniques (*see* Chapter 4) that will establish a good foot profile, because balancing the foot up will help healing and prevent the lesion worsening.

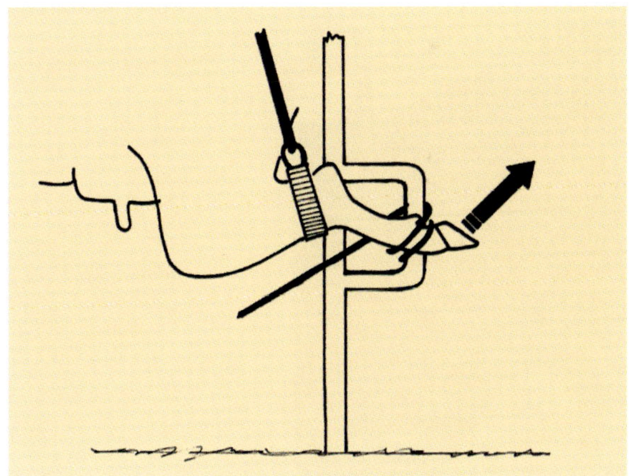

Lifting the foot high brings the sole up more, making it easier to work on.

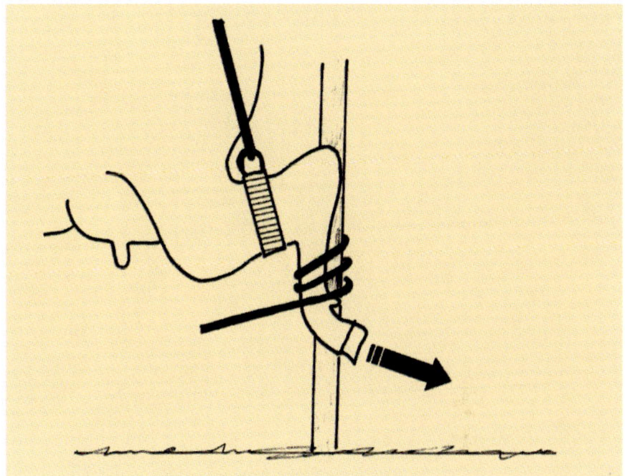

If the foot does not come up enough working can be difficult.

TREATMENT

Techniques for treating feet are primarily based on a specific approach for the particular type of lesion found. However, most cases of lameness need a common approach – to relieve pain and encourage healing. These general techniques can be summarized under the following headings:

- Footbaths.
- Pain control.
- Foot blocks.
- Hospital pens.
- Bandaging.
- Antibiotics.
- Immobilization.

Footbaths

Principles
All dairy herds need some form of footbath. Even beef herds should have access to a foot-bath because with herd sizes increasing the modern beef herd is becoming more prone to 'industrial' lameness.

Footbaths should fulfil certain criteria if they are going to work well:

- They are best sited on the exit side of the parlour so that they will not impede cow movement and the bath fluid will not come into the parlour area. Some herds have sited the baths on the entry side so that the bath fluid will not splash onto the teats after milking and be a mastitis risk.
- They should be far enough away so that a complete side of the milking parlour can be held in the approach to the footbath. This will prevent the exit from the parlour becoming obstructed by cows waiting to go through the bath, which would slow up milking.

The size, shape and design are important. The traditional single-file approach is not the best for larger herds.

- Cows must have reasonably clean feet on entering the 'active' bath. The active agent in the bath must reach the foot tissues.
- There are safety issues for cows and the stock personnel.
- There are safety issues for the environment.

The positioning of the bath dictates how well cattle move through it. On the exit side of a race or a dairy parlour, cattle are more likely to move through the bath without coercion

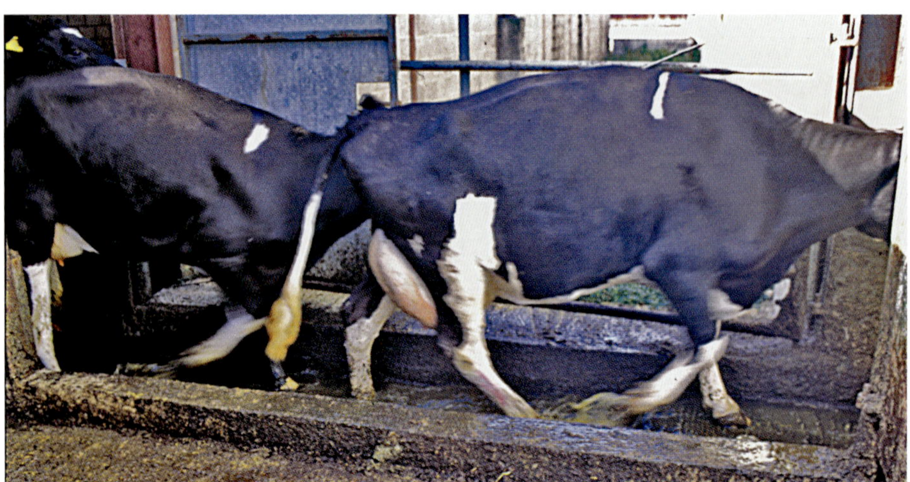

A traditional-style footbath– the cows are often bunched up.

as they make their way back to feeding and bedded areas. The interval when they are restricted, either in the parlour or the race, provokes them to make best use of their freedom and move through quickly. Many of the materials used in footbaths are noxious (formalin) or could cause milk contamination (Lincocin). Therefore, it is best to keep them away from the milking area. Studying cow flow patterns through footbaths indicates that it is best to have two baths side-by-side to allow cows to move through easily without being restricted to single file. A reluctant cow can block the footbath and prevent good cow flow. If cows are not used to a bath, fill it with straw for the first few occasions, as this will give them more confidence to move through it.

Construction

Most footbath systems are designed to have a clean water-filled bath to wash the feet before entering the treatment bath. If the feet are not clean, the footbath chemicals will not come into contact with the foot and will not work as well. In dairy herds this is not necessary if the feet are cleaned in the parlour before going through the bath. However, this will only be feasible for infrequent treatments, and regular use involving a daily walk through the bath is best organized with a wash bath before the treatment area.

The design of the footbath should allow the foot to be covered with the treatment chemical but not so deep as to allow excessive skin contact higher on the leg because this may burn or irritate sensitive skin, especially when using formalin. Baths are often made with a corrugated base so as to spread the claws to try and allow better contact between the digits. This is probably not necessary and from observation it appears to make it difficult to get the cows through the bath as they appear to find it either painful or uncomfortable. The corrugations in the bath may spread the foot too much and damage the cruciate ligaments. The baths should be above the surrounding floor surface and have a drainage hole so that they can be cleaned out easily after use. Plastic footbaths are very useful as they can be moved easily and emptied by tipping up at one side.

The bath soon fills with faecal material and this will quickly inhibit most treatments from working efficiently. It may be necessary to have a top-up policy with some products so that the bath is replenished with active ingredients after a period of use to prevent it deteriorating. Drainage should, if possible, be directed towards the farm dirty-water system so that any active agent can be inactivated by contact with manure and stored to allow it to break down before being spread on the land.

Many footbath treatments are potentially dangerous to cattle, especially if the compounds

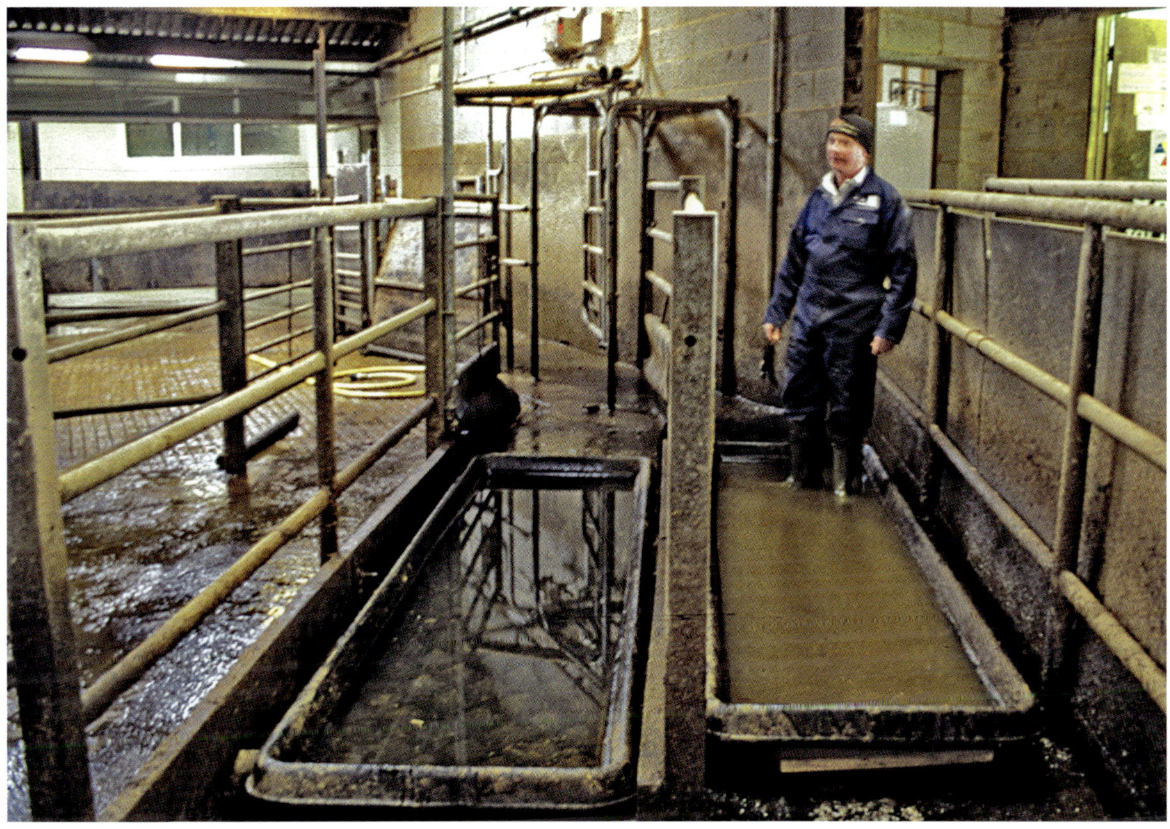

A double system takes the pressure off cow flow through the baths.

used are ingested. Antibiotics will damage the rumen bacteria and severely damage milk production, and copper compounds are toxic. Make sure that the first few cows through a fresh footbath move through without drinking from the bath. As they move through, the first cows will dirty the fluid, so making it less palatable for the next animals.

Compounds to Use

What you use in the footbath depends on what you are trying to achieve. Specific agents such as antibiotics should be restricted for specific conditions that require the use of these expensive products, for example digital dermatitis. However, there is a list of 'general purpose' products for use in footbaths that are mainly aimed at improved horn structure and skin disinfection, both of which could have beneficial effects in many disease situations.

They consist of:

Formalin: Formalin is a very cheap, readily available product that has a proven application for cattle footbaths. The product is supplied as liquid containing 40 per cent formaldehyde in water. The manufacturer's instructions are usually for a 2.5 per cent solution, although it can be used at concentrations between 2.5 and 5 per cent. The product acts as a surface disinfectant for the skin in the interdigital area and at the bulbs of the heels, which are commonly infected in foot disease. It also draws water out from the horn of the foot, so making it harder, although the evidence that this is effective in reducing infection or damage is scant. Formalin is an organic compound and will break down quickly in the presence of manure. It is, however, very unpleasant to handle and great care should be taken for the following reasons:

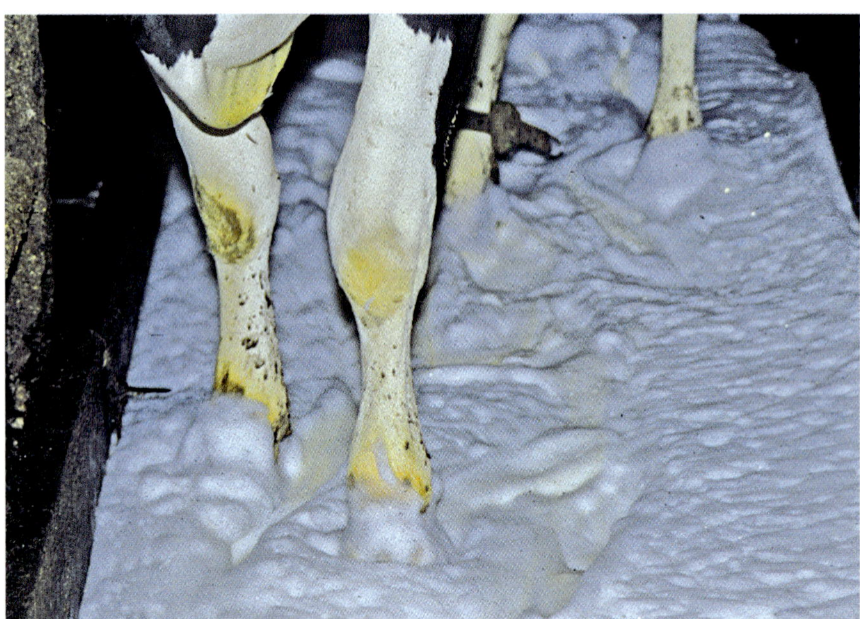

Foam footbaths are now used to try and get the treatment to stick to the feet for longer.

- The fumes are an irritant and it should not be used in a confined space.
- The product may be carcinogenic and toxic so human contact should be prevented.
- It is an irritant on exposed skin lesions and therefore cattle with active infections on the feet (e.g. digital dermatitis) should not be put through the bath.
- It can cause skin irritation on normal, exposed skin, especially in hot weather, so ensure it is not too deep or too concentrated.

Zinc sulphate: This product is much safer to use and acts as a skin disinfectant. It can, in the right conditions, be absorbed through the horn to help strengthen it. Often a dispersant or surfactant agent is used to help it penetrate the horn. The amount that penetrates is probably very low and it is difficult to know if it is effective in producing stronger horn growth. However, it remains a good product to use, although it may be more expensive than some other treatments available. It is generally used as a 10 per cent solution.

Copper sulphate: This compound is a strong surface disinfectant and was commonly used in many footbath preparations for sheep to prevent bacterial growth in the footbath. It is, however, very toxic and poses some problems for disposal because, if used regularly, it will build up on the pasture and potentially produce toxic grazing. It can be used as a 5 per cent solution.

Other disinfectants: There are many other compounds that can be used, most of which act as skin disinfectants. Examples

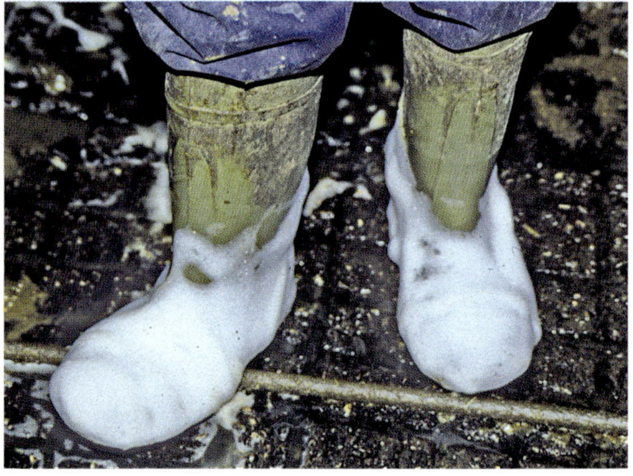

Foam does stick to feet very well.

are benzalkonium, peracetic acid and 'Virkon'; even chemicals discarded after the dairy washing processes are often used. Novel delivery techniques for foot treatments are being developed all the time, for instance a system that allows the use of a disinfectant foam has been introduced recently.

Always be careful to assess the dangers of using other products that do not have a recognized application for cattle footbaths because there may be issues such as:

- The safety of the animals going through the bath.
- The safety of the staff using the baths.
- Disposal of the product after use.

Pain Relief

Modern pain-relieving drugs are now available and are licensed for both beef and dairy cattle. They are very effective and have been shown to have good economic advantages in getting the cow back into production faster.

Localized pain relief is often used when examining a nasty lesion, especially if the treatment has to be invasive or radical. This localized effect is usually achieved with local anaesthetics or powerful analgesic drugs such as xylazine ('Rompun'), which will also make the animal recumbent if required.

There are now many non-steroidal anti-inflammatory drugs (NSAIDs) available with powerful anti-inflammatory actions and excellent pain relief. Even though the length of action may be only short-lived, there appears to be distinct advantages in using these products in the short term. Useful examples are flunixin and ketoprofen.

Foot Blocks

Lameness is caused by pain or discomfort when a foot is weight bearing or touches the floor surface. For this reason, treatment of a diseased claw often involves lifting it up to take it out of contact with the ground. This not only relieves pain but also helps prevent wound contamination and speeds up the healing process. A block applied to the adjacent sound claw will effectively immobilize the affected claw.

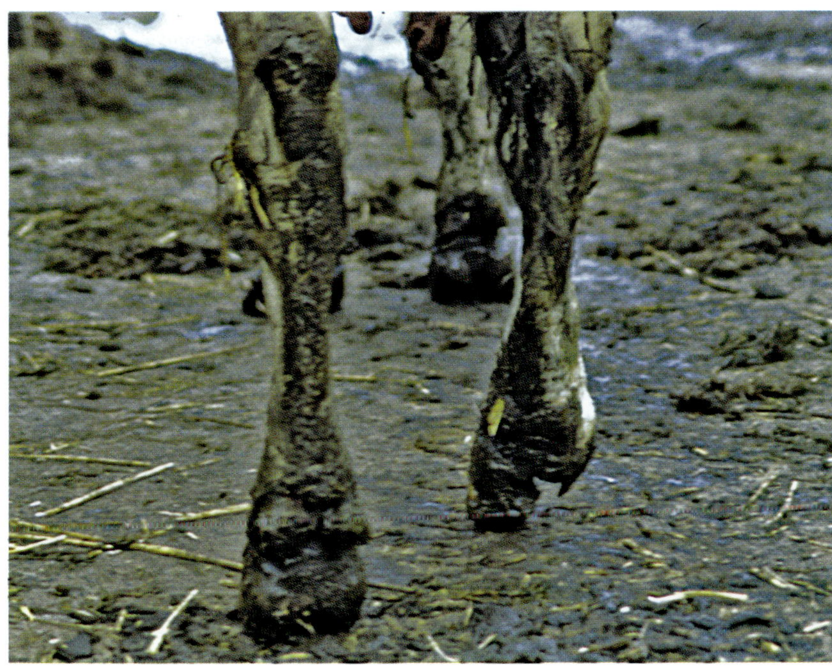

Using foot blocks on the sound claw lifts the affected claw.

In general, an 'ideal' type of block should:

- Be easy and quick to use, and preferably inexpensive. If it meets these requirements, it will be used frequently and not just for the 'special' cases.
- Be thick enough. A good thickness of block is necessary to lift the affected claw well above the floor surface. Diseased claws are often swollen and need a lot of clearance to take them off the ground.
- Be fitted well back on the sole towards the heel. This is the most common mistake made with blocks. If they are too far forward then the foot rotates (drops) backwards, straining the flexor tendons and possibly permanently damaging them. It also concentrates wear on the back of the block, which with time slopes away and exacerbates the problem.
- Be stable and not move.

When and Where Do You Use a Block?
A block can, in general, do no harm as long as it is applied correctly to the sound claw. Therefore, the decision is one of justification, time and the expense involved. The main areas likely to show benefit from the use of a block are:

- Exposed corium. If an area of corium is exposed during treatment, or caused by a lesion, contact with the ground when walking will cause pain and could affect healing, e.g. a solar ulcer.
- Weight bearing. Any disease that produces pain when the foot is weight bearing. In practice, all lameness is due to pain on weight bearing so it must be qualified to mean where pain is excessive or there is the prospect of it being prolonged.
- Immobilization. Any disease of the limb that requires immobilization of the affected claw to help with pain or healing, e.g. septic arthritis.
- Blocks should be used only if the animal is to be housed on, or regularly moved across, a hard surface. Blocks will offer no support in a straw-yard environment.

Acrylic Resin (Methacrylate) and Wooden Block (Demotec/Technovit)
Moderate skill is needed to prepare this block, especially in cold weather. Careful foot preparation is required for best results, which means that the claw to be blocked must be trimmed properly, thoroughly clean, and dry. The application time is reliant on ambient temperature because the reaction between the liquid and the powder in curing into a hard bonding structure is temperature dependent. The reaction is rapid when hot and very slow when cold. The easiest way to speed up the process is to warm the liquid component in a bucket of hot water before use. Slow curing can be problematic as the block will move around whilst it is setting. Any thickness or type of wooden

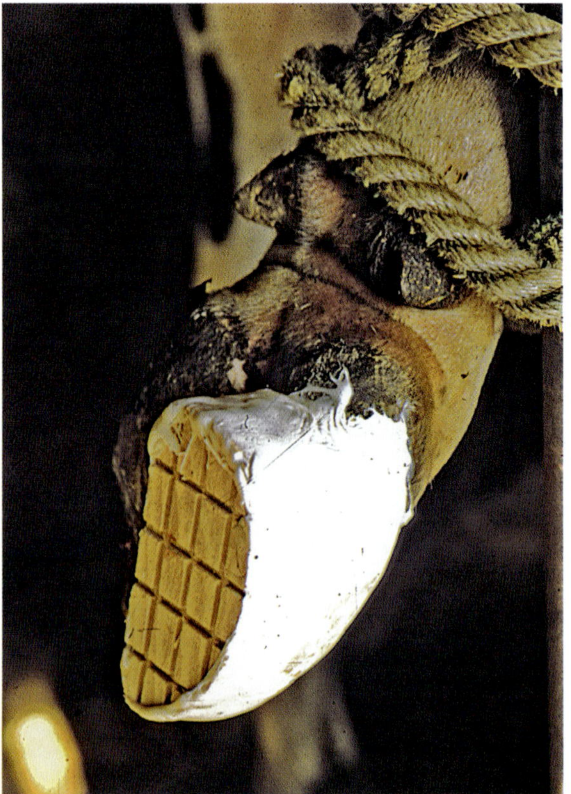

'Demotec' foot block.

48

block can be used and better-quality hardwood blocks can be made easily and used with the commercial packs to give more depth or a better shape. The position of the block is easy to control provided it is adjusted during the curing period. Eventually the block may need removing, especially if the heel has worn down first and produced upward rotation of the toe. However, it is normal for the block to wear off without any interference needed.

Acrylic Resin 'Cowslip' Type
Less preparation is required for this type of block, but the same comments on the speed of application apply as with the above. These blocks require less skill to apply and thus take less time to employ. The size of the block is dependent on the product and cannot be altered, although there are a variety of sizes available. Because the block is slipped over the claw from the front its size and, in particular, its length controls where it is finally positioned. Often on a cow with a long foot the standard block cannot be positioned far enough back and this can cause problems with rotation of the digit as described above. New longer versions are now available. You need to keep a supply of different blocks because they are 'handed' in their shape to fit either left or right claws, as well as being available in different sizes.

Strap-On Blocks
There are two main types of strap-on block. The lace-up whole foot boot, of which the 'Shoof' is an example, comes with half of the sole fitted with a wedge to produce the neces-

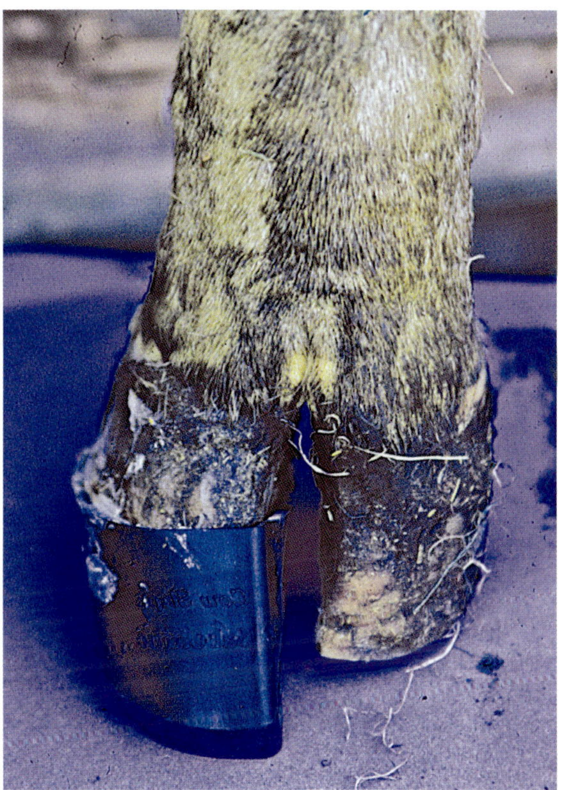
'Cowslip'-type block.

sary lift. It is not now commonly used as it needs to be stocked in a range of foot sizes with the need for a variety of left or right 'lift' to take account of which claw needs to be raised. There are versions of the 'Shoof' with a totally flat sole which, if sealed properly to prevent dirt and slurry getting in, can be used as a protective 'bandage' for the foot if too much corium has been exposed.

Type of foot block	Unit cost (£)*	Application time (min)	Time on foot	Total cost (£)*
Demotec/Technovit block	9	15–25	4–12 weeks	34–45
'Cowslip'	10	10–15	4–8 weeks	26–35
Wood block + bandage	7	10	2–10 days	25
Rubber nail-on block	5	5	2–12 weeks	13

Table 6 Types of block available and comments on their use
Note that these are typical veterinary prices based on 2005 costs

However, a quick method of blocking is to strap a wooden block onto the sound claw using adhesive bandage. This system is very easy to use but does not last long, especially when the cow is walking any distance. It is difficult to get tight and position accurately, but it is cheap and quick. The main advantage with this method is that it can be used to 'assess' which digit to put a more permanent block on if you are not sure of the cause of the lameness – a 'trial block'.

Nail-On Blocks

This product needs much skill and many users are put off after failing with a 'mishap' or two. A nail in the wrong place can do a lot of damage. However, they are cheap and quick to apply. The block thickness is dependent on the product, but it can be positioned anywhere it is required on the foot – forward or backward. A minor problem with these blocks is that they can rotate into the midline after a period of time and can start to rub on the diseased claw, although this is usually after most of the healing has occurred; to correct this problem, remove or 'dish' out the inside edge of the block with a knife. About 10 per cent of rubber blocks need some kind of removal (whether it is the rubber or just the nail remnants) after

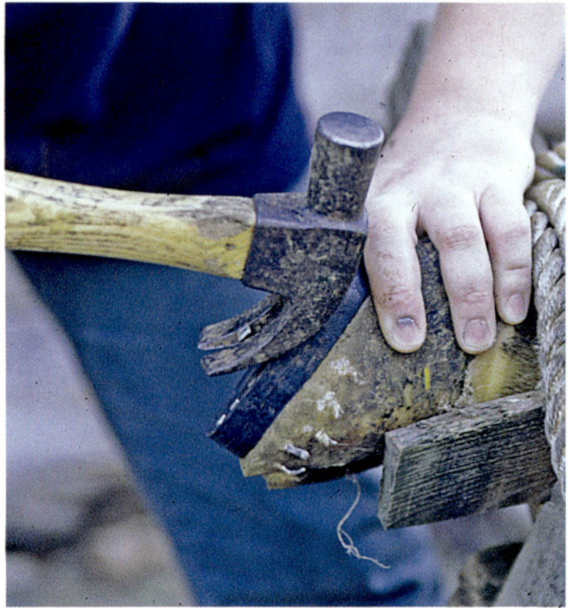

Skills using the equipment are best learnt away from the real thing. Nail-on blocks need a lot of practice to get right.

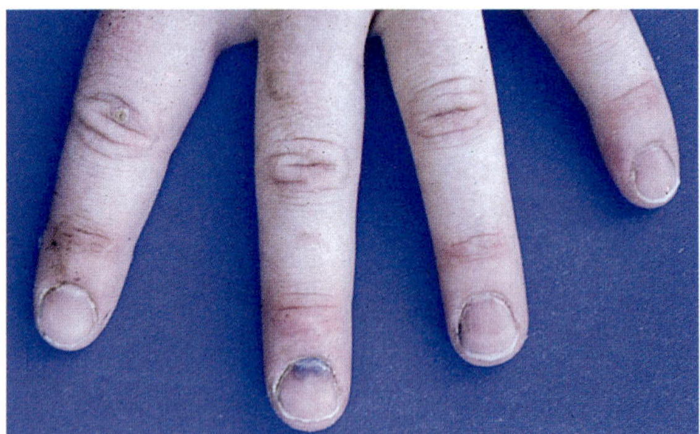

Not all nailing goes to plan – accidents do happen.

a period of time, although complications from leaving them on are very rare.

The best way to become accustomed to any sort of block and its use is to practise. Training courses can be arranged using feet from the local abattoir held in bench clamps or proper training stands to hold the foot steady whilst working. It is much easier to develop skills this way before going near the 'live' cow.

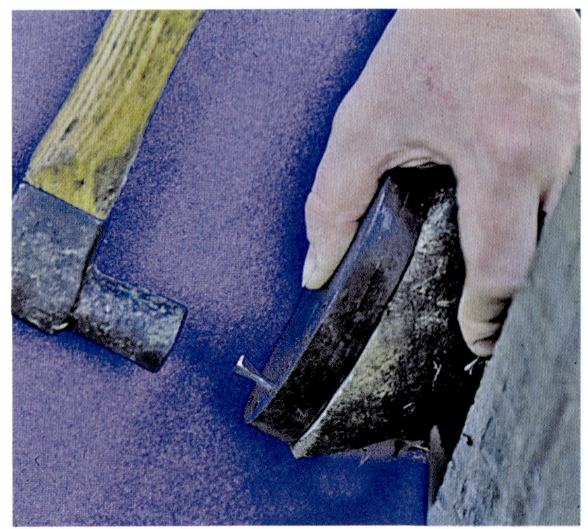

A nail-on block.

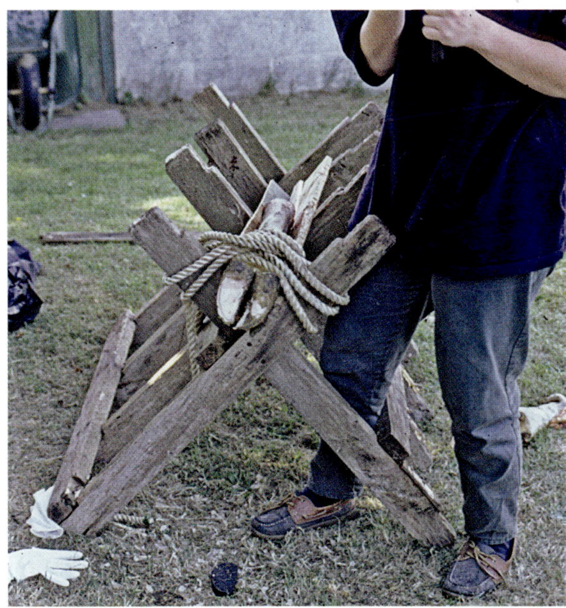

Use abattoir limbs to improve skills with trimming and foot care. This shows a stand being used for teaching.

	Mattress base	Sand base
Normal cows	2.4h	1.7h
Slightly lame cows	4.4h	2.1h
Lame cows	6.1h	1.8h

Table 7 The length of time cows stand in the cubicle

The aim with any block is to reduce the amount of pain for a long enough period of time to allow near-normal movement of the limb. An added benefit is that it should improve the healing process by stopping effective use and preventing irritation and contamination of the affected claw. I now use cheap blocks, such as the nail-on variety, in preference to all other foot dressings.

Hospital Pens

Do we pay enough attention to the type of environment in which we house the lame cow? Research in Wisconsin, USA has indicated that although normal cows may behave similarly in different types of cubicle and on different bedding materials, provided they are of good design and quality, lame cows may not. This is important because to get the best healing rate in lame cows we must ensure that they are given conditions compatible with good recovery.

The work done in the USA looked at sand and mattress-based cubicles or 'free stalls' as they call them. They observed (as shown in Table 7) that there was little difference between normal cows, but the difference was very marked for lame cows. Standing behaviour increased by over 4 hours in the lame cows on mattresses.

Although this work may be specific to USA conditions it highlights the need to treat lame cows in such a way as to prevent this happening. This increased standing behaviour may have relevance to the healing rate of foot lesions in lame cows. The surface material of the cubicle has an effect on the confidence of the cow to lie down and get up so she spends more time standing. Standing behaviour is strongly associated with increased levels of lameness and it is possible that it will delay healing and produce a greater prevalence of lameness, as more cows will be lame for longer periods of time. In the UK it may be that we should be using more sand-based cubicles for dry cows and as a hospital yard, although it would be more common to see a straw yard used for this purpose. Although straw has some drawbacks for other health issues, such as mastitis, it is a good environment for the freshly calved and the lame cow to increase lying times and prevent further damage to the feet.

There is no point in using blocks on claws as treatment if you put the animal back into a straw environment. The block will only have an effect if it is used on cattle on a hard surface where it will support the damaged claw away from the surface.

Bandaging

A common question from herdspersons is whether or not bandaging a foot will have any benefit. On average the answer is no. There is little need to wrap the foot after treatment and

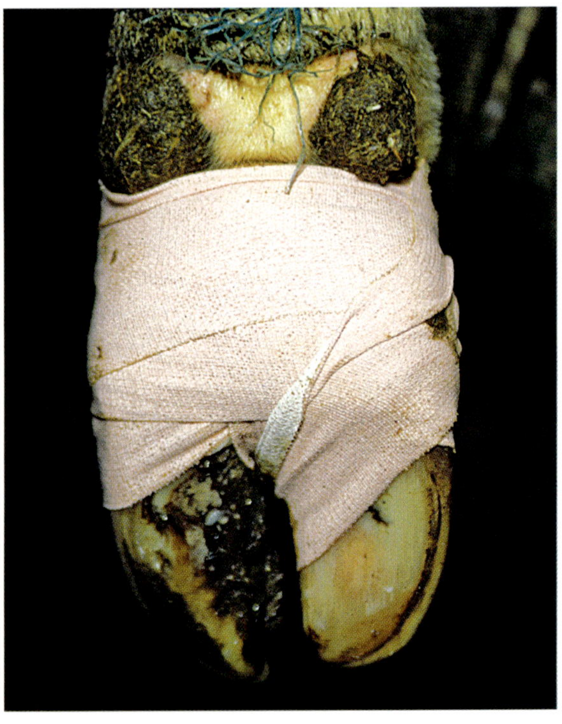

Bandage a foot only when you need to keep treatment on an affected area – digital dermatitis.

usually it is contraindicated because this will prevent drainage of infected material from the site and cause further problems by retaining pus and fluid in the lesions. Bandaging stands proud of the foot surface and will put more pressure on the lesion as the cow walks unless a good foot block is applied to the sound claw to lift it clear.

The only two indications that would require bandaging are:

- If you need to keep a treatment in the area of the lesion for a period of time, for example a chronic digital dermatitis lesion can benefit from wrapping in antibiotic.
- If vital structures have been exposed you may need to protect the foot from being contaminated with slurry or bedding materials. Usually blocking the good claw is sufficient by itself to do this and is much the preferable option.

Antibiotics

Antibiotics should only be used with veterinary guidance. In general they are not of prime importance except in specific conditions such as 'foul'. They can, however, be a useful adjunct to other treatments, but never expect the use of an antibiotic to produce any benefit without diagnosing what is wrong with the foot first.

Most conditions affecting the bovine foot present a very demanding situation for antibiotics. Due to the relatively poor blood supply to some areas of the foot, especially structures such as bone, joints and skin, systemic treatment may not reach the target site in levels sufficient to produce any benefit. Other forms of therapy often heavily influence the choice of antibiotic and they are rarely successful as a primary treatment, usually requiring additional procedures to be fully effective. For instance, it is unrealistic to expect an antibiotic to clear a septic arthritis without first managing to drain the joint thoroughly.

In summary:

- Do not use antibiotics without first finding out what is wrong.
- Do not use as the primary treatment except for 'foul'.
- Always drain septic material before using an antibiotic.
- Get advice on which antibiotics are likely to be most effective.
- Establish good protocols for the use of antibiotics with a veterinary surgeon.

The general use of a 'blue spray' (usually oxytetracycline plus a blue dye) is a good topical treatment after any routine foot care, although how much good it does is unknown. It is good practice to put the cow into a clean, dry area after topical treatment to allow the spray to dry on the foot. This is very important if you are relying on sprays as the front-line treatments for digital dermatitis.

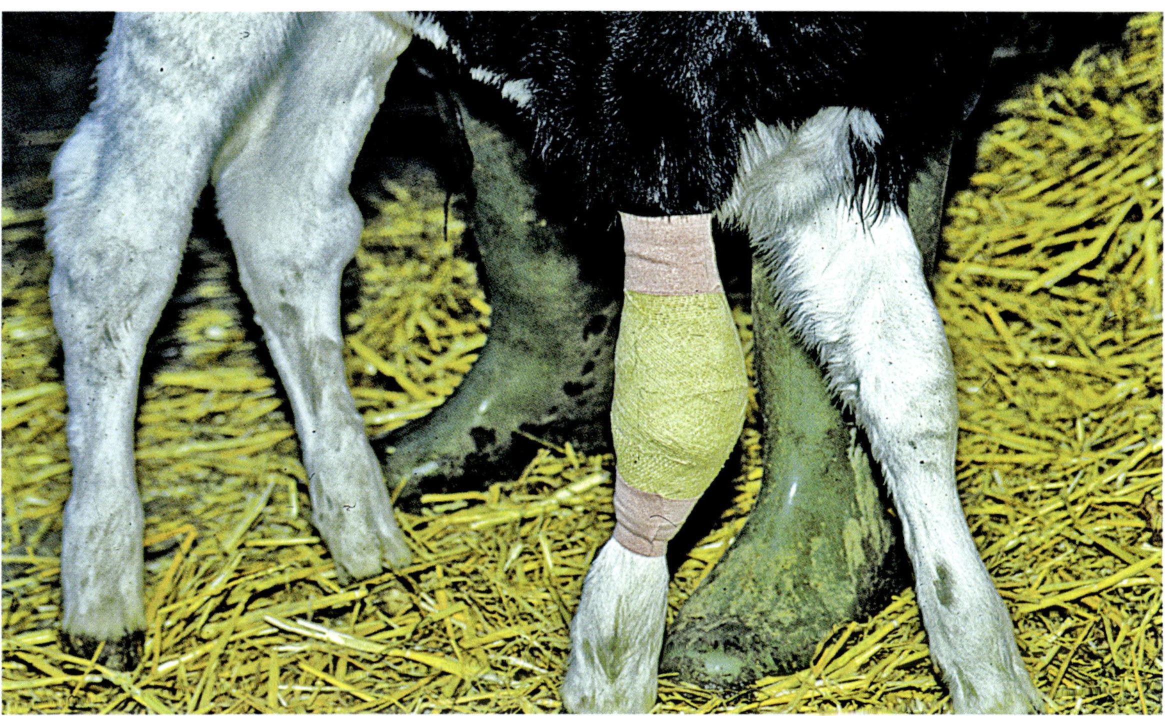

Using plastic casts is very effective. This calf has a joint infection, which is now immobilized making it less painful.

Immobilization

Immobilization was a common last resort 25 years ago for a foot lameness that was getting out of hand. Today, as a general treatment, it has largely been replaced by good blocking techniques. However, it can be useful for a variety of specific and non-specific reasons. Immobilization will aid in pain relief and recovery with any lesion where movement of the joint is likely to make it worse, for example a septic arthritis in the pedal joint (*see* Chapter 7).

What is available?

- Plaster cast materials.
- Plaster in combination with a plastic or other reinforcement.
- Plastic casts.
- Bandages and splinting.

Plaster is cheap and easy to use; however, it does not last long, especially in the normal working conditions of a dairy farm, unless the cow is housed separately. It is heavy in proportion to its strength and soon breaks down in wet conditions. The best way to use it is in conjunction with a plastic reinforcement.

Temperature-sensitive plastic meshing rolls can be used to improve the plaster cast; they add strength and lightness by reducing the amount of plaster required.

Nowadays plastic, cold-water cure, casting bandages are extremely good and becoming less costly. They are easy to apply and incredibly strong for the weight of material applied. One of the biggest problems is actually getting them off after use. You will need to bury a cutting wire into the cast to cut through and remove it. However, some of the newer plastics are so tough that it requires two cuts with the wire at opposite sides of the cast to remove it (you can get your fingers badly trapped trying to open them up from one side only!).

CHAPTER FOUR

Foot Trimming

Foot trimming involves trying to realign the foot through the structured removal of horn so that it represents an ideal form. This should promote a good gait, less lameness and better cow comfort, along with all the benefits that this entails. Trimming a cow's foot should be considered an 'examination and judgement' of the foot, the horn growth and its conformation. The outcome of this examination is that some feet will need attention although many will not. There is no need to trim all feet regardless, as this is likely to produce problems rather than solve them.

There is little evidence that trimming cows' feet has any effect on lameness in a herd. It is difficult to show any major advantage in many of the objective studies that have been done. There are a few studies where there has been some indication that overall locomotion scores are better, along with fewer lame cows, when trimming has been carried out. Common sense tells us that trimming cows' feet must be beneficial, but we need to be careful that we carry out the technique well, choose the right group of cows, and do the job at the right time. If not, many of the potential benefits will be lost.

Whenever a cow is examined for lameness it must be borne in mind that the aim is not only to treat the cause of the lameness but also to return the foot to a better conformation by applying trimming skills. This may help prevent further problems and can improve the comfort of the cow and the rate at which the lesion heals. Foot trimming, however, is also a procedure in its own right that needs to be done regularly to try and prevent lameness lesions occurring.

If done properly, trimming can have several major benefits:

- It allows examination of the foot in a case of lameness.
- It is an integral part of any specific treatment for lameness.
- It prevents irregularities in horn growth.
- It produces good foot conformation.

TECHNIQUE

Restraint of the animal has already been discussed, along with the fact that the requirements for trimming as opposed to lameness examination are very different. Routine trimming can be done using specialist trimming crushes that allow better access around the foot to get a good view of the angle of the claws and the 'balance' between them. Specialized crushes may also be able to handle large numbers of cows more efficiently because they can be specially fitted out with geared or automatic winches and so on. However, for most farms carrying out their own trimming, the same restraint method and the same type of crush as used for lame cows is adequate. Also, if a less experienced operator were carrying out the trimming they would benefit from more secure holding of the foot rather than the freely suspended foot in the trimming

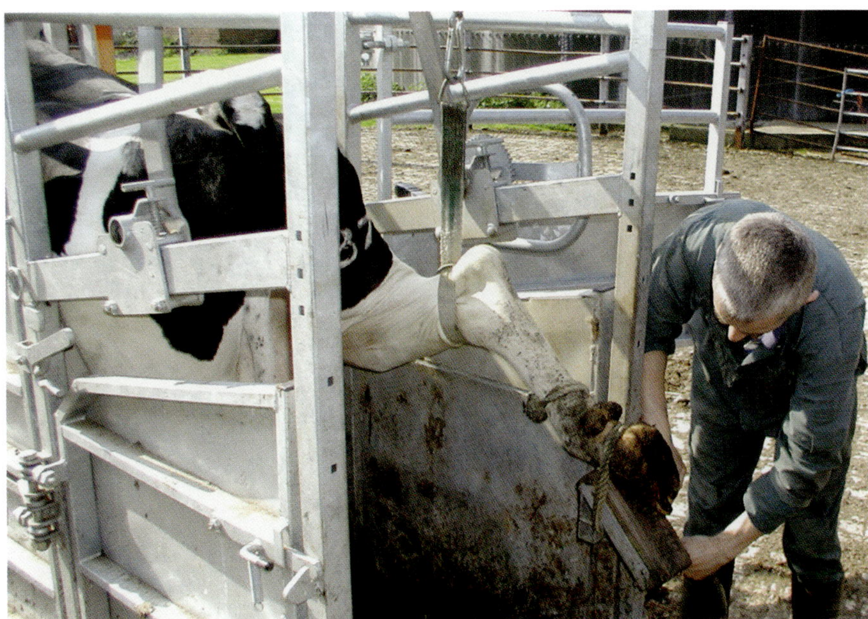

Make sure the leg is anchored well if you are inexperienced or using an ordinary crush.

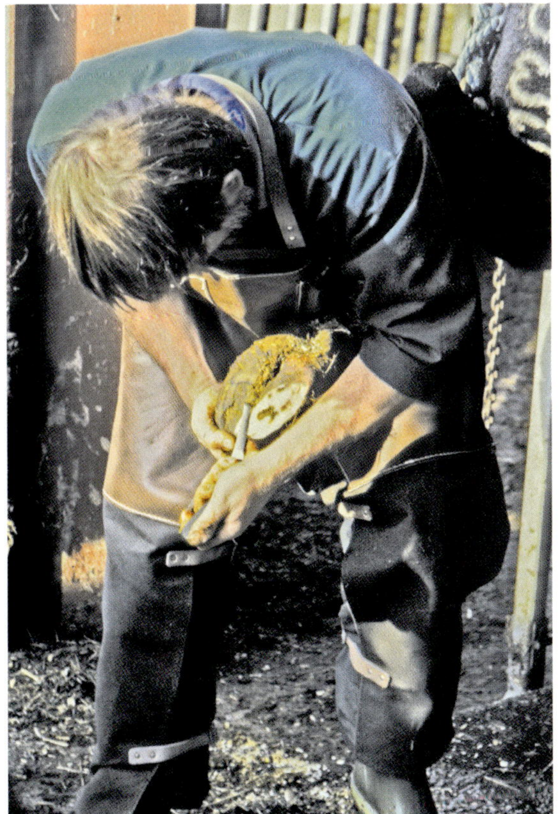

Using a trimming crush means you can work very closely with the foot to see the angles to trim at.

crush. In fact, most veterinarians prefer using a fixed-point type of restraint. It is easier and, in my experience, a lot faster to do the job using this approach.

Clean the foot up in the same way as described in Chapter 3, so that you can see the horn and spot any defects that are present. Remember that the aim with trimming is not to find lesions but to correct conformation and establish correct weight bearing for the whole foot. Do not try and follow every horn defect and forget what the aim of trimming the foot is all about.

The same basics for examining the lame cow apply to the trimming job – good light, a well-restrained cow and sharp tools.

USING THE TOOLS PROPERLY

The tools required are the same, although if large numbers of cows are being trimmed power tools make the job a lot easier. Various cutting discs and grinding wheels are now available, but they need careful use as it is easy to produce too much heat on the horn or simply be too enthusiastic and remove excess horn from the wrong places. This can cause

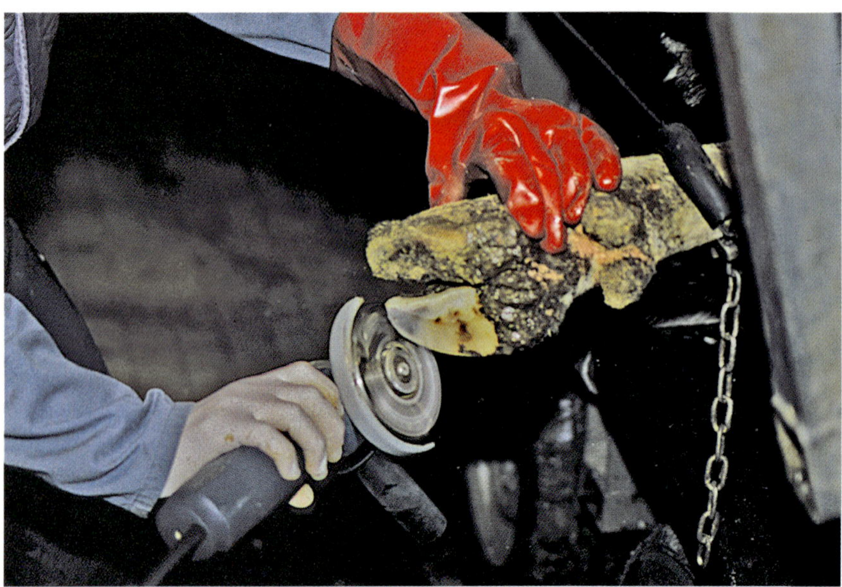

Power tools can make life easy but be sure you can control them.

problems with sore feet or even lameness rather than trimmed feet.

The Clippers or Hoof Shears

Using the clippers is straightforward, especially if a good-quality small design is used (e.g. 'Diamond'). It is essential to try and use them so that the cut is in the same plane as the sole. Any horn removed will then allow the walls of the horn to stay weight bearing in contact with the ground.

Cutting away the wall horn vertically means it cannot bear weight, so more pressure will come to bear on the soles and potentially cause problems. The easiest way to use clippers is from behind, facing the same way as the cow. The foot should be strapped firmly to a vertical support so that it is fully immobilized whilst the clipping is done with both hands. Many foot trimmers use the clippers whilst supporting the foot from the front – facing backwards and putting the leg on the operator's thighs to support it. This allows you to keep a constant eye on the plane of cutting and compare the two claws at the same time by looking down the leg on top of the claws. You will, however, have to use the clippers single-handed, which can be awkward and time-consuming.

The Foot Knife

Whenever possible use two hands on the knife to control the cut and transfer enough power to the blade. Decide which side of the foot you are most comfortable working from; if you are right-handed this will usually be on the right of the foot and the reverse if left-handed. When you are comfortable with the working position, the double-handed action works well for downward cuts on the claw nearest the operator, but the knife will have to be reversed for the inside claw. This means using it single-

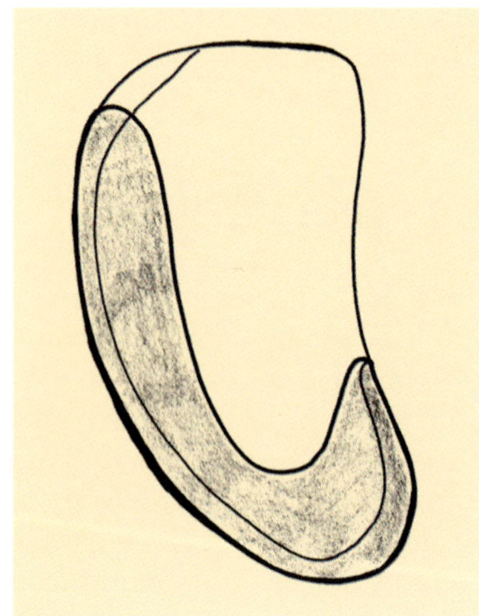

View of the sole with the shaded area indicating weight bearing.

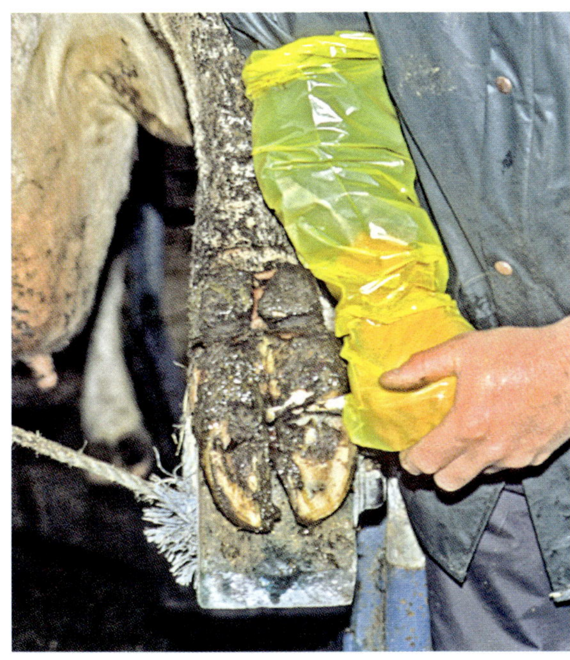

On the nearest claw use both hands for a controlled downward cut.

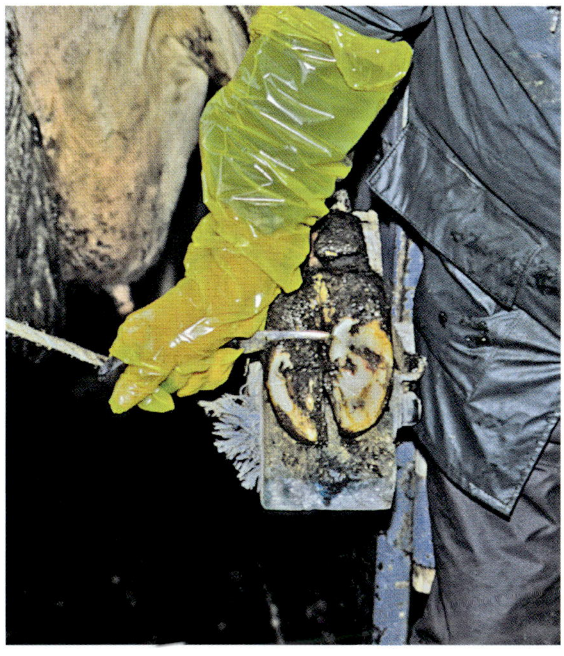

On the farthest claw use one hand, keeping the other out of the way.

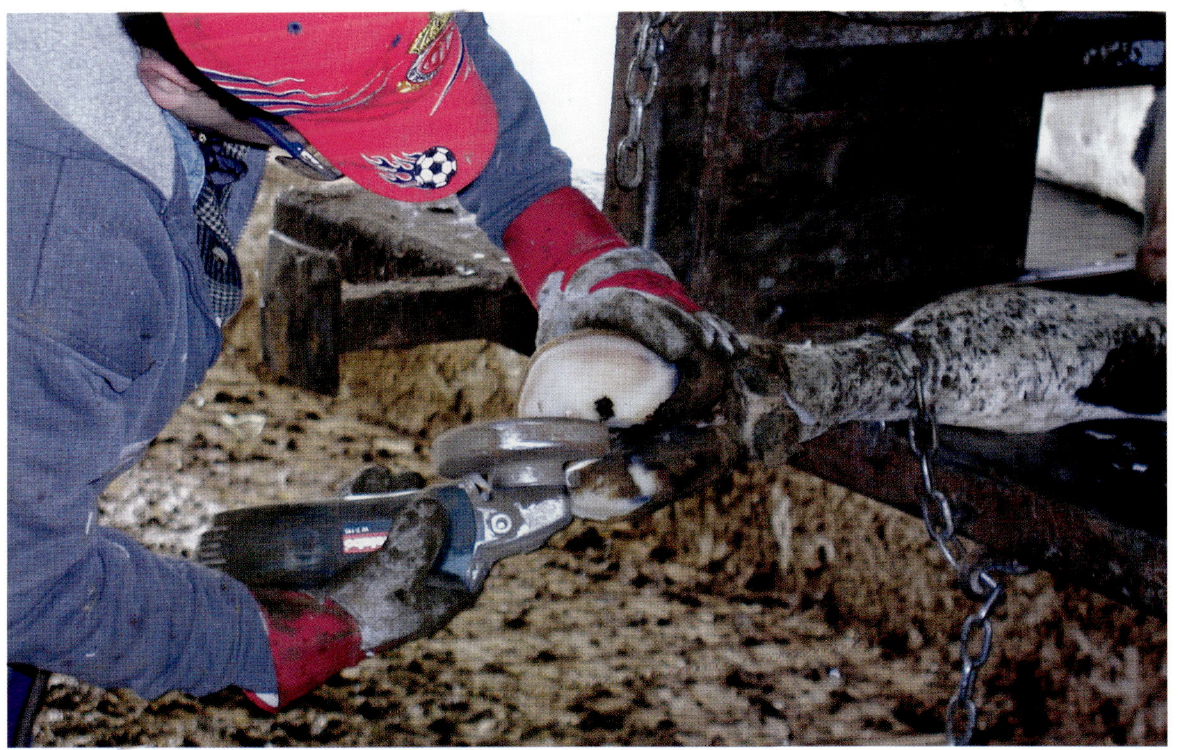

Power tools are used.

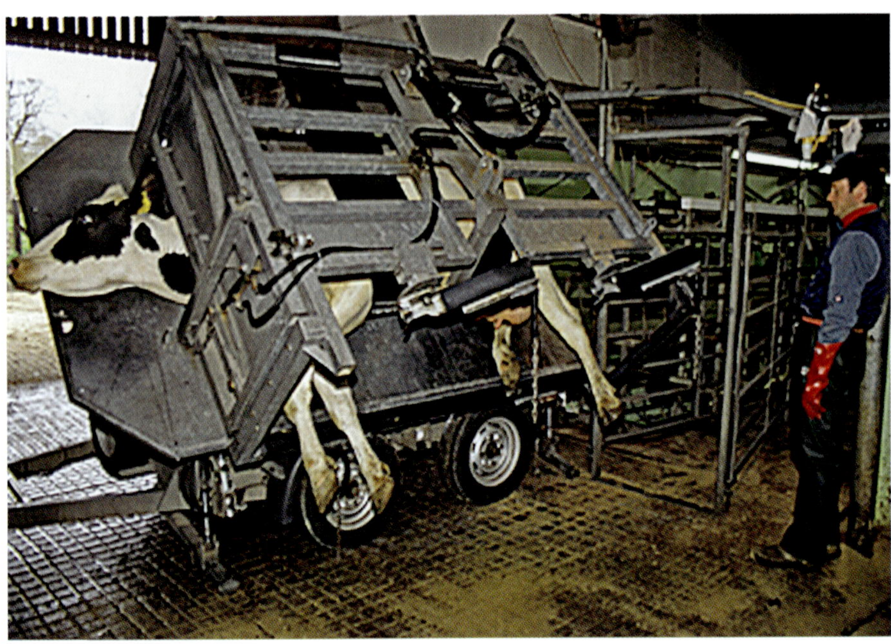

Hydraulic tipping crushes are essential if trimming a lot of cows.

handed as placing two hands on the knife for the farther claw will be awkward and one of the hands will obstruct your view of the claws when leaning across the foot. When using a knife single-handed, keep the other hand behind your back to prevent the temptation to hold the claw whilst trimming. Holding claws with one hand and trimming with the other is very dangerous.

Surforms or hoof files may be useful to finish the job off and make the horn smooth, although a good knife well used will do the job in one step without the need for these tools.

When using the knife it is important to control the angle at which the blade is cutting. If it is angled too deeply, too much horn will be engaged at one time and this will make it difficult to trim. Using shallow angles will make it easier to remove smaller amounts of horn quickly. Changing the angle of the knife during the length of the cut is a skill which allows slivers of horn to be pared off accurately

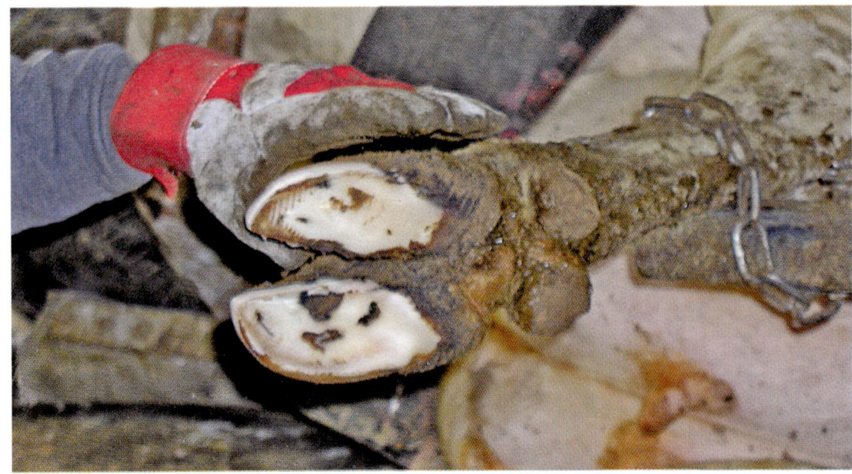

The feet are fastened securely.

rather than getting the knife stuck in the horn or paring off unnecessary amounts of horn.

TRIMMING PROTOCOL

The process of trimming can be based on a set protocol such as the 'Dutch Method' for foot trimming. This is a very successful method, but its widespread success probably represents the fact that it is a protocol that can be taught and followed easily rather than any gold standard that has to be adopted. Many foot trimmers, veterinarians and farmers have developed their own skills that do the job perfectly well but are not written down.

Visual Assessment

Always look at the claws first before diving in with the knife and clippers. Assess the quality of the horn, the shape and distribution of it (especially on the sole) and view the foot from above to get some idea of the comparison between the claws – the so-called 'balance' of the foot. If you put the handle of the knife across both claws, you will see by looking down the leg from the hock whether or not the two claws are even. Evenly placed claws will put weight straight up the leg whereas uneven claws (usually the lateral claw is thicker than the inner claw) tend to make the leg angle

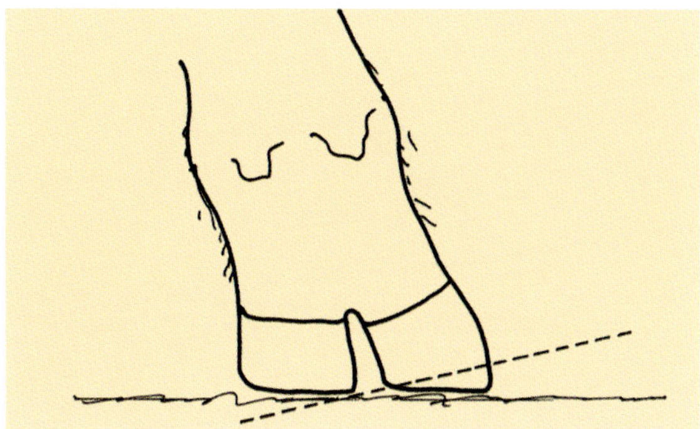

Balancing the foot means trying to keep both soles in the same plane, so it encourages good posture and prevents excess horn pressing on the sole.

outwards as the cow tries to take weight on both soles.

The Inner Claw as a 'Template'

The outside claw on hind feet usually needs most trimming and therefore the inside claw can be used as the template to work to. Quickly neatening up the inside claw will give the dimensions and angles needed for the outer claw, which will take more time and effort. The outer claw should have its sole at the same level as the inner claw and a reasonable effort should be made to try and make the outer claw the same length and angle. The reverse is true when trimming front feet.

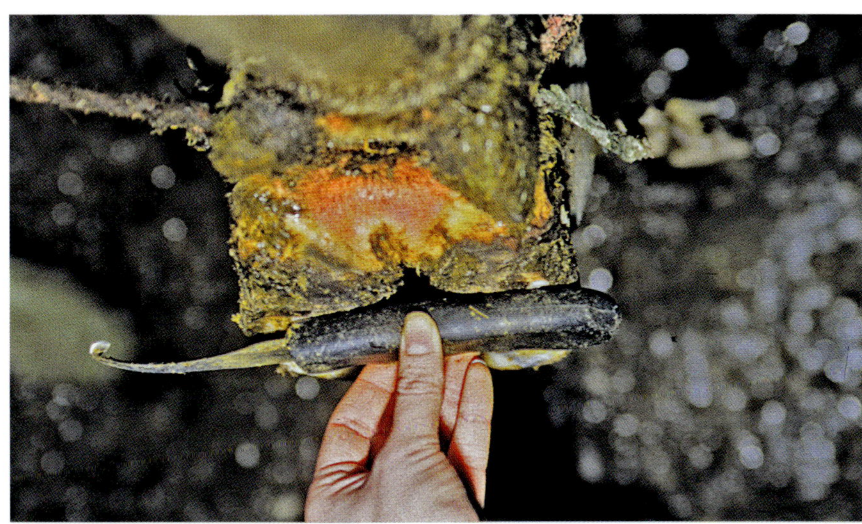

Use the knife handle across both soles and view it down the leg from above. The 'balance' between the claws should be apparent.

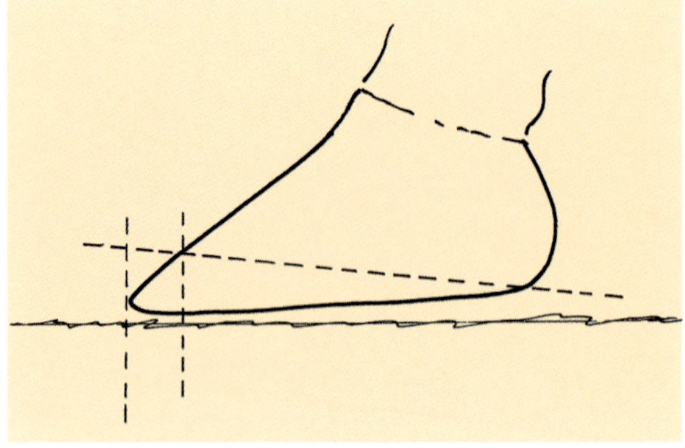

Trimming means taking off horn to shorten the toe and improve the angle of the foot.

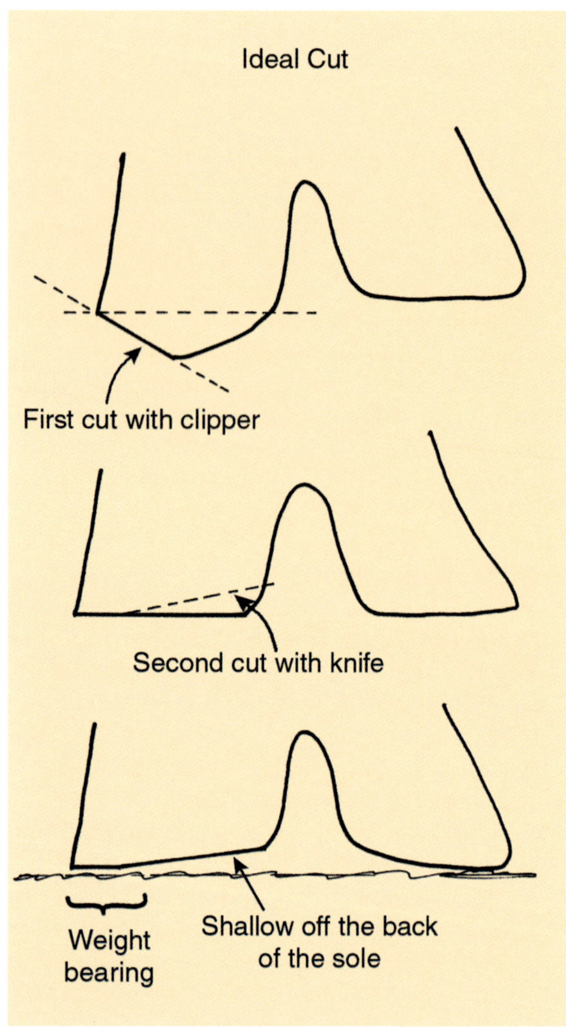

Foot section showing the steps taken to create an ideal cut.

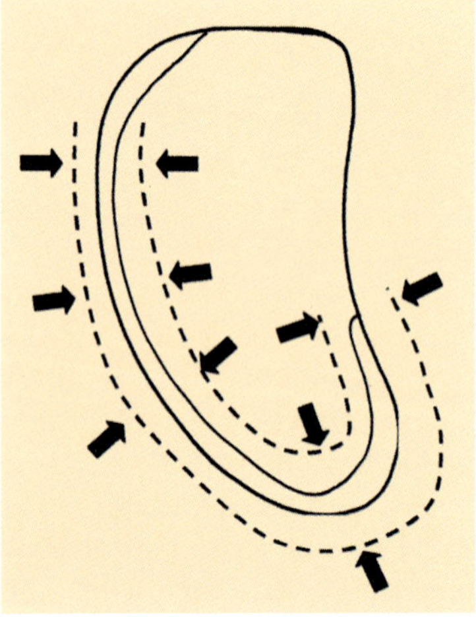

Using the clippers as flat as possible with the sole, clip from the heel towards the toe and up the axial wall.

Removing Horn

You should now have a template to work to and an 'ideal' shape that you want to achieve; mostly this will involve trying to reduce the length of the toe and recreate a steeper hoof angle.

Using the clippers start from the heel and clip away the outside wall. Keep the clippers parallel to the sole of the foot so that all the horn cuts are in the same plane as the sole of the foot, i.e. flat with the sole. This is not easy, as when using the clippers flat like this they tend to skip over the sole horn because the angle of contact with the sole is very shallow.

To counter this make sure the clippers are pushed towards the interdigital space to force the cut into a flat plane. This cutting should progress along the wall, down to the toe and up the interdigital space for approximately two-thirds of the way. The depth of the cut increases as you move from the heel to the toe area; to decrease the length of the toe take progressively more off the wall, which then shortens the toe.

Use a knife to trim the sole down to match the pattern of the outside wall cuts and aim to correct the plane of the sole. First level the sole, then dish it out slightly towards the

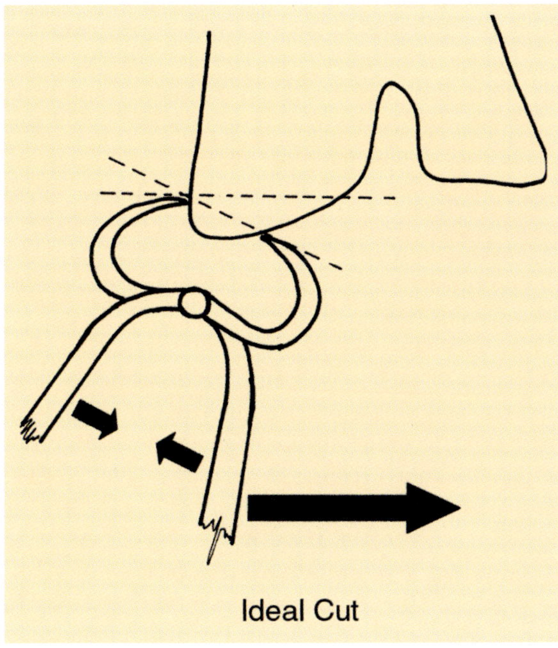

Ideal Cut

The ideal cut is keeping the clippers flat – push them inwards when clipping.

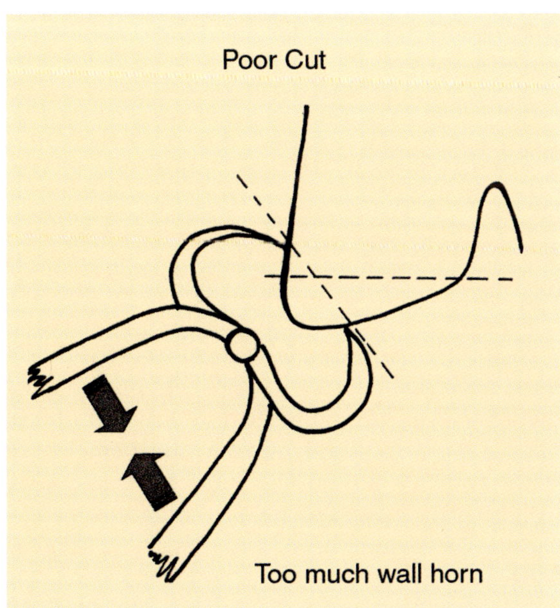

Poor Cut

Too much wall horn

A poor cut with too much wall taken off – the clippers swing outwards.

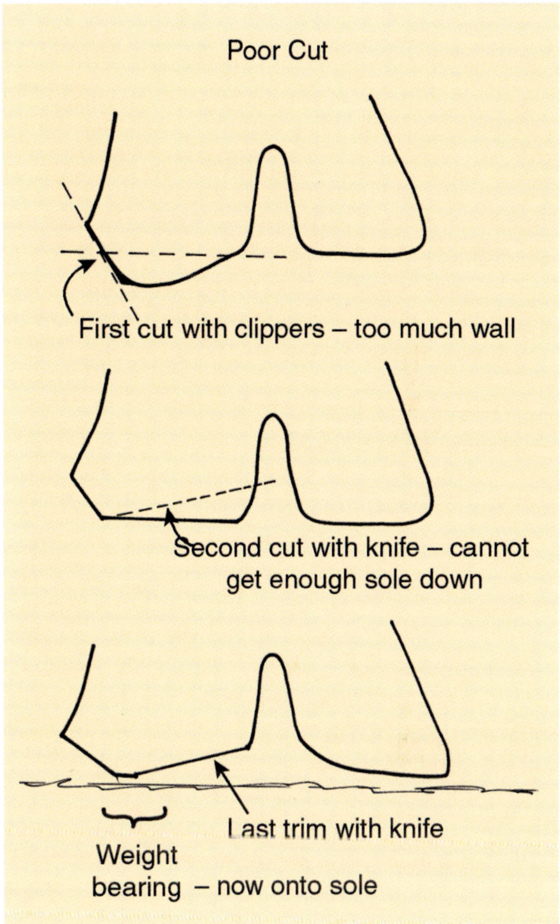

The effect of a poor cut is more weight is taken on the sole.

interdigital space so that the weight bearing is on the wall–sole junction round the entire length of the white line. Do not dish the sole so that the axial wall is reduced; this will prevent the foot from standing level on the ground because the claws will be forced apart, which will put pressure on the cruciate ligaments (*see* diagram in Chapter 1).

Check the conformation of the claws. Look at the balance between them, the length of the toes and the claw overall, the length of the front wall and the angle of the front wall to the flat of the sole. If you are not happy that they are even, the foot may need further trimming.

It may not be possible to achieve the ideal shape at a single trimming session. In some cows the shape of the claw cannot be corrected because there is not enough solar horn to be able to pare it back into shape. These cows will need another session of trimming after there has been more horn growth. Removing too much horn to achieve an ideal pattern is a mistake because it is likely to expose the corium or make the sole too thin. Both of these will make the cow lame or tender on its feet.

WHEN TO TRIM

Fortunately horn continues to grow and this produces the healing we see when lameness lesions are treated. However, this growth in cattle that have been lame often involves developing an abnormal conformation that makes them more prone to further cases of lameness and thus they will, in turn, need more frequent trimming.

For this reason foot trimming should, ideally, be decided on a cow-by-cow basis based on keeping good records (has she had problems before?) or by careful observation of gait, the shape of the foot, and horn growth. This is often apparent when the cow is seen in the milking parlour at eye level. Check for excess horn lifting up one claw and angling the foot outwards (*see* diagram on page 59) and ensure the toes are not too long. With larger herds, however, it is necessary to have set protocols to make sure jobs are done on time rather than relying on stockperson skills. This means setting up a fixed procedure for routine foot trimming that will, on average, give the best benefit. Most protocols are based on trimming the cow at drying off. This has several advantages:

- When trimming at this time the cow is likely to go out into the field or be left in a straw yard for several weeks without any exercise back and forward to the milking parlour. This will help with any excess trimming that may be needed or if a defect has been found that needs extra treatment.
- All the defects that have accumulated from problems during the lactation can be dealt with before the stress period of the next lactation starts. Most lameness occurs at or soon after calving.

For some cows it will not be enough to trim once in the lactation. Recording the results of a trimming can help to highlight which cows will need more frequent attention. Very often some form of routine trimming is needed for certain cows after they have calved. A lot of the damage is done at calving, and soon after, so part of the set protocol should be to trim high-risk cows – those that have been lame before, or shown problems at the routine drying-off trimming. It is unrealistic to think that a single trimming will be sufficient when a cow's foot is growing at a rate of 5mm of horn per month. There is a good case for setting a target of 2–3 months after calving for problem cows to have their feet trimmed or at least examined again.

WHICH COWS TO SELECT

Should all cows be foot trimmed on a routine basis? The answer is probably not if the foot has never been lame and if it has worn well. However, it is essential that all cows be examined if only to clean the foot off and check the horn and the shape of it. If this is normal, the foot should be left alone without any trimming. Many cows will simply need a small amount of trimming to dish out the solar horn and take weight off the centre area of the sole before calving. This may be achieved with as little as a single knife cut.

CHAPTER FIVE

Diseases and Lesions of the Horn

Horn disease is still the most common condition producing lameness in the foot. It is being overtaken rapidly by diseases such as digital dermatitis, but at present between 50 and 60 per cent of all lameness is due to damage involving horn structures of the claw. Horn disease produces the most serious type of damage to the foot, which is often slow to heal and prone to developing complications. The costs, as we have seen in Chapter 2, are the highest of all lameness conditions because horn lesions are difficult and costly to treat and are more likely to have higher indirect costs, such as decreased fertility and an increased risk of being culled. Damage to the horn also tends to leave the animal more prone to further injury and lameness.

Understanding how horn is formed and its relationship to the various structures in the foot is crucial if we are to understand how lesions are produced, how we are going to prevent them, and the best ways of approaching treatment. The general principles of the 'form and function' of the foot have been covered in Chapter 1, but we need to expand on this in order to apply these principles to specific lesions in horn disease.

The likely theory detailed in Chapter 1 is that there are three stages to the process producing damage to the horn. Stages one and two comprise horn disruption and dropping of the pedal bone, conditions which are probably unavoidable and will always occur to some extent. It is at this point that external influences come into play in determining whether stage three occurs, producing damage to the corium and clinical lameness. Most lesions of the horn start internally with external factors acting on the foot to produce clinical effects.

TREATMENT

There are several common principles to follow when treating conditions affecting the horn of the claw.

- Contact with the ground produces pain, lameness, and slows the rate of healing. Try and remove horn in such a way as to prevent the affected area bearing weight and to protect any exposed corium. If too much horn support has been lost or too much corium exposed, blocks must be used.
- Establish good drainage. Remove enough horn to allow the lesion to drain adequately if it is infected or there is a risk of it becoming infected. Do not leave holes or cavities in the horn that can fill with foreign material and cause infections or block drainage of material from the injured area.
- Remove as much 'necrotic' (damaged) horn and tissue as possible without injuring or exposing the corium excessively. It is probably unnecessary to remove every last piece of under-run horn, as it may form a protective covering whilst healing takes place. For instance, a septic lesion of the white

line or sole often produces a double or false sole that can be beneficial. Provided there is adequate drainage and no danger of the lesion becoming impacted and blocked, any covering for the corium or new horn developing underneath must be helpful, so leave it in place.

- Check that the lesion has not extended out from the primary injury site. Infection or necrosis often moves either into deeper structures, especially the pedal joint, or forms a septic track draining out at another site, for example to the heel or coronary band.
- Remove any exposed granulating tissue. Granulating tissue appears as raw strawberry-like growths from the horn injury and is a sign of ongoing irritation to the wound; it needs treatment to prevent it recurring. Irritation will occur if the

edges of the horn are still rubbing onto the exposed corium or there is continuing contact with the ground when the animal moves, i.e. the area of the lesion is still weight bearing.

Horn lesions fall into the following categories:

- Solar ulcers.
- Heel ulcers.
- White line disease.
- Heel erosions – 'slurry heel'.
- Foreign body penetration.
- Fissures – horizontal and vertical.
- Solar haemorrhage.
- Haematoma of the bulb of the heel.

SOLAR ULCERS

Solar ulceration is still the most common cause of lameness in dairy cattle today. This is despite the immense increase in digital dermatitis we have seen over the last 10 years. The most recent estimates show the incidence of solar ulceration to be responsible for between 20 and 25 per cent of all cases of lameness.

Description

Ulceration of the sole is seen when the whole thickness of horn is lost and the underlying corium is exposed. Ulceration can occur anywhere on the sole, but more than 70 per cent of lesions are situated in the central solar area slightly back towards the heel, and often towards the axial edge of the sole. They occur mostly in the outer claw of the hindlimb or the inner claw of the front limb. Solar ulceration can occur at other sites depending on exactly where the pedal bone is pressing down, for example the toe or abaxial sole area (see diagram on page 67).

The corium is the primary tissue affected, which means it will usually take time before the visible effect grows out in the horn and appears at the sole surface. The primary insult to the corium usually occurs at, or just around calving, so it is several weeks before

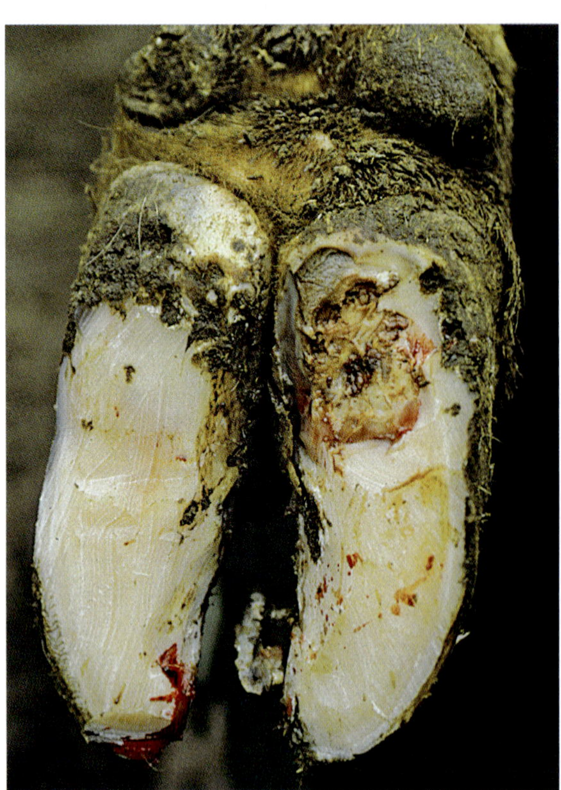

Infection from an ulcer has broken out to the heel.

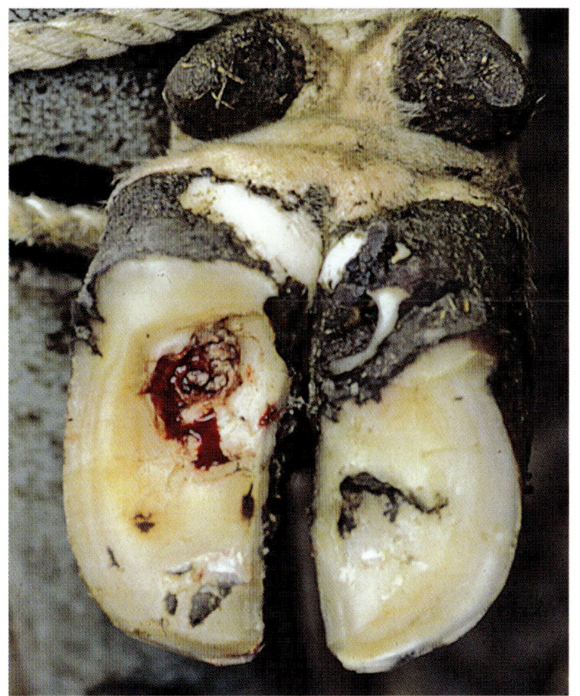

Typical solar ulcer.

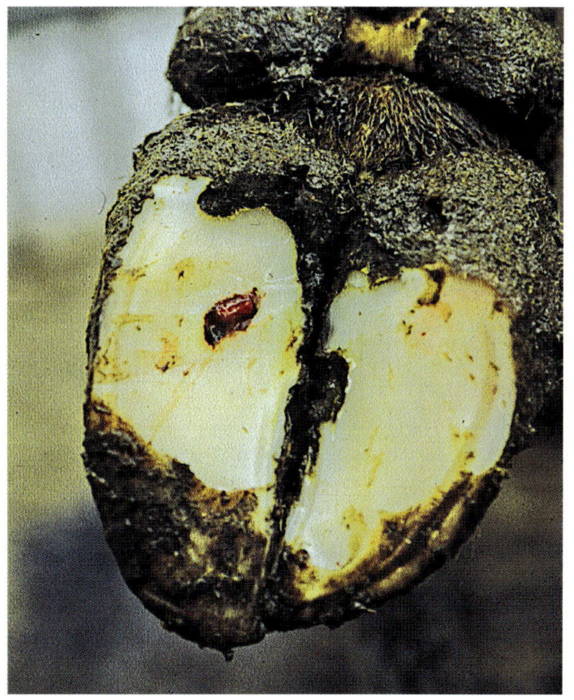

Small solar ulcer.

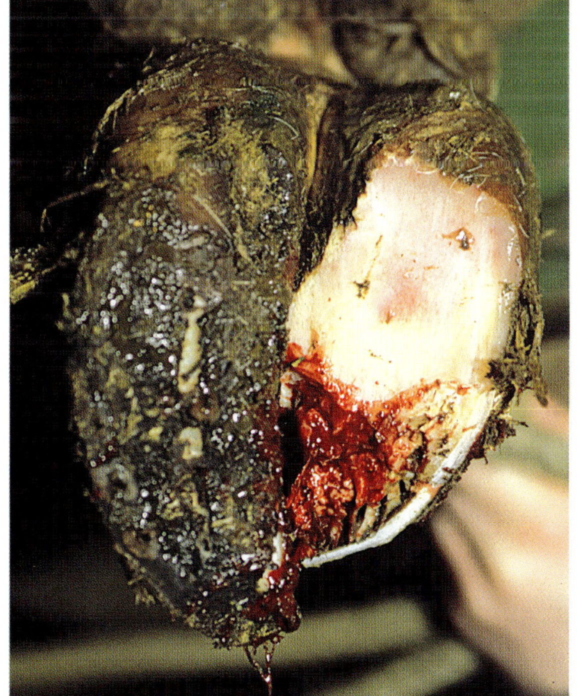

Toe ulcer.

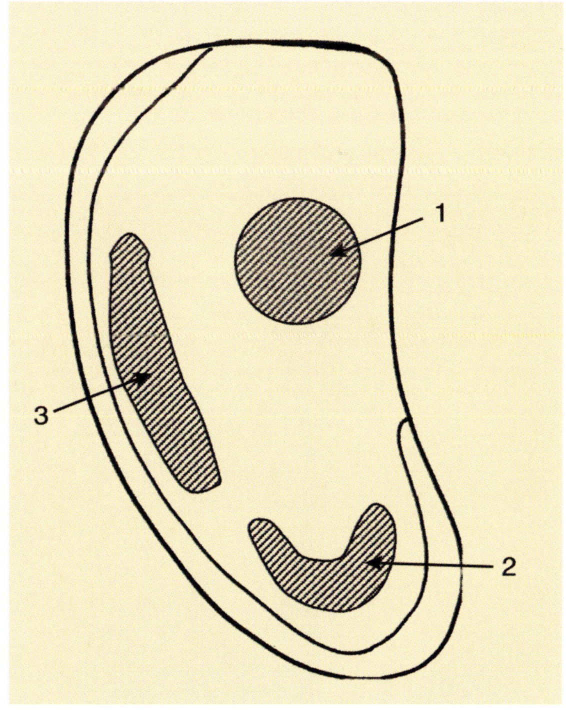

Distribution of solar ulcer lesions in order of likely occurrence.

the typical lesions start to appear. Horn grows about 5mm per month and solar horn is 10–15mm thick; therefore, on average, it could be about 100 days before external damage is seen on the surface. If solar horn thickness was reduced by winter housing conditions, this time span would be markedly reduced.

A typical cow presenting lame with a solar ulcer will already have the fully exposed ulcerated corium present. Often this is immediately beneath a ledge of horn overlying the area extending from the abaxial wall. Removing the ledge reveals the typical raw ulcer with exposed corium. The surrounding horn is often 'layered' like the cut surface of an onion with several separate sheets of horn visible, one on top of the other.

In the early stages of an ulcer lesion you may only see areas of abnormal horn at typical sites on the sole. This horn is often discoloured (yellow), soft (depressed easily) or friable with some areas of haemorrhage. Haemorrhages on the sole of the claw, however, do not always mean that an ulcer is present. Removing the haemorrhagic area may reveal normal horn underneath; in this case the underlying defect has not been severe enough to produce an ulcer lesion.

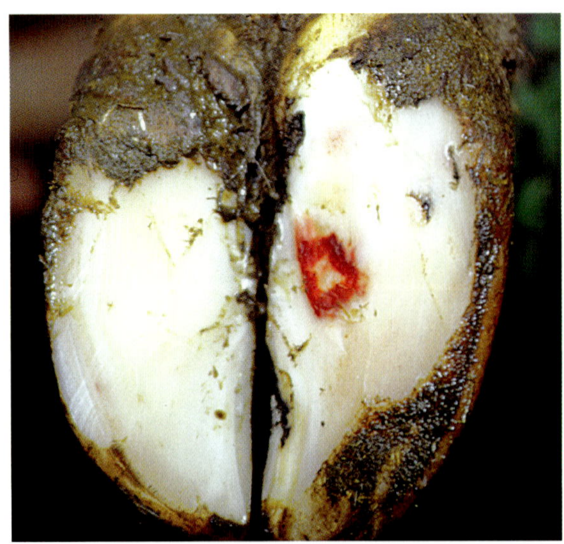

Solar haemorrhage only – no underlying lesion.

The characteristic ulcer appearance of concentric rings of under-run horn ('onion ring' look) is due to defective and damaged horn and inflammatory fluids (serum) being laid down in consecutive layers. These layers weaken and separate the horn to produce sheets of false soles that become exposed as the ulcer erodes to the corium. This process gives it the typical appearance. The presence of false soles means that infection can run along these fault lines and drain to other sites in the claw. An infected ulcer regularly tracks under the surrounding horn and forms a drainage route to the axial edge of the hoof and into the interdigital space. This drainage may also go back and extend to the heel, where a loose flap of periople is seen at the sole–heel junction; this can be lifted with a finger or knife to expose the drainage route or sinus as it is called. The corium can be extensively damaged and exposed, thereby opening up a route for infection to gain access to deeper structures in the foot.

Chronic ulcers produce large amounts of granulation tissue that protrude as strawberry-like lumps from the centre of the ulcer. Granulation tissue is a result of the underlying corium thickening as it responds to irritation caused by rings of horn surrounding the ulcer rubbing on the corium as the claw moves or, more likely, makes contact with the ground on weight bearing.

Cause

Suspension of the pedal bone can become disrupted soon after calving and it is this, along with environmental, nutritional and management influences, that causes the majority of horn disease we see in practice (*see* Chapter 1). In the case of solar ulceration the downward movement of the pedal bone causes it to press down on the underlying corium of the sole, so producing the primary damage. The way the pedal bone impacts on the sole determines where the solar ulceration lesion occurs. If the back edge of the pedal bone hits the corium first, a typical solar ulcer will occur. If the toe impacts first then a toe ulcer

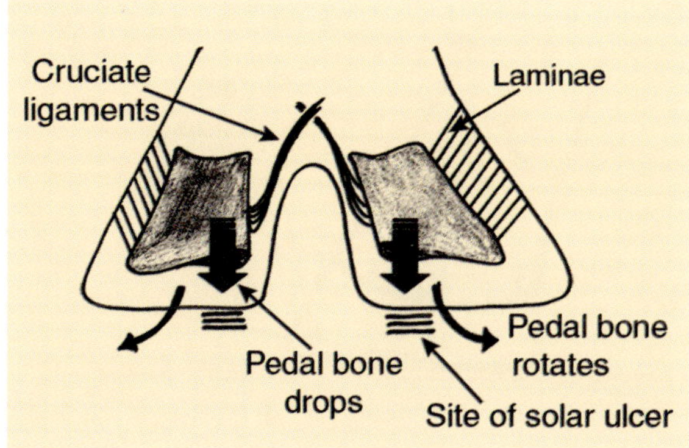

Movement of the pedal bone down, and rotation due to the hammock support, will favour impact on the sole in the typical solar ulcer site.

is produced. The most common site for a solar ulcer is on the caudal edge of the pedal bone due to a protuberance or tuberosity on the bone where the main tendon of the leg – the deep digital flexor tendon – is attached; this tuberosity on the pedal bone presses onto the underlying corium in a limited area, which explains why the majority of ulcers are located in this specific zone of the sole. Another factor in determining the site of the solar ulcer is rotation of the pedal bone; the attachment of the pedal bone is much stronger on the abaxial

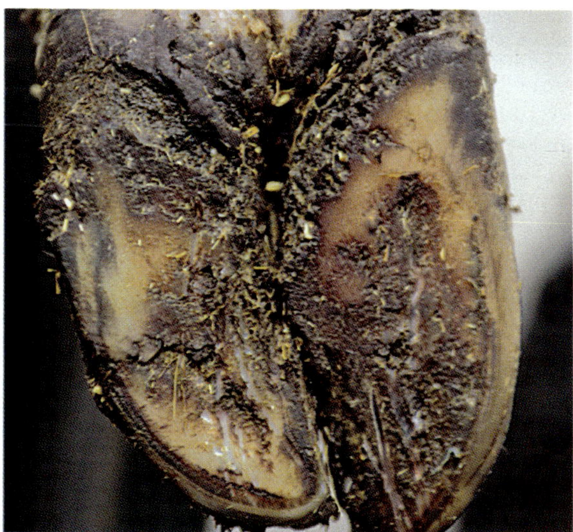

Flap of horn present, thickening the sole of the outer claw.

wall horn (through the laminae) than it is on the axial wall where there are not as many laminae and the cruciate ligaments hold the pedal bone. This causes the pedal bone to rotate as well as sink, especially in the axial area (adjacent to the interdigital space), and compresses the corium more axially.

The fact that solar ulcers are more common on the outer claw of the hindlimb and the inner claw of the forelimb is due to the distribution of weight bearing. More weight is put onto these claws as the animal moves, therefore they will be exposed to more environmental impacts.

As mentioned in Chapter 1, many solar ulcers are found in association with large flaps of horn that have grown out from the wall over the sole area. These horn outgrowths produce increased force on the sole as the animal walks, because weight cannot be distributed evenly along the white line area. This excess horn can cause the pressure from the outside to combine with the pedal bone dropping from the inside. It is difficult to decide whether the primary insult comes from inside the hoof – from pedal bone movement – or whether it is due to external forces. The answer is probably that both are important and that this is another example of external forces capitalizing on the pedal bone movement to magnify the damage and produce lameness.

Conformation of the leg is important in determining the incidence of this disease. The effect of the udder in the freshly calved cow is to push the hindlimbs outwards, so altering the angle of the limb and the way it impacts with the ground. This allows more horn growth from the wall to come over the solar area, which produces the flaps described above.

Diagnosis

The site of the lesion and the type of damage seen is typical enough for an accurate diagnosis.

Secondary Problems

Solar ulceration presents one of the most important risk factors for secondary infection

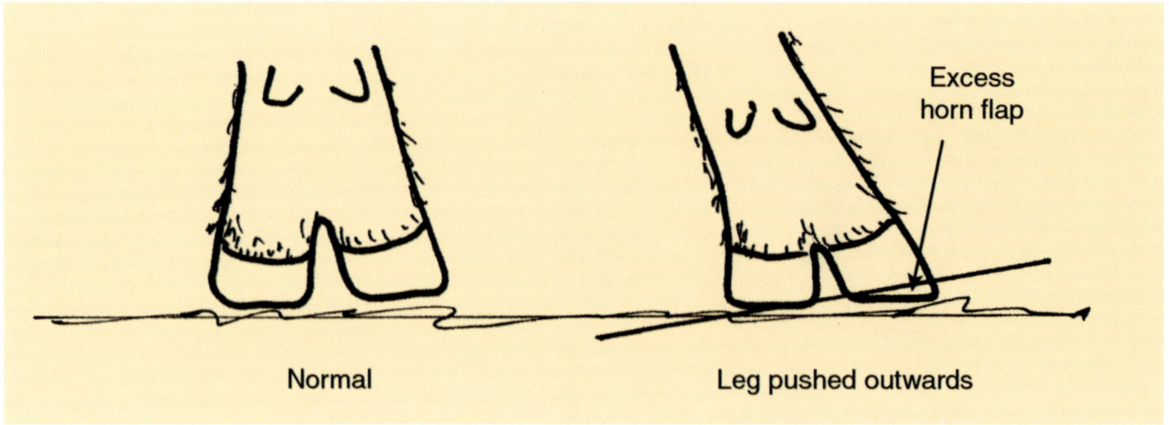

Poor alignment of the hindlimbs will allow a flap of horn to form on the sole.

of the foot. The lesion is adjacent to key structures in the foot and if neglected there is the distinct danger that ulceration will allow infection to extend to both superficial and deeper structures to produce the serious complications often associated with this disease. These complications are:

- Superficial tracts of infection that underrun the sole with drainage outlets at the heel or axial wall.

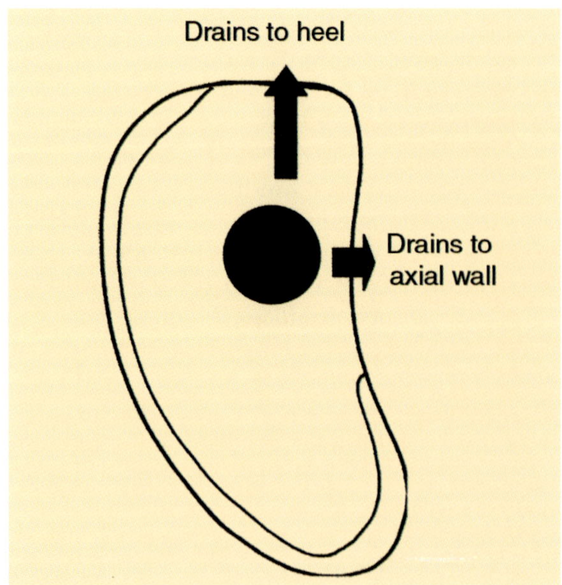

Damaged horn and secondary infection will easily produce drainage tracts.

- Localized abscessation of the sole.
- Extension of the infection caudally to produce an abscess under the bulbs of the heel – the retro-bulbar area; this affects the navicular bone, bursae and flexor tendons.
- Extension to the pedal joint, producing a septic arthritis.

Cows that have suffered a solar ulcer are more likely to experience lameness in subsequent lactations. Once the pedal bone has moved and produced changes to the corium it will not return to its original position and is more likely to be involved in future damage to the foot. Heifers lame from solar ulceration in their first lactation are three to four times as likely to become lame with horn disease in subsequent lactations.

Treatment

The key to treatment is to apply a radical approach at the start and prevent complications occurring. It pays to be brave at the outset!

The aims of treatment are listed below.

- Removal of necrotic tissue and defective horn allows new horn to grow out from the corium normally without being affected by surrounding damage. It will be deformed or become disrupted if infection or damaged material is present. Pare away

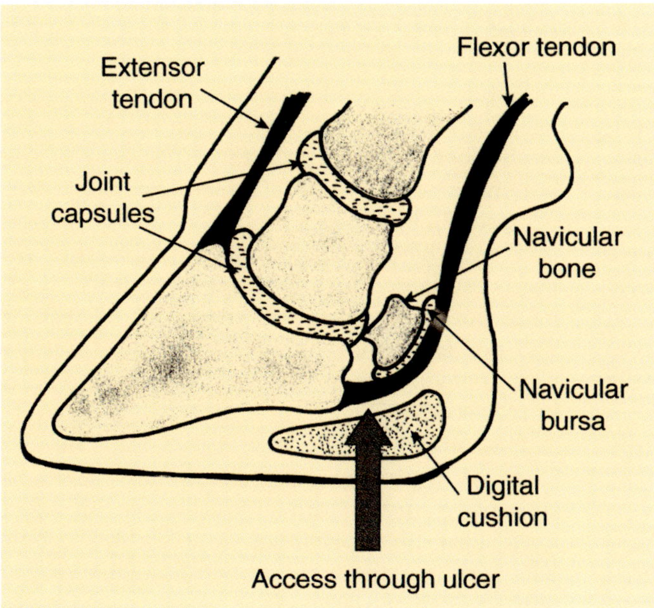

If infection goes deeper, it can easily reach the vital structures at the back of the foot.

the horn, but be careful because the lesion involves the sensitive corium and will be very painful if this layer is damaged.

- Establishing drainage by paring away the lesion is a basic principle of any foot treatment, but there is a difference between drainage and exposing a lesion. Too much paring and the sensitive layers will become exposed, so producing a lot of pain. Too little and infection will fail to drain and will build up to produce an abscess. This raises the question of whether ulcer lesions ought to be bandaged. On the one hand, it will protect the lesion and can be used as a support to keep a mildly caustic material in place to 'dry up' the ulcer. On the other hand, you have just established drainage, so to bandage it is surely nonsense. Do not use bandages on solar ulcers unless the environmental conditions are very bad or there is a need to keep a medication in contact with the ulcer.
- Small ulcers are pared back easily and the sole 'dished' to make sure that the lesion is not weight bearing and painful. However, larger lesions can be difficult to dish out and require some artificial means of

removing the lesion from weight bearing. This involves the use of blocks.
- Granulation tissue indicates that the lesion is being irritated constantly, causing the underlying corium to produce excessive tissue as it tries to 'distance' itself from the irritation. Removing the claw from weight

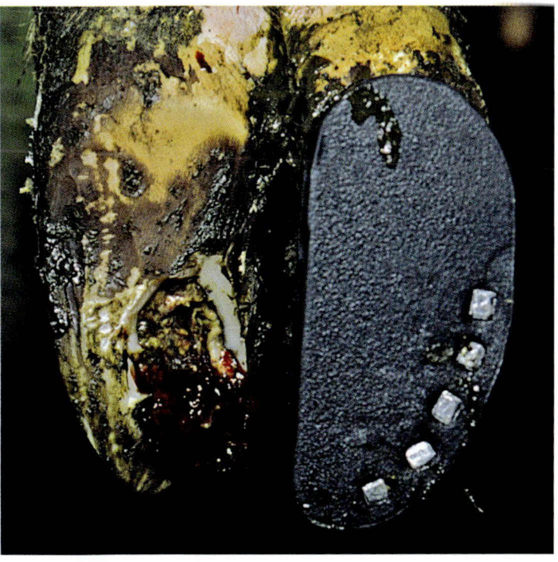

A toe ulcer with a nail-on block in place.

bearing is usually all that is required to prevent it forming or re-forming. Many people use mildly cauterizing substances to dry up the lesion and encourage healing without the formation of granulation tissue. Copper sulphate or mixtures containing formalin can be used, but they will burn the corium and prevent healing. Nowadays good blocking is all that is recommended. If granulation tissue is present, it has to be removed. This nearly always involves trimming the underlying corium, which is painful and may require anaesthesia.

- It is essential to investigate the lesion fully at an early stage and assess what secondary problems may be present. Prompt treatment is essential. If secondary infection or abscessation is neglected or not observed it will establish and become a major issue.

One issue frequently overlooked in treatment is what to do with the cow after you release it from the crush. Does it go back into the herd or should we be more specific about the environment in which we place the cow in order to produce the best cure rate? Work in the USA has looked at the problems for lame cows in cubicles and found that the cubicle surface can affect the rate of healing.[6] A soft surface with good grip, such as sand, can mean the cow spends longer lying in the cubicle and can accelerate the healing process. Cows in some types of mattress cubicles spent longer standing after treatment for lameness and this depressed the healing rate. Be careful not to give the sand option too much importance; in the UK a straw yard may well produce the same benefits. Interestingly, we have found in some of our herds that cows with solar ulceration can spend too long lying in a cubicle, which may produce pressure sores and other complications. If the cow can stand up easily and get in and out of the cubicle without causing too much pain it will do so; if not it may lie down all the time.

If blocks are used, the aim must be to keep the cow on a hard surface, as the benefit of the treatment will be wasted in a straw yard.

HEEL ULCERS

This term has been proposed for an ulcer-like lesion affecting a specific site in the heel area of the foot. It accounted for 6 per cent of the lameness seen in the Gloucester study (*see* Chapter 2), but this is probably due to the high incidence of the condition in one of the five herds studied. The condition is variable, with most herds having a low incidence of around 2–3 per cent and the occasional herd with a high incidence (nearly 20 per cent in one herd in this study).[7]

The origin of the heel ulcer may be the same as any other solar ulcer – an insult to the underlying corium that produces damaged horn and haemorrhage, which then grows out to the surface. However, the cause of the damage and the area affected differ.

One theory is that the damage is caused by the back edge of the pedal bone pressing down. However, recent work has suggested that the pressure on the corium in this case may be coming from the pedal bone squeezing the digital cushion (especially the central pad), which has undergone changes making it more fibrous and cartilage-like. The pedal bone could easily compress the hardened pad and produce damage in this area.

As the horn growth at the heel is oblique, the pathway of the infection and damage is angled back towards the bulb of the heel. The

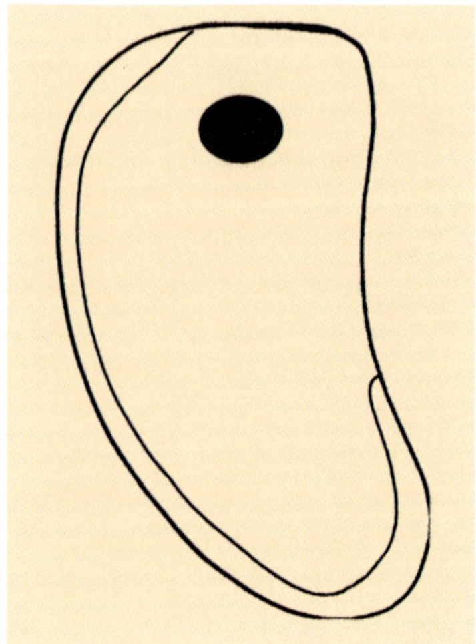

Typical site of occurrence for heel ulcer.

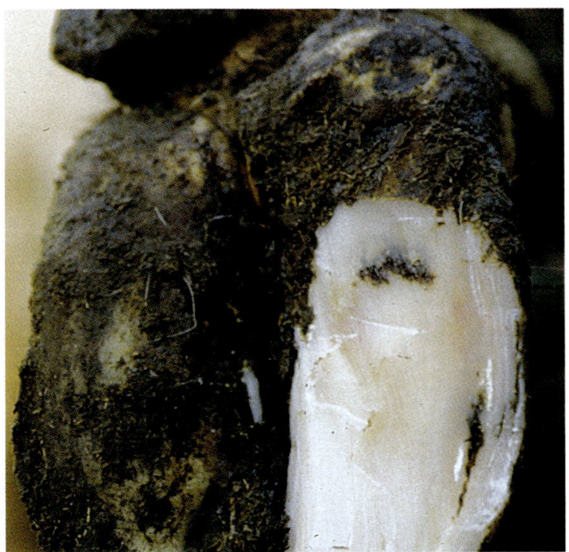

Typical curved black mark of a heel ulcer.

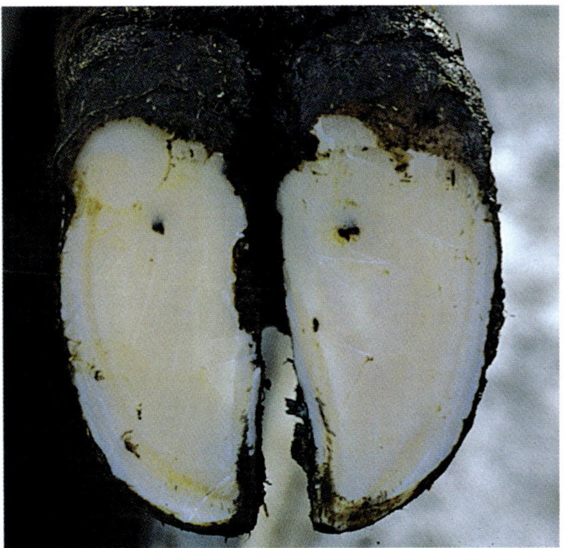

Heel ulcers often occur on both claws.

lesion shows superficially as a small black area placed centrally at the back edge of the sole. Sometimes the initial mark is a single black spot and in other cases it may appear as a crescent. When investigating this small spot the lesion tracks backwards at an oblique angle towards the bulb of the heel along the 'grain' of the horn in this area. The track often goes right back to reveal a haemorrhagic area of the corium, often with infection present. The difference between this and a solar ulceration is the distribution of the lesions and the way the horn is arranged at this site. It is often present on the medial claw of the front foot, but on the hind feet it affects both the outer and inner claw alike, in contrast to solar ulceration. In these lesions use the same principles as for treating a solar ulcer.

WHITE LINE DISEASE

There is an inherent weakness in the white line junction between the horn of the sole and that of the wall of the claw. Unlike the horn of the hoof wall, the white line horn has no structure to reinforce it. The white line consists of the leaflet horn, which lubricates the wall as it moves over the laminae, and the interdigi-

tating horn produced from the papillae of the sole. White line horn is some of the softest horn in the foot. It allows the foot to move slightly to produce some 'give' between the sole and the wall during weight bearing. Its susceptibility to

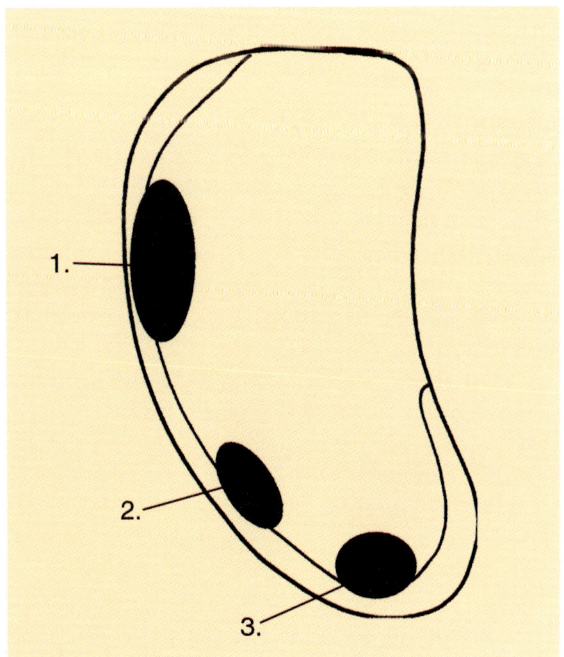

Distribution of white line lesions in order of occurrence.

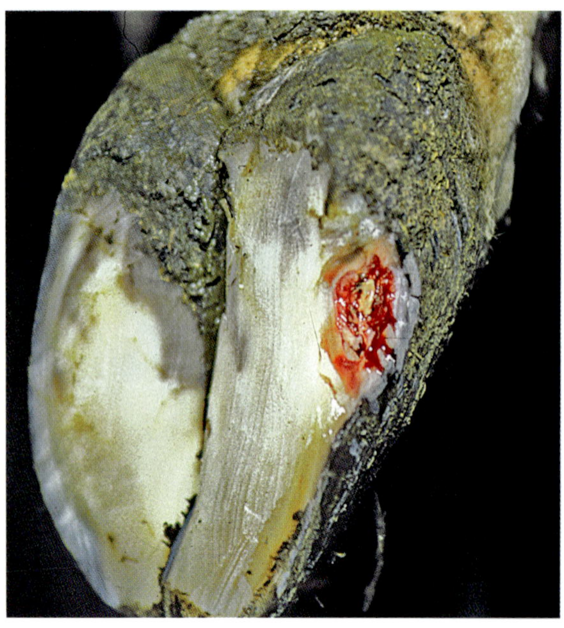

Typical white line disease opened up to show septic focus under the white line.

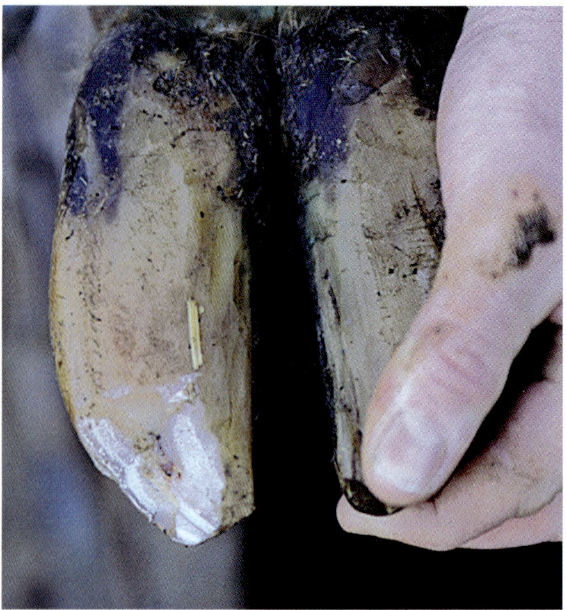

White line lesion at the toe – often very small lesions.

changes in horn structure and the movement placed on it makes it a prime site for fissures to form and foreign material to enter, producing infection.

Description

There are three classic sites for white lesions to become involved – the posterior abaxial wall, the anterior abaxial wall and the toe. This characteristic positioning probably reflects movement in the white line in these specific areas, making them more prone to this lesion.

Often there are early warning signs of the disease in the horn of the white line:

- Yellowing.
- Haemorrhage.
- Widening.
- Softening.

The presenting lesion in the lame cow is a dark area on the white line at one of the typical sites outlined above. This area may be a single spot, but it is usually a more diffuse black line on the junction. When paring the lesion the cow shows pain when pressure is applied, and the black mark tracks down to the corium at the same angle as the wall of the hoof – along the growth lines of the laminae. Diagnosis is

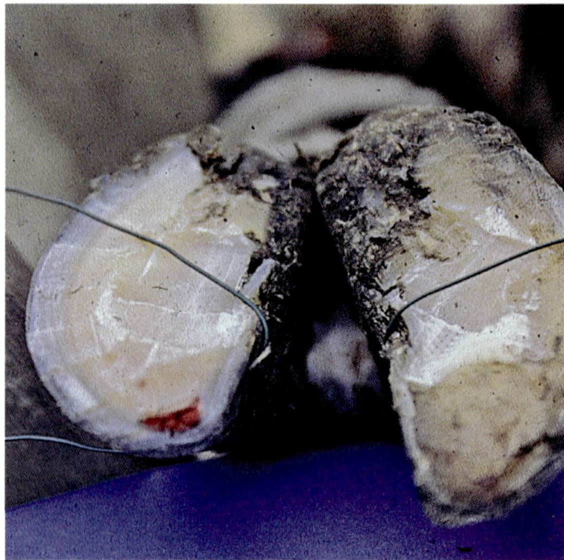

White line lesion at the toe – note the pink swollen area in the interdigital space.

usually straightforward, but when the toe is affected the penetration point is often difficult to see. In this case a good practical tip is to look for a swelling in the soft tissue at the front of the interdigital space, on the side of the infected claw.

Always check for an exit route when paring the foot. Pus follows the course of least resistance and can break out at the heel or coronary band.

Cause

There is evidence that the main factor for white line disease is the quality of the horn at the white line junction. If this is weakened, weight bearing will cause distortion of the white line, especially in the central/posterior abaxial wall area, which is the most typical site for a white line lesion. However, this inherent weakness is probably due to several factors of which the main considerations are:

- Changes occurring within the foot at, or around, calving. The same issues that were involved with solar ulceration may play a part in white line disease. Movement of the pedal bone may produce abnormal horn at the wall–sole junction, which makes the site weaker and more likely to form fissures.
- The pedal bone is supported in a hammock-like arrangement with the ligaments and laminae on either side. As we have mentioned in the descriptions of solar ulceration, as the pedal bone drops it may also rotate in an abaxial direction due to the difference in the strength of attachments on either side. This axial rotation allows the abaxial outer edge to move outwards and strike the horn of the wall, especially at the white line junction. This produces haemorrhages in this area and damages the white line junction.
- Calving will present the lactating cow with increased demands for nutrients, which are absorbed from feed. Milk production will take the dominant role in the requirement for nutrients. Some nutrients, such

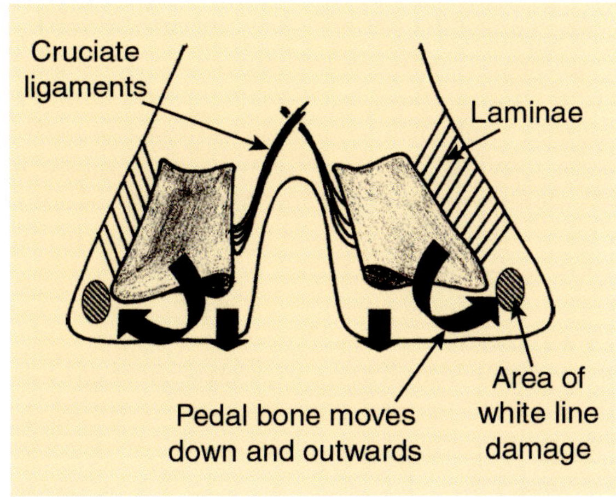

Movement of the pedal bone can damage the white line area and produce an inherent weakness for infection to enter.

as biotin, could become limiting, possibly producing inherently weaker horn, especially at the white line junction.

When the white line is damaged, normal movement of the foot will place more pressure on the joint, especially in the central abaxial area where most white line lesions occur. Excess movement of the joint can then open up fissures and encourage more weak horn production that is penetrated easily by foreign material.

Biotin has been shown to have a significant effect on the incidence of white line disease and it may be that external environmental factors do not play such an important role in producing this disease as they do in solar ulceration of the horn. Certainly, when environmental factors are addressed, there is often a failure of white line disease to respond to these improvements. In a 1000-cow trial in Gloucestershire, there was an almost four-fold reduction in white line abscesses in older cows that was associated with feeding biotin at 20mg per day.[5] This amounted to a 50 per cent reduction in the disease as a result of improving the horn quality. The other 50 per cent of cases may well involve other environmental issues (*see* Chapter 9).

In summary, there are certain circumstances that could allow white line disease to occur; mainly poor horn strength and damage such as haemorrhages as a result of the pedal bone moving. This, along with movement of the wall away from the sole on weight bearing, widens the white line and opens up fissures to allow infection in.

Treatment

The prime aims in therapy are the same as those for the general treatment of horn disease. The main points to emphasize with white line disease are:

- Ensure the lesion is fully opened up to allow drainage and prevent it becoming clogged up with foreign material as the cow walks. To do this, take out a wedge of the wall horn so that a cavity is not produced.
- Only take out sufficient wall to drain the area. The wall and the white line are essential weight-bearing structures so only trim and remove what is necessary to allow access to infection. Use blocks if a lot of the white line is affected.
- If the white line at the toe is affected, a section from the front will need to be removed in order to establish drainage.
- If a false sole is present, leave it in place as long as there is adequate drainage.
- When treating white line abscessation involving a sinus at the coronary band,

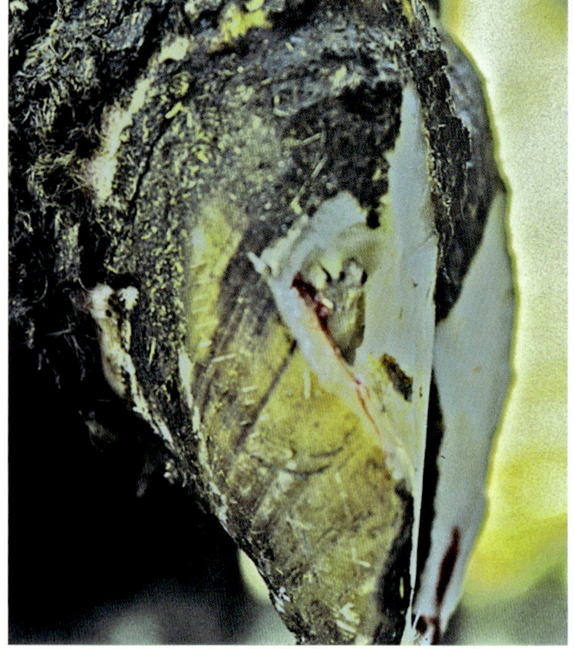

A white line lesion with part of the wall removed to allow drainage.

do not remove the whole length of the infected tract. Open up the top and bottom of the lesion but not the full length, as this will create a vertical fissure. If a vertical fissure is created, the sections of the horn wall either side will move independently, making it difficult for healing to occur. Leave a bridge of horn in place.

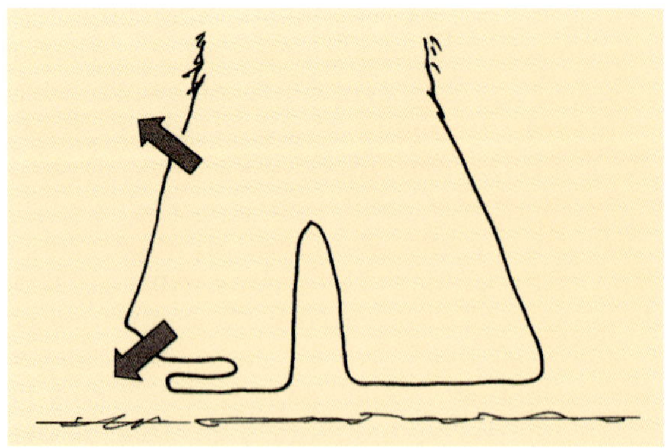

Establishing drainage is the key to success.

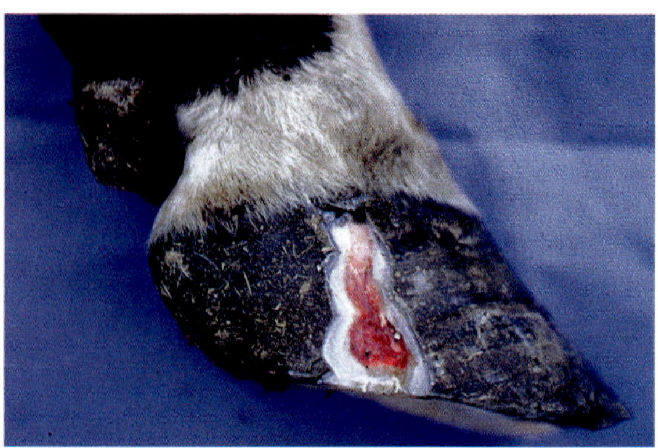

Do not remove the whole wall if the infection tracks up to the coronary band.

- Check for a discharging sinus at the heel. If this is present, it will need to be followed back along the abaxial wall to the original entry site on the white line.

HEEL EROSIONS – 'SLURRY HEEL'

These are common in housed cattle and are thought to be primarily due to the effects of slurry, wet conditions and harsh concrete surfaces. The horn at the bulbs of the heel should be a smooth transition between the sole and the skin junction at the periople. In slurry heel this bulbar horn is pitted and rough with erosions producing irregular cavities and channels across the heel area.

These erosions are found at the end of the winter housing period and are due to prolonged exposure to environmental conditions. Although there is no doubt that slurry heel has been around longer than digital dermatitis has, there is much evidence that digital dermatitis can, nowadays, be involved in this condition in many herds. Digital dermatitis will liquefy horn and, if present as a chronic infection on the bulbs of the heel, it will erode the bulbar horn to produce cavities and ledges (*see* Chapter 6).

Eroded heels unbalance the foot and will cause it to drop at the heel, as the bulbar horn is worn away. The strain on the flexor tendons and the poor foot angle can lead to other problems. Do not routinely trim out the grooves, but try and increase the angle of the foot (anterior rotation) or use blocks placed well back on the claw to preserve the angle of the foot. It is possible that drying agents such as formalin may help as they will harden the horn of the sole and may make it more resistant to erosion. Unfortunately there is no evidence for this. If digital dermatitis is present in the herd, good control of this disease to prevent chronic and established infection should be the main approach.

Improvement in slurry and moisture conditions in the housing environment will benefit both erosion and digital dermatitis control.

FOREIGN BODY PENETRATION

The usual site of penetration is the sole because it offers the biggest target. By definition a foreign body in the white line is a separate disease involving an inherent site of weakness and a 'natural' fissure through the horn.

Foreign body disease occurs when a sharp object penetrates normal solar horn. The most common foreign bodies are sharp stones and felt nails, although surprisingly common foreign 'objects' are cast teeth, which have spiked roots. Outbreaks sometimes occur during winter housing due to stones being brought into the housing area by tractors. Foreign bodies produce most damage when they are on a solid surface, such as concrete, as the weight of the cow forces them through the solar horn. An incident involving a foreign body penetrating the sole will show as a sudden lameness due to immediate contact with the corium. At this stage, infection may not be present, but treatment must establish drainage because infection

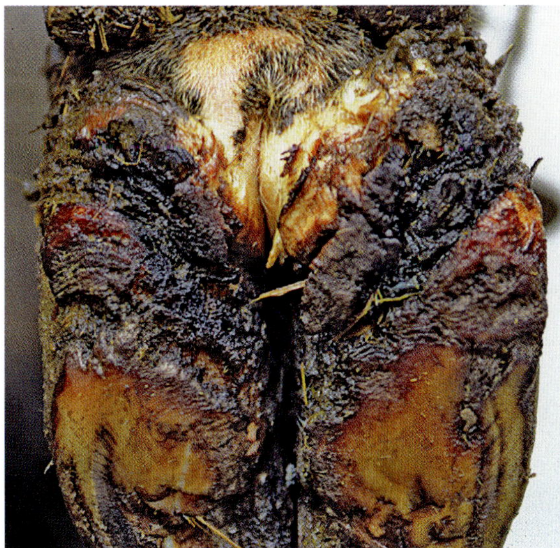

Slurry heel with damaged and pitted horn at the heels.

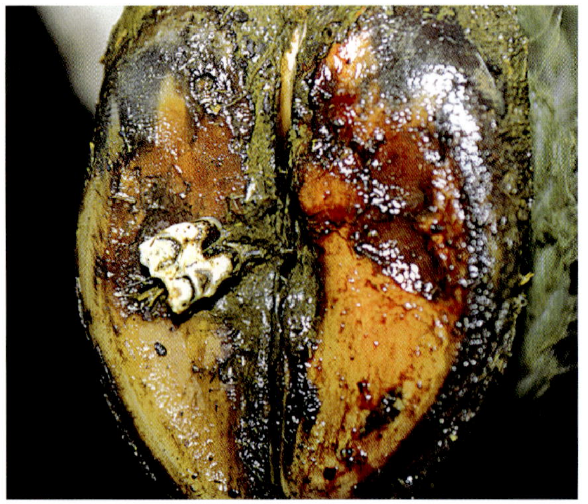

Foreign body penetrating the sole – in this case a cast tooth.

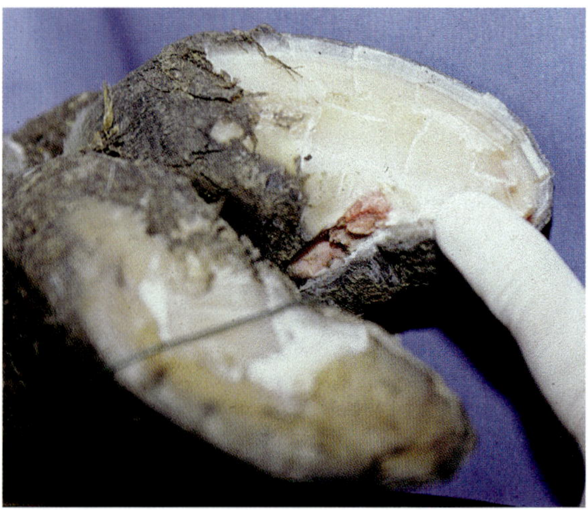

A fissure in the axial groove.

will surely develop from the contamination introduced.

If the penetration has been present for some time, there will be infection or abscessation with a false sole commonly produced. The general principles outlined above for treating horn disease are all that is required to treat this condition successfully.

FISSURES

Growth abnormalities are often seen in the horn of the wall, but only a few develop into cracks or fault lines. If these then start to open up and expose the tissues under the horn they are called fissures. They can be classified as either vertical fissures running from the coronary band down the wall of the hoof, or horizontal fissures running across the wall in line with the 'plane of growth' of the horn wall, i.e. they are parallel to the coronary band as they grow out from it. If the wall horn dries out excessively it becomes brittle and may crack from the solar surface upward, again producing a vertical fissure (commonly referred to as sandcracks). These lesions have been found in cows on very dry (sandy) grazing during hot weather and are possibly due to the waxy coat produced by the periople being lost.

Vertical fissures also form when the horn at the coronary band is damaged. This damage is usually localized and affects only a limited area of the horn. The horn growing out from this area is defective and the weakness soon opens up as a crack or fissure. The most common vertical fissures seen are:

- From the coronary band. Presumably localized damage to the periople produces

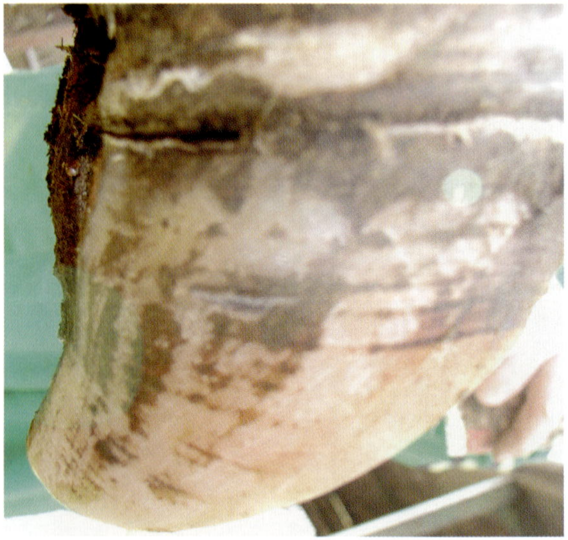

This foot shows distinct hardship lines and one of these is starting to form a horizontal fissure.

a focal weakness and allows a crack to occur at this point. Nowadays a vertical fissure is usually associated with digital dermatitis damage. Chronic digital dermatitis damage on the coronary band (usually at the front near to the interdigital space) produces liquefaction of the horn as it is formed or dissolves away the existing horn. Very often a vertical defect in the horn grows out from the site of the digital dermatitis infection, which makes it very difficult to treat.

- In the axial groove. There is a typical oblique fold in the axial wall as it rounds into the interdigital space and runs down to meet the sole. This often becomes affected and is a slow, difficult lesion to heal.

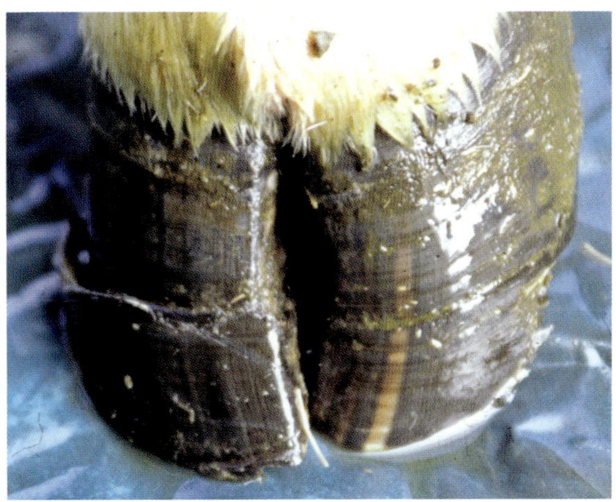

Horizontal fissures affecting both claws. The toe has started to loosen producing a 'thimble' of horn.

The most common horizontal fissure is the 'stress' line that works its way down the wall from the coronary band; these lines reflect past exposure to a generalized infection or 'difficult' time (they are called 'hardship lines'). Hardship lines or grooves are commonly seen in the horn of the wall and most remain fully intact and cause no problems as they grow out. The act of calving can cause a stress line due to temporary disruption to horn growth, and severe cases of mastitis or uterine infection will cause enough effect on the body to disrupt many processes, including horn production. As the fault line works its way down the horn wall it may start to move and crack open. Some of these grooves are severe enough to start opening up and form open fault lines as they grow out. This forms a loose flap or 'thimble' of horn that can be seen to open up when the cow is walking, allowing foreign material in and producing an infection. Be very careful removing these thimbles of loose horn, as there is often a large area of corium exposed.

Treatment
Vertical fissures:

- If digital dermatitis is causing the problem, treat this first and remove damaged horn from the area. These lesions can be very difficult to treat (*see* Chapter 6 on digital dermatitis).
- It is theoretically possible to groove out these cracks and staple them together as is done with horses. In cattle this is probably impractical.
- Blocking the foot for long periods of time will effectively seal the crack together and cover it whilst new horn forms from the coronary band and grows out. This will need to be long-term treatment as complete horn growth of the wall will take around 15 months, although enough new growth to hold it in place may be present after a few months.

SOLAR HAEMORRHAGE

It is difficult to decide when areas of haemorrhage are just a casual occurrence involved with trauma or injury and when they reflect problems occurring within the foot. When the haemorrhages are aligned in the crescent of the pedal bone or at the toe or solar ulcer area it is highly likely that they are due to pedal bone pressure. They indicate the possibility that solar horn disease could follow. Haemorrhages are an early indicator of damage to the corium

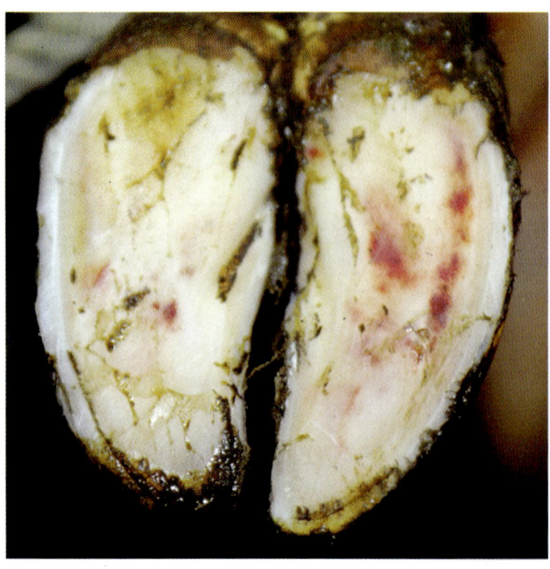

Haemorrhages on the sole indicate damage from the pedal bone. They may or may not progress.

that may only affect individual animals, or it may indicate a herd problem, especially if environmental factors start to make these lesions worse.

HAEMATOMA OF THE BULB OF THE HEEL

A large blood-filled cavity is found at the junction of the sole and skin at the bulbs of the heel. The cavity only causes mild lameness despite the fact that the hole, when opened, is often extensive. Even though it is a relatively rare condition, it may occur more often than is recognized because the lameness it produces is so mild it can pass unnoticed. It has been reported in cows subject to a lot of walking, possibly over rough or hard ground, and therefore is probably associated with trauma. The lesion could be due to pedal bone movement, although this is unlikely as it occurs so far back in the heel. It is more likely to be due to local injuries as the heel is involved in impact control during movement (*see* Chapter 1).

Conservative treatment with drainage and blocking is all that is required.

CHAPTER SIX

Diseases of the Skin

INTRODUCTION

Diseases involving the skin of the foot account for nearly 40 per cent of all cases of lameness found in the dairy cow. Their importance over recent years has been increased greatly by the introduction of digital dermatitis and its rapid spread within the UK and the rest of the world. The arrival of this 'new' disease has altered the relative incidence of lameness and made skin disease a much larger proportion of the total lameness now seen. It is likely that without digital dermatitis the overall incidence of lameness would have declined, indicating that we may be making progress in reducing the overall level of lameness in the dairy herd.

Why should the skin of the foot be such an important area for disease and so frequently produce lameness? The skin of the leg merges with the horn of the claw at the periople; this junction is very prone to disease and damage, either due to its position or some inherent structural weakness. Skin in this area is more exposed to the rigours of modern life, especially in the housed dairy cow. The environmental effects producing damage include:

- Wet yards.
- Slurry contamination.
- Trauma from concrete surfaces.

Diseases of the skin that produce lameness are:

- Digital dermatitis.
- Interdigital necrobacillosis (interdigital phlegmon) – 'foul'.
- Per-acute interdigital necrobacillosis – 'super-foul'.
- Interdigital hyperplasia.
- Mud fever.

DIGITAL DERMATITIS

The Disease

Digital dermatitis (DD) is now one of the most frequently diagnosed causes of lameness in cows in many countries. There is often confusion recognizing or deciding what lesions are involved in DD because the variation and distribution of them is so great. Yet it is likely that the whole disease is based on a single type of lesion and pathology, which varies according to the site affected and the circumstances present in the herd, therefore producing the varied clinical appearance in cattle. It is most likely that a combination of environment, length of exposure to infection and the site infected dictates the type of lesion seen on the foot. The primary lesion is a clear-cut superficial erosion, but more complicated lesions occur with continued exposure.

There is some confusion concerning the names and definitions used to describe the lesions associated with DD. In the USA there is abundant reference to 'hairy warts', whilst in the UK this form of the disease is not common. There is also reference to interdigital dermatitis and dermatitis affecting other areas of the foot. There is most likely only one standard lesion. A severe form of DD has also been seen in sheep, where the disease is referred to as CODD – contagious ovine digital dermatitis.

Estimates of the current level of DD are difficult to assess because most farms are now well used to diagnosing and dealing with the problem themselves without the need for veterinary attention. DD now ranks as one of the most common conditions causing lameness in housed dairy cattle. Clarkson, in 1989 (soon after it was first found in the UK), recorded DD at around 8 per cent of the cow cases recorded in his study. Estimates of the level of the disease in the late 1990s showed that the incidence was around 20 per cent. In recent years, however, the incidence is almost certainly higher than this and a figure of 25 per cent has been suggested. Confusion with other foot lesions could make this figure even higher, as will be explained later in the chapter. In the USA, in cows that are constantly housed, there are reports of the disease now accounting for over 50 per cent of the total lameness seen.[8] This is perhaps a warning for our industry if the trend towards total housing continues in the UK.

This disease is so widespread that it has now become closely involved with many other skin diseases of the foot. It is becoming increasingly difficult to distinguish between typical diseases involving the skin around the foot and the complications or involvement that DD produces. Previous chapters have referred to DD being involved with heel erosion and vertical fissures.

Cause

Since it was first described in Italy in 1972 this disease has become recognized throughout Europe, the USA, Japan and Australia. DD is an infectious disease and current work indicates that the causal organism is a spirochaete. Spirochaetes are a type of bacteria that take their name from their characteristic spiral shape. They are active and motile organisms that move rapidly in a wet environment. Drying rapidly kills them; consequently they are usually associated with water or moist areas of the body. Spirochaetes commonly produce disease in the gut and the urinary system as well as the uterus. These organisms have a predilection for keratin and this helps to explain the type of damage they do on skin surfaces and the horn of the foot. They are difficult to isolate and grow artificially, which means that a precise diagnosis is difficult. There are also many species of spirochaetes that are commensal or environmental, i.e. they are free living in the environment and commonly found in wet areas such as the foot but may not produce any disease. They may even be opportunistic organisms, only producing damage when they are allowed to enter the skin, for example due to damage or weakness, which often occurs when an area remains moist or wet for any length of time. This has made it difficult to ascertain which specific organisms are involved with DD. However, the particular spirochaetes involved are possibly related to ones that are commonly found in the mouth of humans and are responsible for oral and gum ulceration. These particular spirochaetes are called Treponemes (e.g. *Treponema brennaborense, Treponema denticola*).

Symptoms

Clinically, DD can produce a profound lameness because the skin lesions are often very painful depending on where they are located and how extensive they are. There may be suspicions of DD in a herd with cows showing wet tufted hairs at the back of the heel and frequently picking up the leg and shaking it as if trying to throw something off the foot. Some stockpersons can detect a smell associated with DD lesions – this is doubtless like 'foul', due to secondary infection and necrosis of the skin in badly affected lesions.

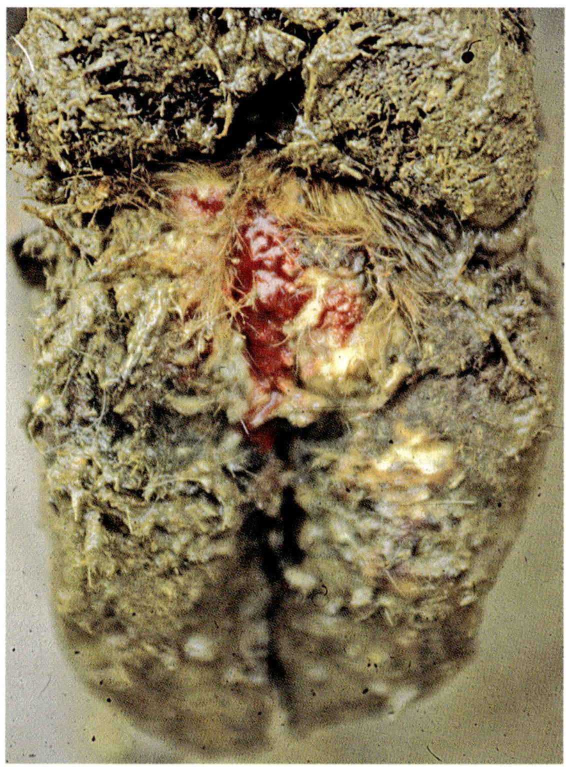

Digital dermatitis affecting the bulbs of the heels as it looks before being cleaned off.

Primary Lesion

DD is primarily a superficial lesion. The characteristic stages of this initial lesion are given below.

Liquefaction

The infection has a predilection for keratin and liquefies the superficial epidermis – stratum corneum and granulosum – to produce the typical 'wet' lesion on the skin surface. Often one of the first signs is a characteristic smell and observation of the overlying hairs clumping together due to the liquefied material on the skin surface.

Superficial Erosion and Invasion

Loss of the superficial epidermis by this process soon exposes the underlying dermis, which shows as a reddened layer. Some invasion of the stratum spinosum and papillary dermis occurs, which produces an inflammatory response of the epidermis and dermis.

Mild Proliferation

Irritation of the exposed germinal layers produces hypertrophy and hyperplasia – excess production of skin material and enlargement of parts of it. This is usually seen as small keratin 'pins' in the early lesion, giving it a typical stippled effect or a strawberry-like appearance. It has a coarse 'gritty' feel when overlying material is scraped off.

The combination of liquefaction, superficial erosion, inflammation with mild hypertrophy and hyperplasia is typical of lesions seen in the UK. These key features of the disease enable it to be recognized in less typical areas and in conjunction with other foot lesions.

Secondary Lesion

More advanced stages can occur that give the more chronic form of the disease. These can be seen in combination with the earlier signs above or appear to have taken over the lesion entirely.

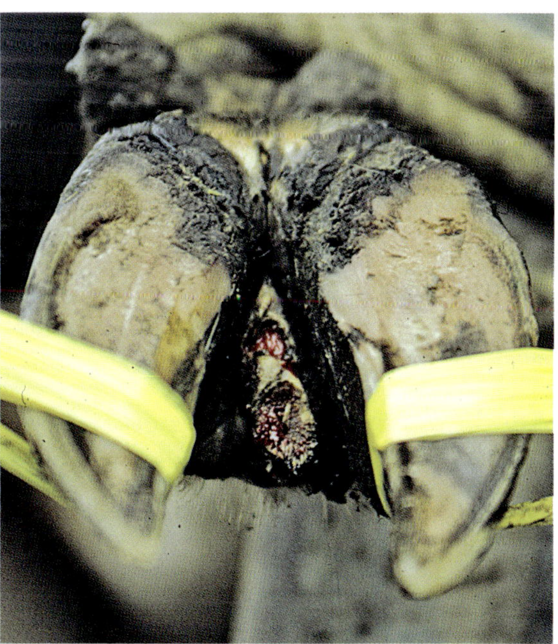

Digital dermatitis affecting the interdigital space – a very common form.

Extensive Proliferation

Proliferation continues as the uncovered dermis is exposed to protracted or extensive irritation. The keratin pins become elongated so that they appear as 'hairs' of keratin. These produce the 'hairy wart' appearance commonly described in the USA, which is perhaps starting to become more common in the UK. Some countries describe other types of proliferation, such as scabeous or solid plaques of keratin tissue. These have not been reported in the UK.

Deep Erosion

Erosion continues, not only removing superficial cover but also deeper layers. This is usually seen as deep areas of tissue loss, although flat or raised granulomatous lesions (large areas of granulation tissue) have been described.

Horn Erosion

Any horn adjacent to a DD lesion can dissolve away exposing the underlying corium. Sometimes the corium responds by producing excess horn, which takes on a layered appearance like slurry heel. Exposure of the corium can produce infection, which tracks under the surrounding horn, like pus from a septic focus.

Deep Invasion

Extensive invasion of the dermis allows entry to secondary infection. This allows other lesions to be created or produced synergistically with DD, for example some types of 'foul' or infected vertical fissures in the horn wall.

Acute Lesions Seen in Practice

The appearance of the lesion and the area of the foot that is affected can describe the type of DD lesions seen in practice.

Bulbar

Bulbar lesions affect the skin at the bulbs of the heels. The lesions are characteristically horseshoe-shaped and extend between the bulbs of the heels across the skin at the back of the interdigital space. In the UK the skin lesion is primarily a 'wet' lesion with erosion and some hypertrophy/hyperplasia producing the classic strawberry-like appearance.

Interdigital

The same typical lesion occurs between the claws on the skin of the interdigital space. The lesion is usually circular and clearly outlined, unlike the ragged split seen in a 'foul'. Also, the surrounding tissues are not swollen with DD. Often there is skin hyperplasia present (frequently called 'corns') with DD on the plantar surface. Is DD producing the hyperplasia by constant irritation or is an existing hyperplastic lesion predisposing to DD infection? Certainly corns are more common in dairy herds that are infected with DD. This suggests that DD may be causing the problem.

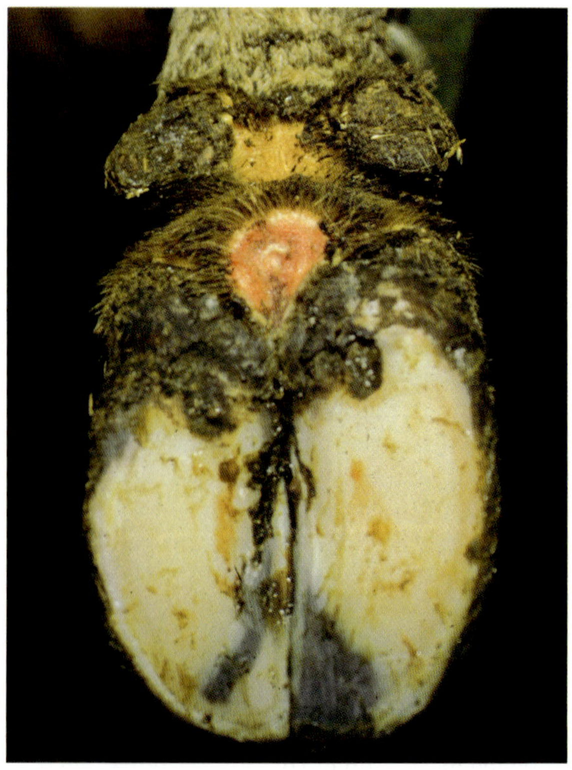

Typical digital dermatitis affecting the heels – bulbar digital dermatitis.

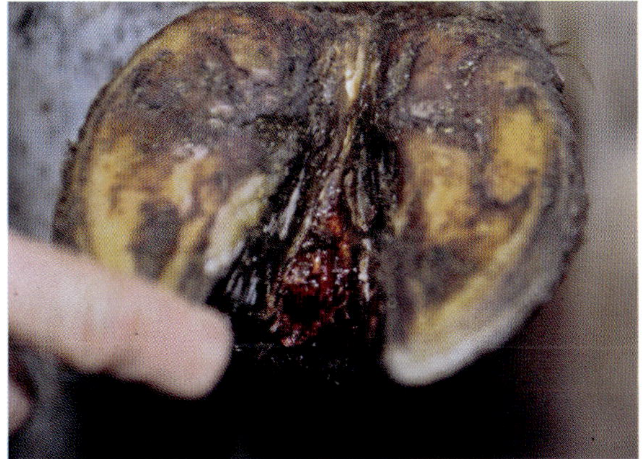

Interdigital digital dermatitis.

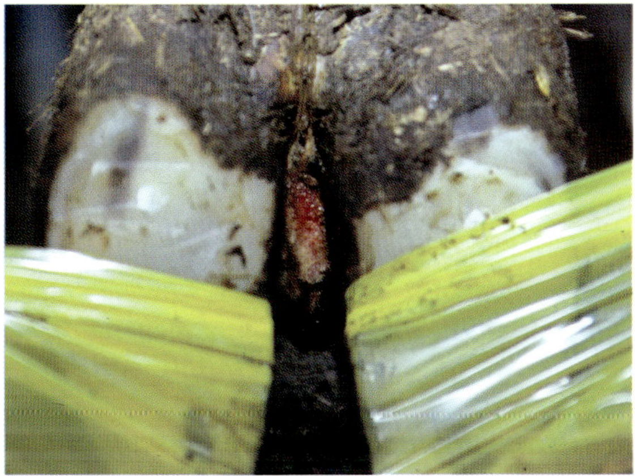

Interdigital digital dermatitis.

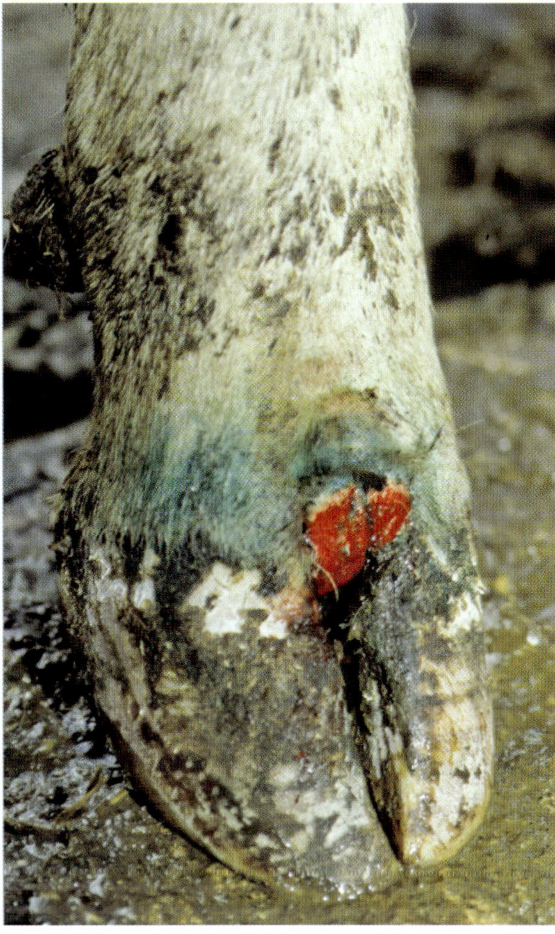

Digital dermatitis affecting the coronary band – it is usually found at this spot.

Anterior Coronary Band/Dorsal Wall
Any DD lesion at this site quickly produces liquefaction of the adjacent horn. A deep erosive lesion is seen as the process extends or tracks down under the horn and eventually a vertical fissure is produced. These lesions are usually adjacent to the interdigital space and as there is often extensive damage due to secondary infection they are very difficult to treat. Typical sites are on the anterior aspect of the coronary band adjacent to the inter-digital space and more medially on the axial surface at the top of the axial groove.

Solar
Very occasionally a typical DD lesion is seen on the solar surface. This may be opportunist extension under the solar horn from the bulbs of the heel or interdigital space, or it may be due to the fact that ulceration or sepsis has exposed the solar corium to DD infection.

Other Sites
Any DD lesion affecting another site shows the typical reactions in the skin. A typical DD lesion can occasionally be seen affecting the accessory digit. Just as with any skin–horn junction, the accessory digit can show the same sort of lesions.

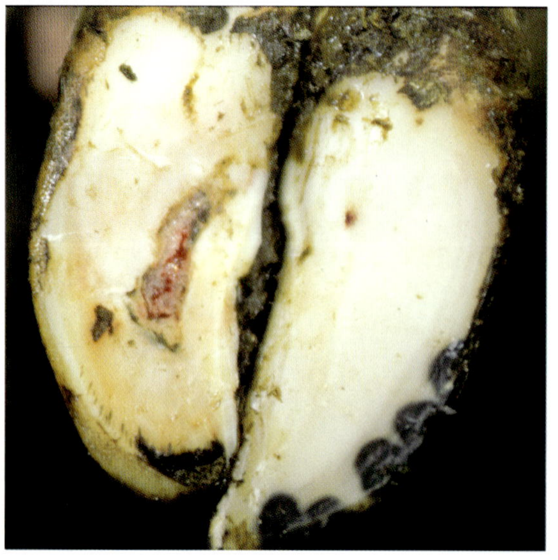

Digital dermatitis is an opportunist and can affect other areas such as the sole.

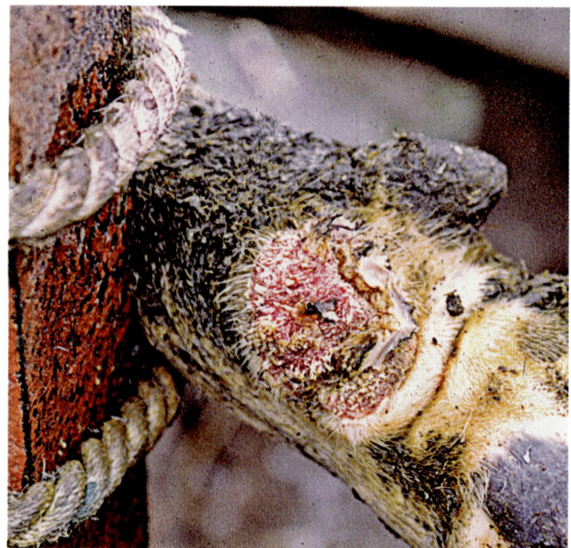

Digital dermatitis sometimes affects other areas of skin such as the accessory digits.

Ulceration in front of the udder can occur. A lesion similar to necrotic dermatitis (udder seborrhoea or intertrigo) can occur, and there is enough clinical evidence to suggest that this may, in some cases, be a DD lesion. It is easy to speculate that when the cow is recumbent the foot often comes to lie against the area of skin just in front of the forequarters. If the foot is infected with DD, this area of skin could become infected by direct, close and repeated contact. It is also possible that contamination from the ground occurs in this site.

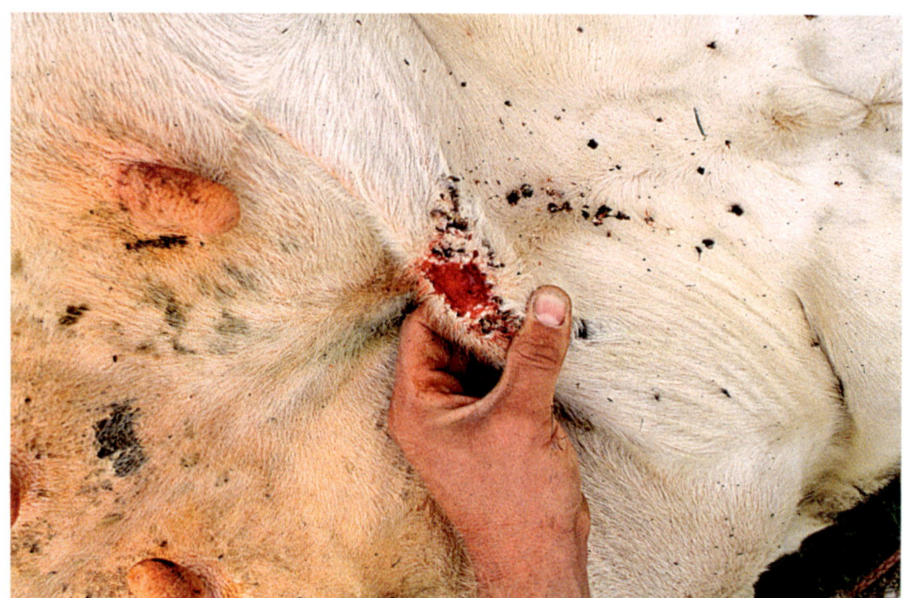

Digital dermatitis can also affect the udder by producing a sore area just in front very like intertrigo.

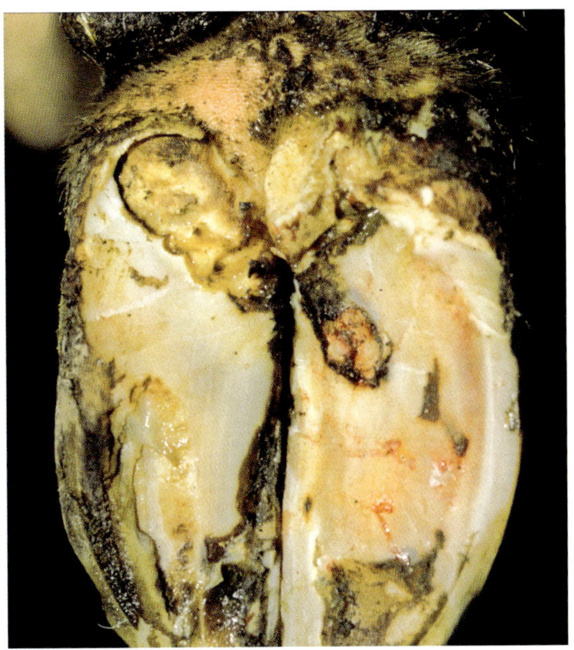

Digital dermatitis can be involved in lesions around the edge of the heels, like slurry heel.

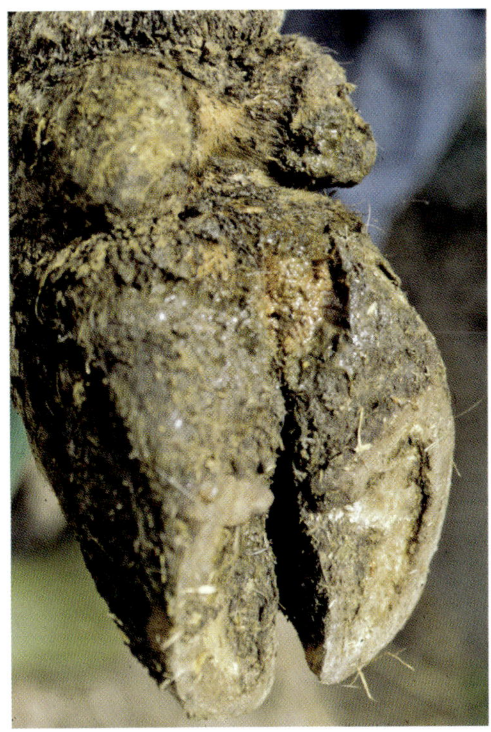

You can see the ledge of horn being produced as the digital dermatitis erodes further into the heel. These lesions often carry the infection through the summer to contaminate the housing next winter.

Chronic Infection

Horn Erosion

Horn erosion can occur at any site where a DD skin lesion lies adjacent to horn. The usual sites are at the heels, at the hoof wall on the anterior coronary band, and at the axial groove. The lesion at the heels can be either a deep fissure, similar if not indistinguishable from slurry heel, or simply loss of the horn so that the corium is exposed. (There is a suggestion that slurry heel is a consequence of DD, although, as mentioned before, slurry heel has been around longer than DD so this is not always the case.) There is some evidence that horn erosion produces a layered type of lesion with several platforms of horn exposed.

Deep Invasion

Any lesion that allows deep invasion of the dermis will suffer complications due to infection. This is especially true with interdigital DD infections. These will allow secondary infection to enter and produce complications

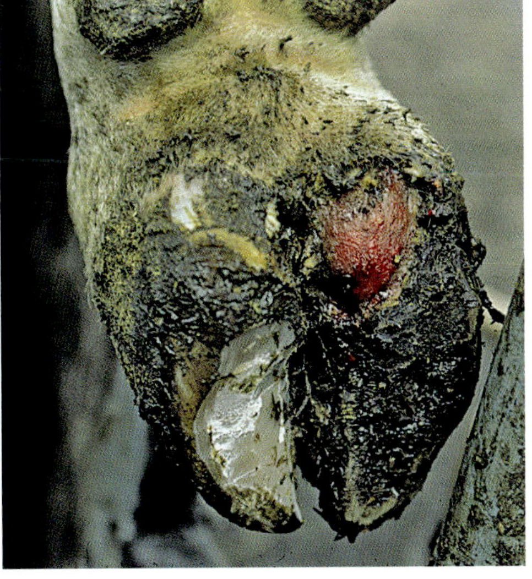

A deep chronic digital dermatitis lesion.

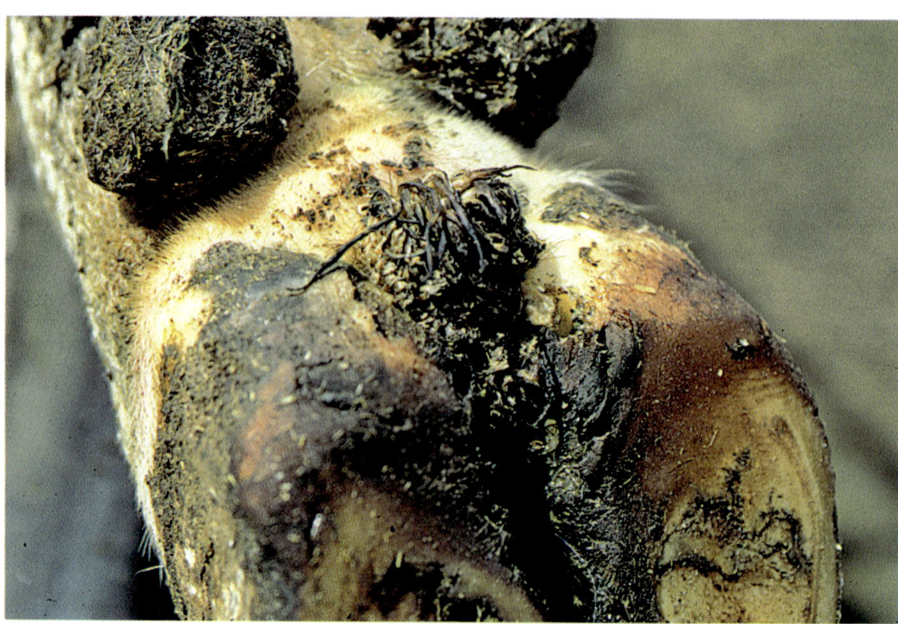

Chronic heel lesion producing a 'hairy wart'.

such as a severe foul or even a peracute foul ('superfoul'). However, this disease is not always associated with DD.

Proliferative Disease
Any prolonged irritation of the germinal layer will stimulate excess keratin production. This is usually seen as the chronic, proliferative 'hairy wart' lesion that is often described in the USA. It is now more commonly seen in the UK.

Skin Erosion
Very deep erosive lesions that produce excess tissue loss can occur in the skin.

Clinical Variation
What causes the variations seen? Are they different types of infection or simply different expressions of the same disease? The pathology seen in the various lesions is consistent, which indicates that there is uniformity in the disease.

It appears that the variation seen in practice is due to the nature of the disease cycle, either acute or chronic, and which area of the foot is affected. The difference between acute and chronic infection is largely down to how long the disease has been allowed to develop. Are control measures being applied; how frequently or how diligently are they being carried out? The next factor is the site of infection in the affected foot. We are only starting to understand why the disease has, in one herd, a predilection for one site and in another herd a different area. Ultimately it is likely that this will be down to environmental factors and the way the organism interacts with them.

Epidemiology
The general pattern with infection is for most outbreaks to occur during the winter housing periods when the disease can express itself and spread. The key feature is the way that the disease carries over from one housing period to the next. Work at ADAS Bridget's experimental husbandry farm has shown that the level of subclinical or chronic infection in the cows at the start of the housing period is the single most important factor affecting the level of disease that occurs in that group of animals.[9] It is more important than the effect of any preventative or therapeutic regime imposed on the group. DD is carried in chronic lesions and in low-grade scab-type areas on the foot. There is also some evidence that

pockets of infection can be carried in a small pouch often found at the back of the interdigital space.

Other key features of the way this disease occurs are:

- DD is more prevalent during housing periods when cows are more likely to be in wet slurry conditions that favour the spread of the organism and predispose the skin of the feet to infection.
- Some aspects of cubical design appear to be related to incidence. This is perhaps due to cows getting up and lying down and standing with their feet in the dung passage. The key feature may be exposure to slurry in the passageways.
- Some slurry handling systems seem to favour DD. Automatic scrapers that produce 'bow waves' of slurry down the passageways or lakes of slurry at the ends of the scraper run, which the cows can stand in, are more likely to result in DD outbreaks if the disease is present in the herd.
- It is infectious. Often outbreaks are related to bringing in infected stock (and possibly due to infected foot-trimming equipment). If the herd is free of the disease make sure all incoming stock are isolated and put through a footbath at least twice before joining the main herd. Also all foot-trimming equipment must be thoroughly cleansed between cows to prevent infection spreading.
- There is almost certainly a chronic or carrier state. Pockets at the back of the interdigital space hold infection and act as a reservoir for fresh outbreaks. Low-grade infected lesions are also a possible source of infection in the herd. They may not produce any lameness and so are easily missed. Evidence suggests that there is no immunity to the disease and therefore control is unlikely to rely on vaccination. At present, immunity is unlikely to help with long-term control in the herd.

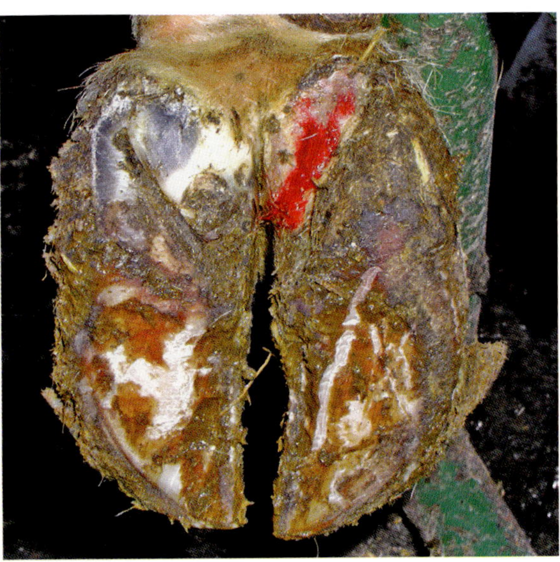

Chronic digital dermatitis at the heel.

- Attempts to spread the disease have largely been unsuccessful unless moisture is applied to the feet for long periods of time. This has been done experimentally through applying constantly wet bandages at the site of inoculation of DD material scraped from an infected lesion. This implies that to acquire the disease the cow's foot needs to be exposed to long periods of wet conditions. Work in the USA has shown that in cattle housing conditions that produce high levels of slurry and wet areas DD problems are twenty times as likely to occur.[10, 11]
- Diet plays a major role because the feeding system determines the type of slurry produced. Work in Israel has shown the possible effect of diets with high protein levels on outbreaks of DD.[12] Some diets with high levels of maize produce 'sticky' faeces, which form a coat on the foot and may help to produce a moist microclimate that enables infection to establish.
- The use of loose housing minimizes spread of the disease, and lameness due to DD is very uncommon in straw yards. This is probably related to moisture levels and faecal contamination.

Treatment

There are two basic approaches to treating DD; each is important and has a role to play:

1. Treating the individual, which is still an essential part of herd control; although time consuming it is more accurate and thorough.
2. Herd treatments save time by applying treatment to many cows in a short space of time, which is essential in a herd outbreak.

There are two basic types of agent that can be used for treatment:

1. Skin disinfectants such as formalin, copper sulphate etc.
2. Specific antibiotics with action against spirochaetes.

In general, when an outbreak of DD occurs in a herd it will usually need treatment with an antibiotic product to control the disease. General-purpose skin disinfectants can then be used preventatively as a routine herd health approach to control the long-term level of disease. The disinfectant products will need prolonged, often daily, use to be effective. The application of these products through foot-baths is covered in Chapter 3.

Systemic treatment by injection or oral treatment is of little use because it is difficult to achieve therapeutic levels in the superficial layers of the skin. There is little evidence that systemically injected or administered antibiotics have any effect on the disease. Antibiotics are best used topically in conjunction with removal of dead overlying tissue from the affected area. This means either individual attention or trying to wash off the feet thoroughly before footbathing the whole herd. Systemically injected antibiotics are only indicated if there are signs of secondary bacterial infection of the DD lesions. The single most important point is to ensure that treatment reaches the infected area.

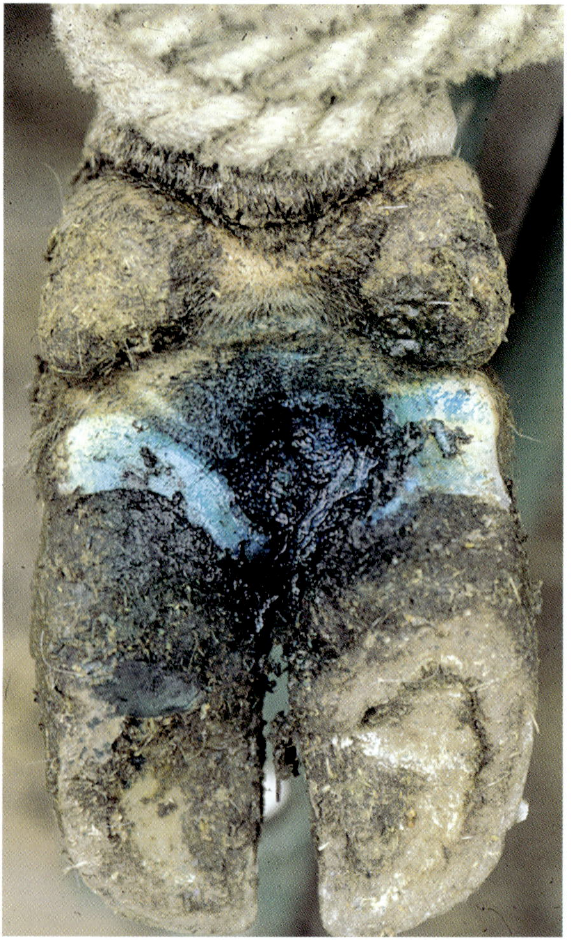

Individual spray works well but it needs to dry onto the lesion.

Difficulty in reaching the infected site with treatments is often due to:

*   Overlying liquefied material.
*   Necrotic epidermis.
*   Hypertrophied or hyperplasic tissue.
*   Foreign material – manure contamination.

In practice, this means that any treatment must be used in combination with an efficient application system to enable it to reach the affected area.

Individual Treatment

Treatment of the individual clinical case presents no great technical problem. Remove as much of the overlying material as possible. Be careful because DD is one of the most painful lesions of the foot. Debridement or curettage are techniques that simply remove the dead and liquefied surface of the lesion to allow the treatment drug to reach the active area; this technique can involve a great deal of pain for the cow. After removal, topical treatment with an antibacterial spray is very effective; there is some indication that with aerosol sprays (usually oxytetracycline) two applications give best results. A double aerosol layer – allowing the first to dry before application of a second – increases the effectiveness of the treatment by making sure that the topical treatment is sealed onto the surface and not washed off by the first bit of slurry or water the cow walks through after treatment. Allowing treated cows to stand in a clean yard for a while after therapy to allow the spray to dry is well worthwhile.

If the overlying tissue is excessive, as with the 'hairy wart'-type lesions, there needs to be a more radical approach to 'debridement', and it may need application of a dressing soaked in antibacterial solution to ensure good prolonged penetration into the lesion. The same bandaging technique will also produce better results in other more chronic forms of DD, such as coronary band lesions or interdigital lesions.

Herd Treatment

Herd treatments involve the use of products through a footbath, the principles of which are described in Chapter 3. There are basically two types of product available for use in footbaths to treat DD: antibiotics and skin disinfectants. Skin disinfectants are compounds such as formalin, copper sulphate, zinc sulphate, peracetic acid, Virkon, benzalkonium and dairy wash effluent (after cleaning the milking plant).

Details about each of these products are described in Chapter 3. However, in general, skin disinfectants will need to be used on a regular basis in order to maintain effectiveness at controlling DD. For instance, formalin should be used at least 5 days per week,

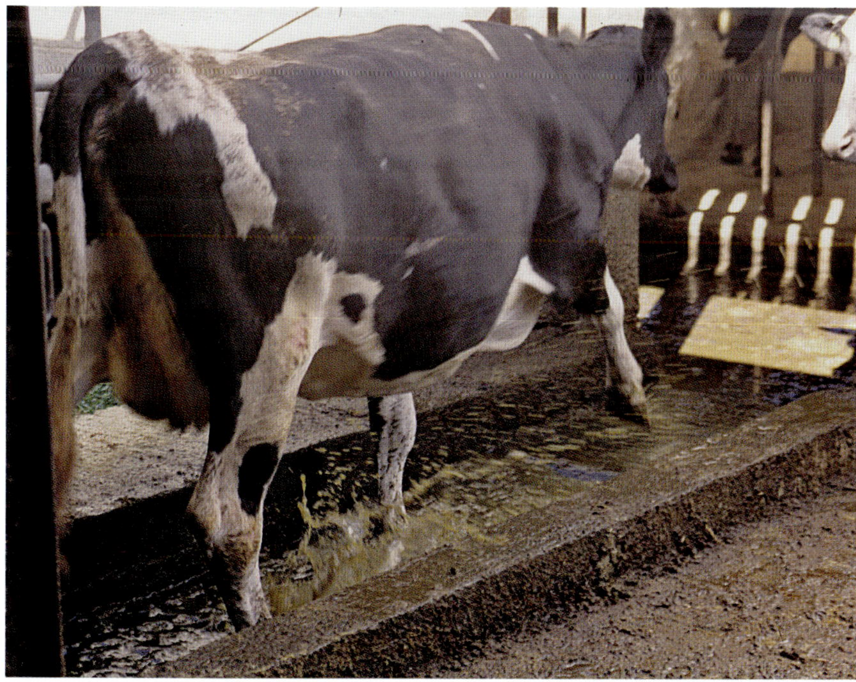

Footbaths are still the main treatment for digital dermatitis.

although most herds adopt a daily routine to keep on top of infection. Formalin is probably the most widely used compound for herd treatment of DD and is usually applied at concentrations between 3 and 5 per cent, although some herds do use higher concentrations.

An extensive choice of antibiotics is available, but the same principles apply to treating the herd as for the individual: choose the correct treatment and make sure it can reach the infected site. This is usually achieved by either putting the cows through a footbath on consecutive milkings for three or four milkings – a 'multipass' system – or by using a single passage through the bath after first cleaning the feet thoroughly and increasing the concentration of the agent in the bath.

The single system is now almost certainly the best advice as it reduces the amount of antibacterial used and, even though washing the feet off in the parlour entails more work on the single occasion, overall it takes less time than repeated footbathing (*see* Table 8).

Drug	Single passage (%)
Oxytetracycline	0.6–0.8
(Dimetridazole)	0.5–1
Erythromycin	0.03–0.04
Lincocin	0.03
Lincomycin/Spectinomycin	0.05
Tylosin	0.05
Tiamulin	0.06

Table 8 Typical agents used in footbaths. *Note that dimetridazole is no longer approved for use in food-producing animals and is no longer available. The concentrations are shown as per cent of the active ingredient in the footbath*

In terms of the actual drugs used, Table 9 shows how this equates to products and dilution rates.

All the products described in Table 9 are prescription-only medicines and must be obtained under veterinary guidance. These types of product are often expensive and it is essential that you get good professional advice

on which one to use, the best method for using it and the safety aspects of the product for animals, humans and the environment. There are anecdotal reports of various other products being used for footbath treatments, but the list in Table 9 represents the common choices.

If these agents are used for multiple passage ('multipass'), the concentration can be halved and fresh footbaths prepared for at least three consecutive milkings. As there has been very little work done on the specific dose required for DD treatment, the dose levels indicated in Table 9 are purely empirical.

For active treatment in an outbreak of the disease it will usually be necessary to use an antibiotic product as listed in Table 9 opposite. Once the disease is under control, there are other options available, such as skin disinfectants, to keep infection levels down and lameness in the herd under control. In general, the choice for ongoing control comes down to using cheaper skin disinfectants every day or using a specific antibiotic less frequently, say every 6–8 weeks. Even though the antibiotic is more expensive than the disinfectant, the reduced frequency of application means less time and effort so there is little to choose between them on cost.

There are safety aspects to consider when using footbaths with antibacterials:

- The footbath must be disposed of safely, immediately after use. The slurry pit or the catchment pit is the best option.
- Make sure the cows do not drink from the footbath. Walk through the bath with some dirty boots on to make sure that the first cows out of the parlour are put off drinking it. Alternatively, have a stocksperson present to ensure the first batch of cows do not drink from the bath. Many of the agents used will greatly upset rumen flora and produce a severe milk drop.
- Do not use the footbath on entry into the parlour. This will avoid any possible teat and thus milk contamination.

Drug	Pack size	Dilution
Oxytetracycline	Various generic products available – usually 800g of oxytetracycline per 1kg pack of soluble powder	1 pack (800g) per 100ltr
Erythromycin	70g sachets of soluble powder containing 11.56g of active erythromycin	3 sachets per 100ltr
Lincocin	150g pots of soluble powder containing 60g of lincocin	1 pot per 200ltr
Lincomycin/Spectinomycin	150g pots containing 33g of lincomycin and 66g of spectinomycin	1 pot per 200ltr
Tylosin	Comes in pots containing 100g of active tylosin	1 pot per 200ltr
Tiamulin	Usually supplied as a 12.5% solution in 1ltr packs for addition to water	1 pack per 200ltr

Table 9 Typical footbath mixes. *All the above mixes refer to water in the footbath. A typical footbath is around 200ltr*

- Be accurate with the dilution rates and measure the quantity of water added.
- Some products, such as formalin, produce fumes which are noxious and possibly dangerous. Therefore, siting the footbath away from the parlour and safe mixing of the products is essential.

Problems

Over recent winter housing periods DD has, in some herds, become more difficult to control. There is no one specific reason for this but there are some options:

- Is the organism resistant to the drugs? This is unlikely. It is more likely that the weight of infection and the conditions during autumn and winter (very mild and wet) have allowed levels of the disease to build up and produce a problem that is much more difficult to control. In herds where treatment has been changed there has been no improvement in the control of the condition.
- Herds that have taken more care about treatment have been successful, although it has entailed a lot of extra work over and above what they would normally have put in. Examples include more individual treatment by lifting the foot and cleaning, curettage and spraying the affected areas over a period of several days, which is very time consuming; also paying more attention to herd treatments by improving the cleaning of feet in the parlour to improve the treatment effect.
- There have been signs of a more chronic form of the disease on the foot. Interdigital growths (corns) have become more common in several herds, with the dependent surface eroded with DD. In my opinion it is more likely that the chronic ongoing irritation from DD is producing proliferation of the interdigital skin to form these growths.

Many stock handlers are becoming weary of the constant daily battle with DD and it is only natural that some aspects of control are being carried out less thoroughly; this results in build up of infection levels and the disease will be even more difficult to treat as more chronic lesions develop. There is no known way to eradicate this disease and prevention will, for the present, always be based on continual control measures. The recent trend of wetter, milder winters has increased the potential for more heavy levels of infection on farms and this is more likely to be the factor increasing the need for meticulous, thorough treatment.

Control

Control concerns the long-term management of the risk factors that allow disease to spread within the herd.

- Work at ADAS Bridget's has shown that, if there is a high level of carrier animals, treatment during the housing period is less effective.[9] These carriers may have obvious lesions, but many are holding the organism in the interdigital pouch or in low-grade lesions. Identify and treat carrier animals or make sure there is more frequent treatment of the cattle, especially at the start or before the beginning of the housing season.
- Cows with chronic proliferative lesions are becoming more common and serve as a reservoir of infection. These types of lesion tend to hold DD for long periods of time because treatments cannot reach the depths of the lesion. These cows need to be singled out for individual treatment. Remember to treat both the dry cows and the in-calf heifers because they are often forgotten when it comes to herd control and they will bring chronic lesions back into the main herd when they calve.
- The environment is very important for the survival and spread of the disease. DD needs moisture to produce infection. Avoid a large build-up of slurry and manure by ensuring all cow areas are well scraped. Be sure that the scraping system on the farm is efficient at preventing large areas of slurry accumulating; this is especially important with automatic systems. A wide passageway is a definite advantage as it minimizes the risk of deep slurry forming. Adequate quantities of straw should be used for bedding in order to keep the feet dry and clean.

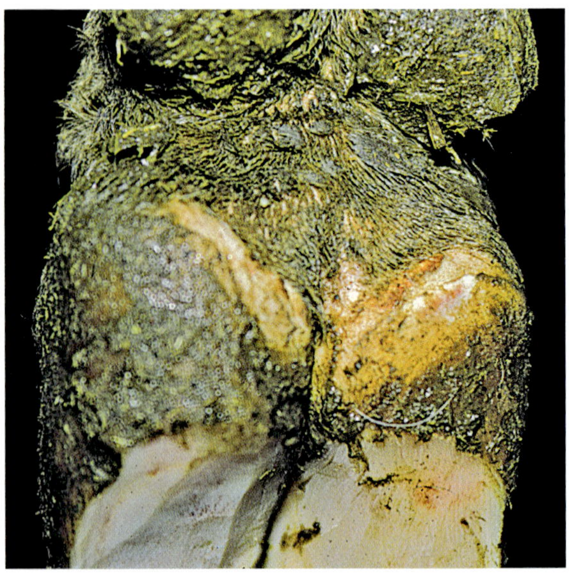

Very early signs of digital dermatitis infection.

- Some feeds may produce more 'sticky' faeces than others. Many practitioners feel that high maize diets are particularly troublesome. As maize diets are so common, it is difficult to suggest any practical improvements here.
- Make sure the footbath is used effectively. The feet must be well cleaned in the parlour before passing through the footbath. Double footbaths run as a consecutive pair, with the first filled with water, will not clean the feet well enough to ensure good application in the treatment bath.
- Long-term control can either be by using an antibiotic product at intervals of around 6–8 weeks during the winter housing period or using a skin disinfectant product on a more regular basis. For instance, formalin is not effective as a one-off treatment for DD and it can make things worse by damaging the skin of actively infected DD cows because it is too harsh on the skin. To be effective, formalin needs consistent use at least 5 days per week or a regular system of daily use. Many herds adopt this regular daily routine during the winter housing periods, as described in Chapter 3.

- Check the dilution rate of the agent used in the footbath. Consider using a higher strength of agent in the footbath at difficult times but only in conjunction with good foot cleaning – not instead of it.
- Increase the frequency of treatment, either by using the footbath more often or by using a handheld spray (using the same agent as in the footbath freshly mixed every couple of days) on the cows after washing the foot. Problem or suspect cows can then be targeted more often. The use of antibiotic products in the parlour is dangerous due to the risk of milk contamination and they should only be used if there is no other way round the problem.

INTERDIGITAL NECROBACILLOSIS (INTERDIGITAL PHLEGMON) – 'FOUL'

This condition is typically due to *Fusobacterium necrophorum*, but other bacteria may also be involved, for example *Dichelobacter nodosus* (Bacteroides) and possibly other *Bacteroides* spp. The lesion is characterized by swelling of the bulbs of the heels and a ragged split of the interdigital skin, which then sloughs to expose the dermis. There is always necrosis of tissues in the wound, which produces the characteristic 'foul' smell that gives the disease its name. Sometimes there is no apparent split or fissure present – only a swelling. The classic textbooks refer to these as 'blind fouls'. When this sort of interdigital swelling is scraped with a knife, the skin often opens to reveal underlying necrotic material. The condition is primarily one of necrosis and does not produce pus unless there is secondary infection.

Treatment

Unless neglected, the condition usually responds well to most antibiotics used for short periods of time. Sulphonamides, although still useful, seem to be less effective in practice and are now restricted in choice (due to loss of products in registration) and nearly all carry a minimum 2-day milk withdrawal. Other agents are now perhaps more useful – synthetic penicillins, oxytetracycline, and so on.

The most common therapy for adult dairy cows is to use nil milk withdrawal products, such as ceftiofur, usually as a single dose,

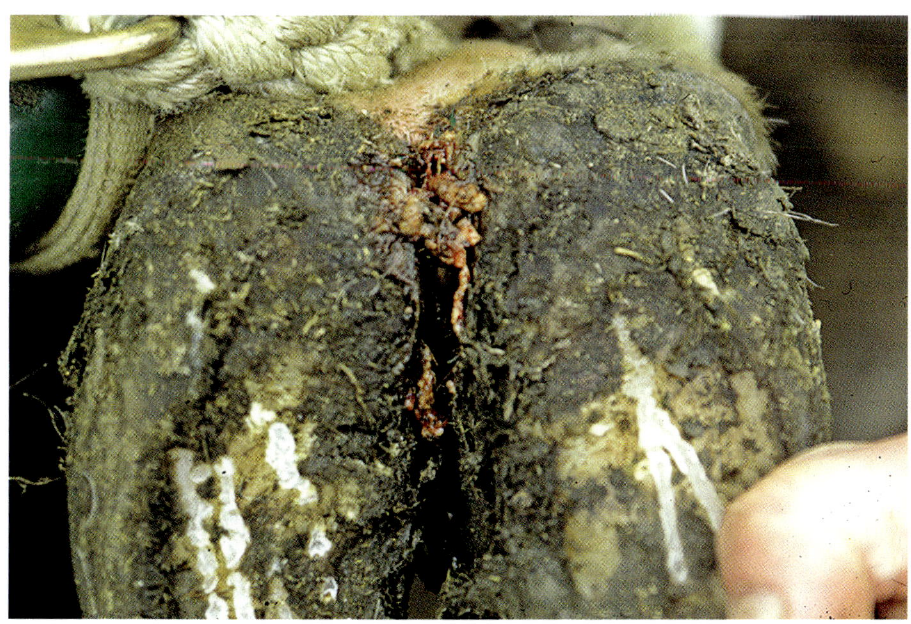

Typical 'foul' infection. Rotten tissue is coming out from the interdigital space.

although sometimes a 2-day treatment regime is required. Other classes of stock do not need to be restricted to nil milk withdrawals and other products may be used. Ampicillin as a 4.5g single dose (24 hours or less withdrawal for milk depending on formulation) is also very effective and oxytetracycline still remains an assured choice with good activity, especially if there is a suspicion of 'super foul' being involved (*see* below).

This condition responds better to antimicrobials if the foot is cleaned off, checked for foreign bodies, necrotic tissue removed and the area cleansed with a topical application of copper sulphate or oxytetracycline spray. If this is done effectively, in some mild cases it is sufficient to affect a cure without the need for parental therapy. This makes it possible to wait 24–48 hours to see if there is an improvement before resorting to injectable treatment.

Loose horn wall is often seen in the interdigital space at the axial margins of the necrotic split; this may be caused by inflammation and necrosis undermining the adjacent horn. Loose horn forms an irritant edge that can damage interdigital tissue and prolong healing. It can even predispose to the formation of a 'corn'. Horn growth at the axial border of the sole can retain foreign material, allowing it to become wedged between the claws. Trimming this horn could improve the healing rate.

To summarize the clinical approach:

- Clean the interdigital space.
- Check for foreign bodies.
- Open up the skin splits.
- Scrape out the necrotic tissue.
- Remove any loose or under-run horn on the axial margins.
- Remove a wedge of horn from the axial edge of the sole.
- Apply topical treatment.
- Apply parental treatment, if required.

Recent trends with DD sometimes make it difficult to assess exactly what lesion is present in the interdigital space and, if both are present, which came first? Be careful to check for

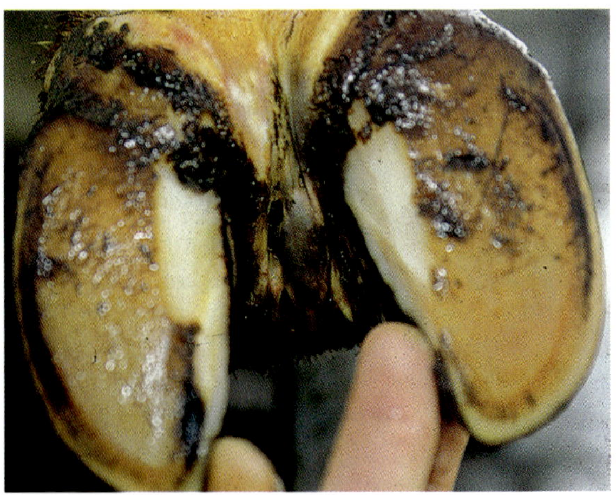

Try to remove a wedge of horn on the axial surfaces to allow the interdigital space to empty.

the typical DD strawberry-like appearance, as interdigital DD is almost certainly more common than the classic bulbar form. It is necessary to know the difference in order to decide whether systemic treatment is necessary and also to plan what herd preventative measures to adopt.

Prevention

A MAFF (Ministry of Agriculture, Fisheries and Food as it was then) survey of footbath use in dairy herds showed that the commonly used agents at that time (primarily formalin, although occasionally copper and zinc sulphate) could only be positively proven to be effective against one foot disease – 'foul'. Footbaths containing formalin used weekly during high-risk periods are very effective in controlling early mild cases and preventing the disease.

Outbreaks tend to occur typically in the autumn in wet, muddy weather. *Fusobacterium* thrive in faeces and mud, making the traditional autumn and spring gateway a haven for infection. Penetration of the skin may be triggered by stones or perhaps the wet conditions. The organism then penetrates the interdigital skin and produces infection. This is often the case with cows going through poorly maintained gateways where trauma will trigger the disease.

PER-ACUTE INTERDIGITAL NECROBACILLOSIS – 'SUPER-FOUL'

'Super-foul' was first reported in 1993 and, although there have been several outbreaks since then, it has not escalated to the scale that was feared at the time. However, although uncommon, it is still seen in some dairy areas and is a very severe disease. It is essential to recognize it, assess its severity and take immediate radical action. Any delay will result in the cow being culled.

It is a particularly severe interdigital necrobacillosis. A necrotic split in the skin rapidly forms a deep fissure up into the soft tissue between the claws. As the infection becomes chronic, large masses of granulated dermal tissue quickly protrude from the fissure. The important feature of this condition is the speed with which the infection becomes established and the severity of the lesions produced. It

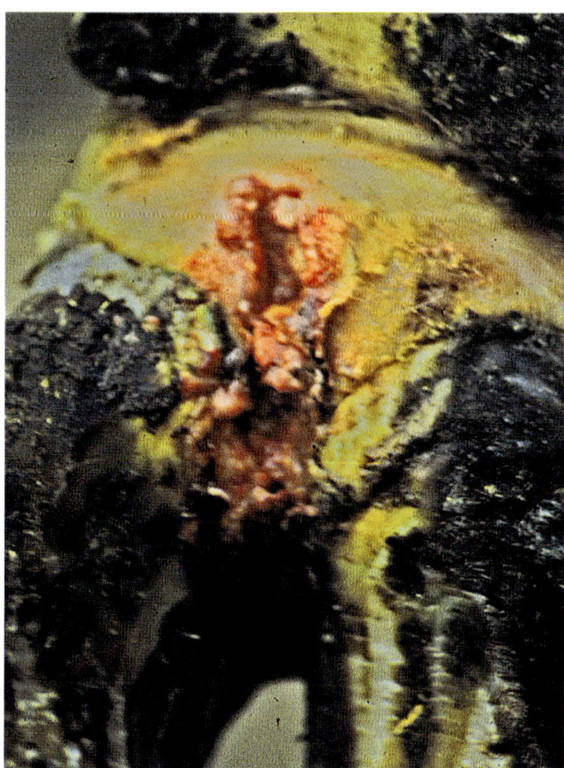

'Super foul'.

often progresses into secondary infection such as pedal joint arthritis or a cellulitis (infection) of the soft tissues of the leg.

The fact that the disease will progress rapidly to a septic arthritis if not diagnosed makes it crucial to assess the case at the outset. Prompt action can be effective if one pedal joint is affected. If both pedal joints are affected, cull immediately (no collateral support during treatment).

Affected herds often have a history of DD and it is unclear whether DD is related to 'super-foul'. Possibly a DD infection may predispose to the disease or, on the other hand, DD may simply make early recognition of the condition difficult. There is some evidence that importations from abroad or purchases of animals from other herds may be involved with outbreaks of the disease. The first outbreaks in Gloucestershire were associated with imported cattle and recent cases seem to follow purchases from other herds.

Most veterinary practitioners who have seen this condition think it is sufficiently distinct to be able to recognize and distinguish it from traditional 'foul'. Unlike the ordinary necrobacillosis, once established the infection is refractory to treatment due to the extensive tissue damage and infection.

Treatment

Early cases present few problems and respond to the usual drugs used for interdigital necrobacillosis. Oxytetracycline at a dose of 6g as a single dose of mixed long- and short-acting formulation is sufficient for early cases. However, cattle are usually presented when there is already considerable extension from the primary lesion. In more advanced cases, aggressive therapy using tylosin at an initial dose of 8g (4g twice on the first day) and then 4g daily is needed along with topical applications of clindamycin. The rational is to produce high tissue levels of tylosin and use a drug such as clindamycin for its activity in an anaerobic environment. Combinations of spiromycin and metronidazole (not licensed for food animals) used topically could have improved action because this product may perform better in the presence of necrotic tissue.

There are reports of the use of regional intravenous antibiotics to achieve higher tissue levels of antibiotic in the affected area.[13] The technique involves regional haemostasis of the affected leg by tourniquet and infusion of large doses of antibiotic into the digital vein. The same reports indicate that the method is very effective, but beware because there are also reports of sloughing and gangrene as a result of clots forming in the veins; this is presumably due to irritation by some antibiotics or their use at such locally high doses. It is unlikely that this technique would be recommended by veterinarians, due to the potential side effects and difficulty in carrying it out.

Prevention

The use of DD footbath regimes is successful at lowering the incidence and preventing outbreaks. However, the footbath may be acting as a general skin disinfectant rather than assuming any association with DD. There was evidence from the first outbreaks of the disease that the use of low-volume footbaths for DD (sponge-based baths etc.) could be associated with outbreaks of peracute necrobaccillosis. It was thought that these baths were easily contaminated and could spread infection because there was not enough active agent in them to cope with slurry contamination from the feet. The evidence for this is purely anecdotal and at present more work is needed to verify this hypothesis.

Be sure to inspect and treat all purchased or incoming animals routinely.

INTERDIGITAL HYPERPLASIA

Proliferation of interdigital skin (hyperplasia) is well known to most stockpersons, who usually refer to it as a 'corn'. Some breeds of cow are more prone to this disease (it is called 'Hereford disease' in some parts of the country because this breed is very susceptible) because they have more open claws that allow

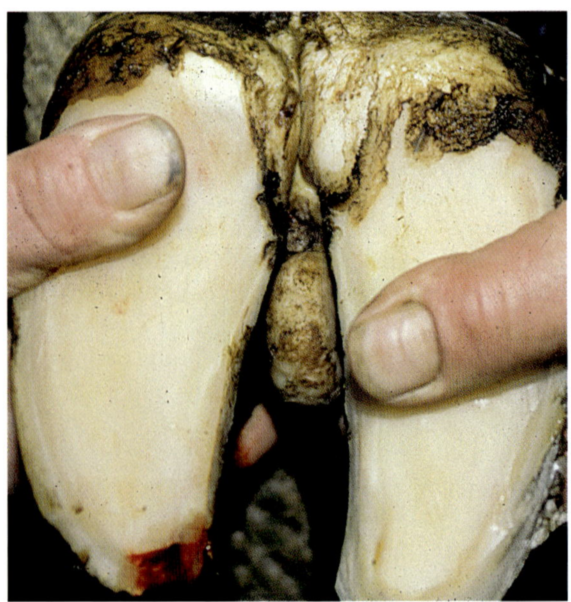

Interdigital hyperplasia.

stretching of the interdigital skin. The skin then forms a large fold, which is compressed when the foot is lifted off the ground, causing pain and discomfort. Skin folds are not usually a problem until there is irritation or infection, which then produces lameness. DD may cause complications in diagnosis and aetiology. DD of the interdigital space is probably now the most common form of DD and one by-product of this may be involvement with interdigital hyperplasia. It is likely that DD is producing the hyperplastic response in this area, and chronic infection with DD gives rise to corns, usually with a typical DD lesion on the plantar surface. Corns can form after any chronic interdigital disease, but with DD becoming so common they are being found more often in dairy herds.

Treatment

Treat the basic cause first. If DD or necrobacillosis is involved, treat this and the skin fold will reduce in size and should be no further problem. If there is secondary infection and necrosis, again primary treatment should be aimed at removing dead tissue and treating the infection.

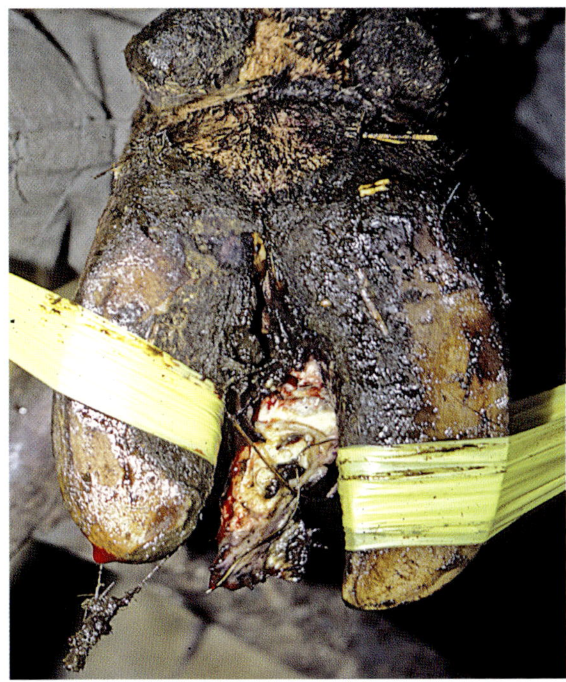

Interdigital hyperplasia that has become infected. This will need removal.

Should a corn be removed surgically? Small hyperplastic folds are not a problem if complications such as DD or necrosis are resolved. Larger folds may predispose to future problems, but removal might not be the answer. Removal often results in the condition reappearing and the granulation tissue replacing the corn is much weaker and more prone to problems. There may be a case for minimum interference. As with necrobacillosis, removing a section of solar horn on the axial or interdigital edge prevents any hyperplasia being pinched, which is often the cause of pain and lameness. Look for loose horn at the margins of the wall in the interdigital space because this will produce enough chronic irritation to form a hyperplasia.

MUD FEVER

If mud or slurry coats the skin of the legs there is danger that it will promote skin irri-

tation and possibly infection. This condition is referred to as 'mud fever'. The leg often swells and the overlying hair is lost. The skin is usually reddened and the swelling may produce folds in the skin with cracks and fissures present. Secondary infection soon causes complications in cases such as these.

Treatment consists of:

- Moving cattle to a cleaner, drier environment immediately.
- Washing off any mud or slurry.
- Applying skin emollients and topical antibacterial products.
- Injecting with systemic antibiotics if there is a lot of skin infection.

Lameness is not severe unless there is a lot of skin infection.

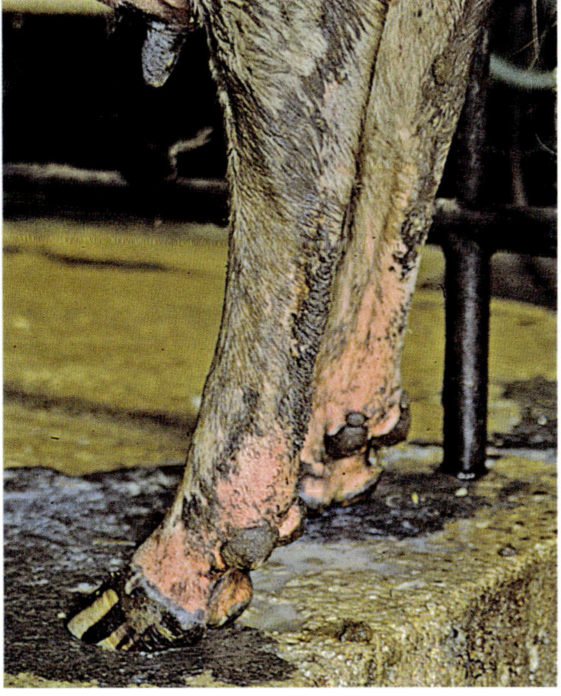

Mud fever.

CHAPTER SEVEN

Diseases of the Joints and Bones

The joints and bones of the leg are well protected from damage and are not often primarily involved in lameness. However, accidents do occur, especially with housed cattle in concrete yards, and any cause of lameness in the foot can progress to involve deeper structures. Both of these events can involve the joints and bones of the leg, producing lameness.

Most of the techniques and treatments discussed in this chapter are based on skilled professional help because, unfortunately, there is often little the stockperson can do themselves. However, it is necessary to be familiar with problems and be aware what treatments are required. Everyone working with lameness in cattle needs to recognize the conditions that cause lameness and know the options for treatment, even if they need help with applying some of them.

JOINT INFECTION – SEPTIC ARTHRITIS

Most joint diseases in the adult cow are due to infection of the pedal joint. Infection occurs when an initial lesion elsewhere in the foot physically extends to involve other structures, of which the pedal joint is the most common. Only rarely is disease due to infection being brought to the joint from the bloodstream; this is more common in calves, where the disease is called 'joint ill'.

An initial lameness injury can, in some cases, progress to produce a variety of lesions affecting deeper structures of the foot and leg. This extension usually occurs because of the anatomical relationship of lesions such as solar ulceration and white line disease with key structures such as the pedal joint, tendons, tendon sheaths and bursae of the leg. This extension may primarily involve soft tissues such as the tendons and bursae, but often the process is rapidly complicated by extension into the joints and bones of the foot (*see* diagrams of solar ulcer on page 69).

Infection and sepsis of a joint in an adult bovine presents one of the most difficult situations for the practitioner and the herdsperson to treat successfully and indeed many of these animals are ultimately culled from the herd. Often the temptation is to be conservative with initial treatment for joint disease, but simply injecting antibiotics will not be enough to resolve the situation; radical treatment early in the course of the disease is essential to produce results. Joints that are infected effectively become abscesses, which ultimately will require prolonged and systematic drainage techniques if they are to stand any chance of healing.

In practice the most common presentation is of a cow treated for an initial lameness injury that has progressed, often due to lack of prompt effective treatment, into a complicated lameness involving joints, bones and related soft tissues. Poor initial treatments and the lack of a positive approach early in the course of the lameness can drastically increase the chances of complications such as joint infection occurring.

The Disease

Joint infection is due to invasion of the joint with an infectious organism or their products (antigenic or 'foreign' material is often enough). The joint initiates a profound inflammatory response, producing changes in the structures of the joint. This quickly results in damage to the cartilage, alterations in joint fluid, thickening and swelling of the joint capsule, and changes in the bone itself such as deep infection, formation of extra bone as the joint tries to stabilize itself (exostoses) and even complete union of the joint to form a solid structure (ankylosis). If left, the joint becomes an abscess with large accumulations of septic material.

In calves, infectious arthritis is due to bacteria in the bloodstream (bacteraemia) 'seeding out' in the joints. In adult cattle this rarely occurs. Infections producing abscesses on the heart valves (vegetative endocarditis) can easily shed material into the bloodstream that may occasionally (especially if it affects the left side of the heart) 'seed out' in the joints. *Mycoplasma bovis* is a bacterial infection that can also produce an infectious arthritis. It is seen occasionally in adult cattle and is often associated with decreased immunity due to disease or calving. Joint infections from this sort of spread can affect any joint and frequently the main distinguishing feature is a swollen hock or fetlock joint in adult animals.

The most common infectious or septic arthritis in the adult animal occurs as a result of direct extension of a local wound or injury into the adjacent joint. Any septic lesion in the foot that fails to drain to the outside may penetrate, affecting deeper structures and eventually the joint itself.

Examples of foot lesions that often progress to joint infection are:

- Solar ulceration.
- Foreign body penetration.
- White line lesions.
- Peracute interdigital necrobacillosis ('super foul').

If the original lameness extends, ligaments, tendons, sheaths, bursae and other bones (e.g. navicular) are involved, as well as the joint itself. It is as important to resolve infection in these structures as it is in the joint itself. As it is very close to the site of many foot lesions, such as a solar ulcer, the joint most likely to be affected is the pedal joint. The pedal joint has little normal movement other than to 'give' under weight so the shock of the animal's weight is dispersed. Therefore, normal joint function is not essential and resolution can involve ankylosis or even amputation to return the animal to normal production and resolve the lameness.

The combinations of clinical signs that indicate a septic arthritis are:

- A discreet ring of swelling at the coronary band.
- A severe lameness.
- Unresponsive to more usual conservative treatment.
- Eventual gross enlargement of the whole area.

Treatment

Before starting treatment it is essential to assess the animal and the farm situation. Welfare of the animal is paramount and all decisions regarding treatment, and even whether to treat, must take this into consideration.

- How much work is the stockperson prepared to put in?
- Can the farm cope with nursing management – is there a straw yard?
- Is the cow going to be able to cope with treatment – is she too old?
- Is there a realistic prospect of the animal returning to production?

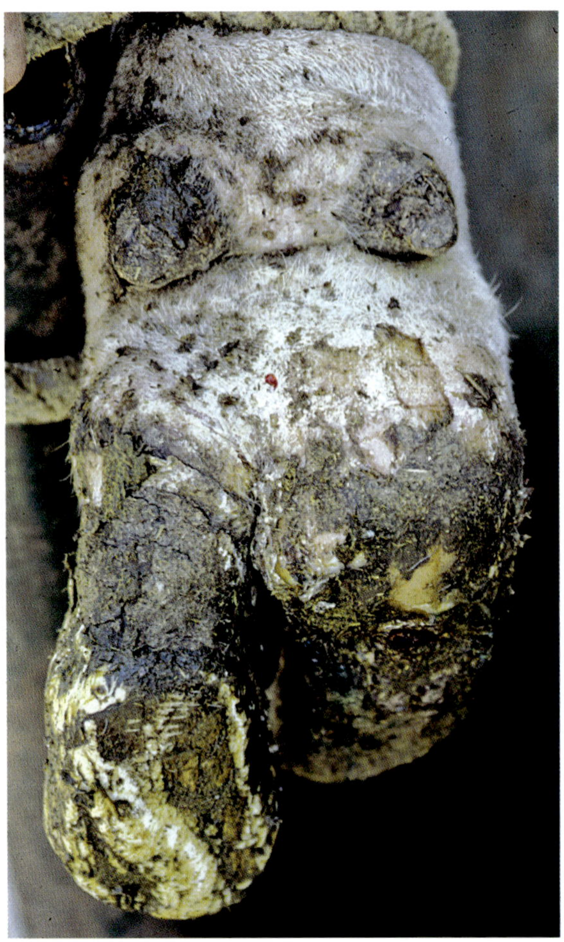

Septic arthritis – note the swollen joint. This cow has been treated unsuccessfully for solar ulceration.

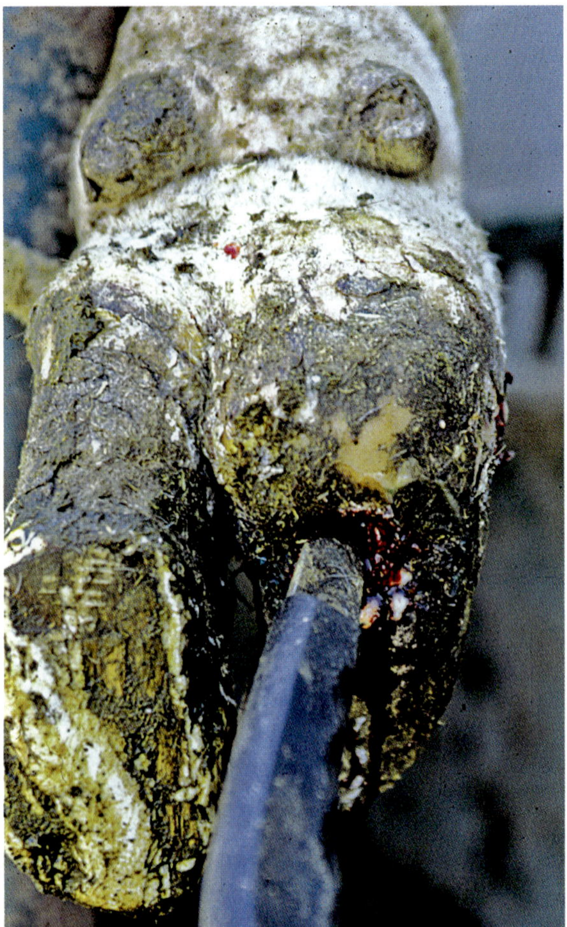

Coring the original lesion open to produce better drainage.

Assess the level of joint involvement and make an early decision about treatment, which will be in order of priority: drainage, supportive therapy and the use of antibiotics.

Drainage

All procedures involving gaining access to drain the joint will require anaesthesia of the foot. This can only be achieved through an effective regional, local or, in extreme cases, a full anaesthetic technique. The approach to the joint is difficult because the pedal joint is normally fully enclosed within the confines of the hoof itself. Therefore, prompt radical treatment should involve skilled veterinary intervention.

The options used in practice are given below.

'Coring': The technique involves opening up the original infected tract through to the joint and all other affected structures. It involves using a foot knife under local or regional anaesthesia to open up a hole big enough to drain the affected areas. If the original defect was a solar ulcer, use the knife to open up the ulcer and bore deeper towards the retro bulbar area. If there is an abscess in this area, the knife will bore in easily and pus will be seen to drain out.

Summary: Easy to perform and gives instant drainage. However, the core hole heals up too quickly and requires regular maintenance to

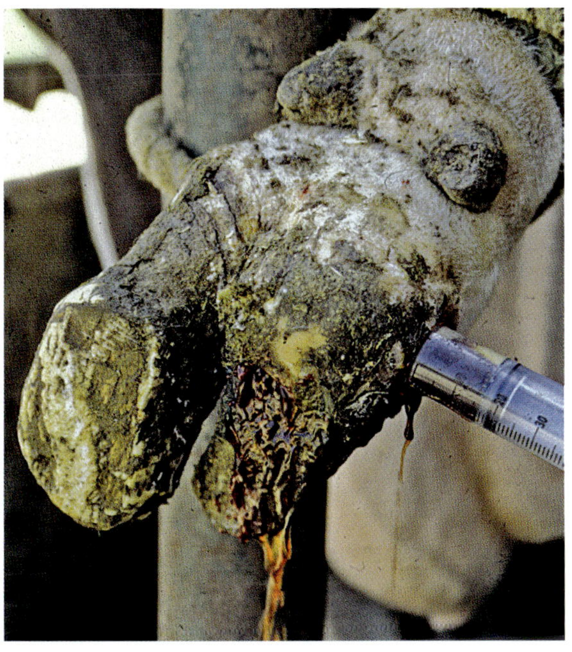

Flushing fluid through the infected joint from an incision on the coronary band.

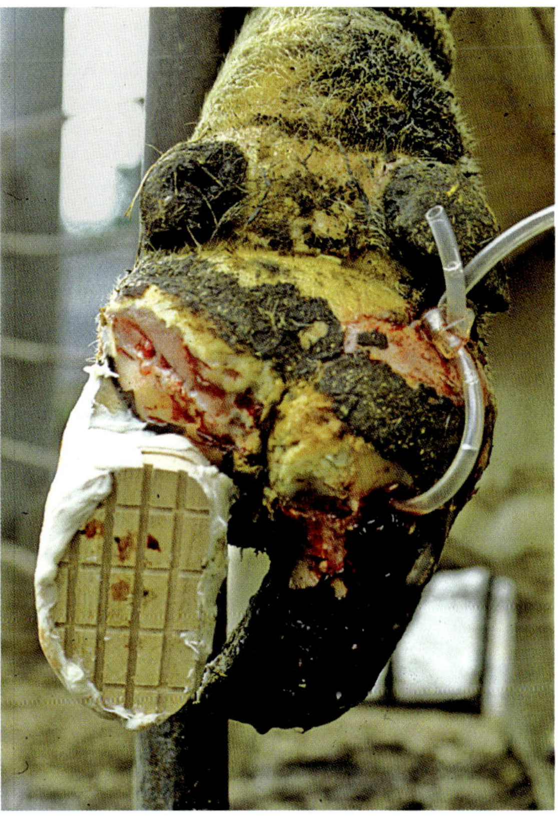

Establishing a drainage tube through the joint using the original wound.

keep it open and draining. It is inaccurate and not usually efficient at draining the joint. It works better when there is an abscess affecting purely the retro bulbar area.

Flushing: An incision is made into the joint capsule, usually from the lateral or posterior aspect of the coronary band, and the original defect line is opened up or 'cored' to allow drainage as described above. The joint is then flushed by pumping fluid in from the incision wound on the coronary band and out through the original defect.

Summary: This is a good method to remove infected material from the joint, but it needs maintenance to keep the flushing and drainage hole established. It will need to be repeated frequently, which may cause problems for the stockperson because it is not the easiest technique to use without help.

Insert a drainage tube: A tube placed through or into the joint has two main benefits; first, it keeps the drainage holes open because it sits in the drainage tract permanently during treatment. Second, it allows much

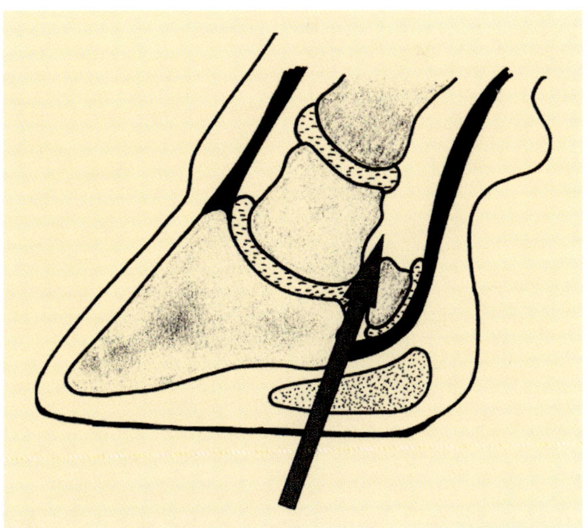

Section through a foot to show the line of drainage with the original line technique.

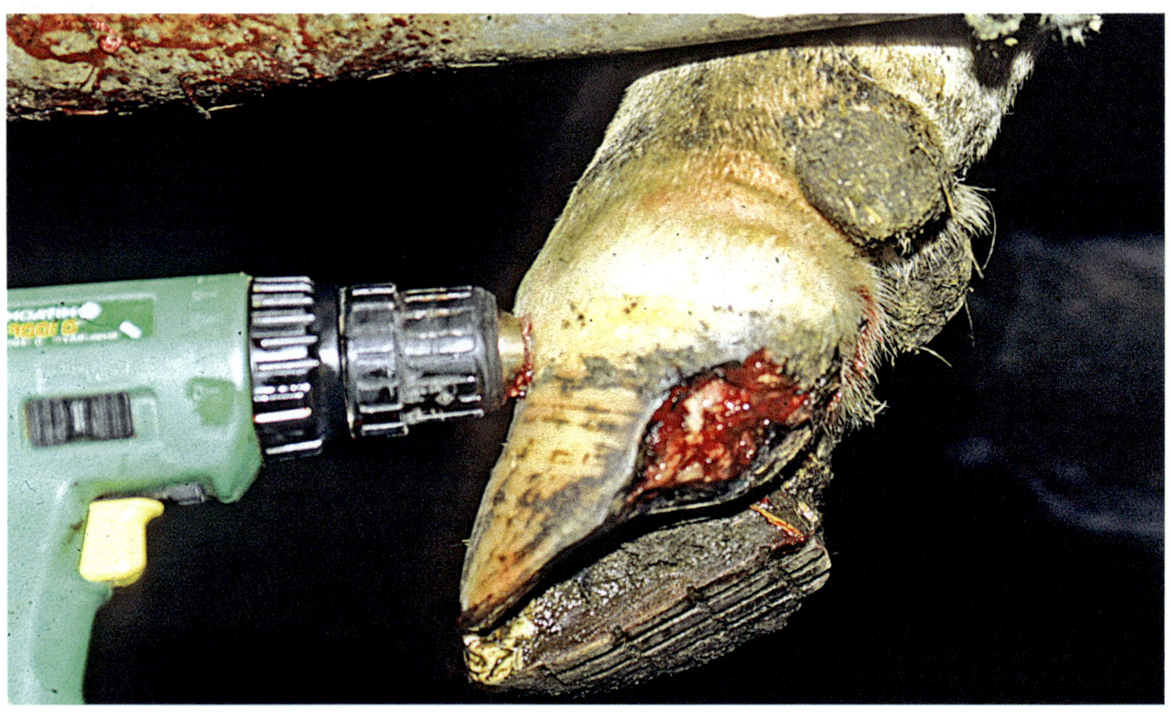

A battery drill is powerful enough to drill a drainage hole in this septic joint.

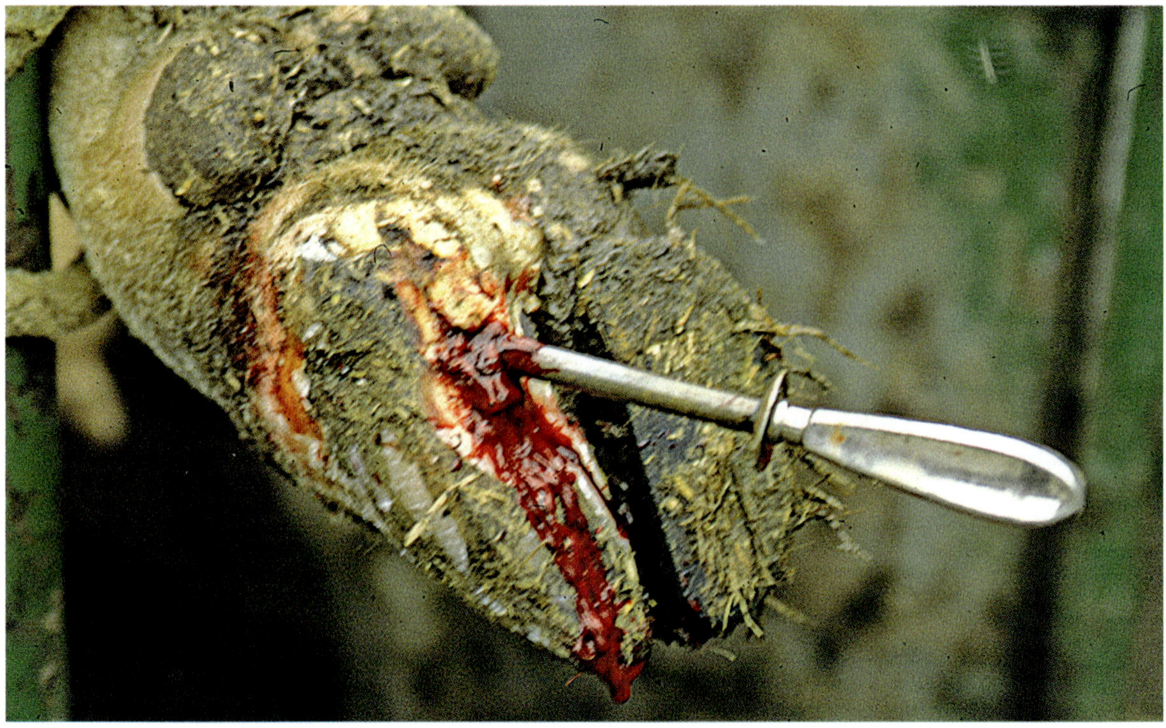

A trochar can be used to gain access to the joint through the original wound – a solar ulcer.

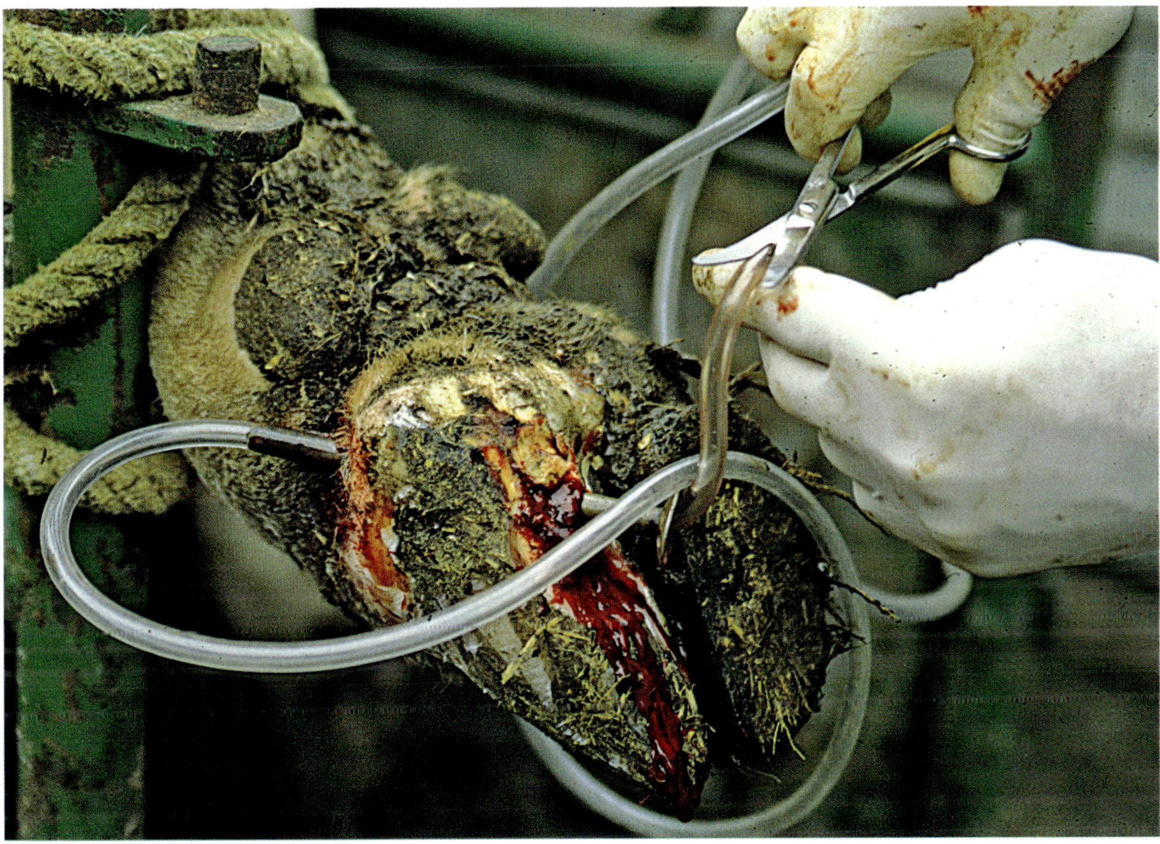

Tubes are threaded through and tied off to enable drainage and flushing.

easier flushing of the joint and surrounding area.

The drainage tube can be inserted by either using the original defect line that drains out at the joint line, or by creating a completely new drainage hole transecting the joint. A drain through the original fault line has the advantage of being easy to do, but it does not allow healing of the original lesion. It may be difficult to get it fully into the joint space because it is more likely merely to touch the back edge of the joint capsule; however, it will not drastically damage the joint. This may seem to be an advantage, but it cannot produce a good drainage line through the joint surfaces and may not flush the joint fully. A new line drilled through the joint allows the original wound to heal, but it does produce extensive damage to the joint

and means that ankylosis will usually be the outcome.

Methods:

Original line: Use blunt-ended scissors or a large-bore trochar and cannula (rumen trochar) to enter through the original defect line (ulcer etc.) and probe deep into the underlying structures. By aiming laterally and backwards you come up under the coronary band area and you can feel the instrument below the skin here. Incise down onto the blunt probe or trochar with a scalpel and create an exit hole in the coronary area. Thread the tube onto the end of the scissors or trochar, or pass the tube down the centre of the cannula. A full drainage tube will then be in place.

New line transecting the joint: Again use a trochar and cannula or a cordless drill, with a suitably sized drill bit, to bore through

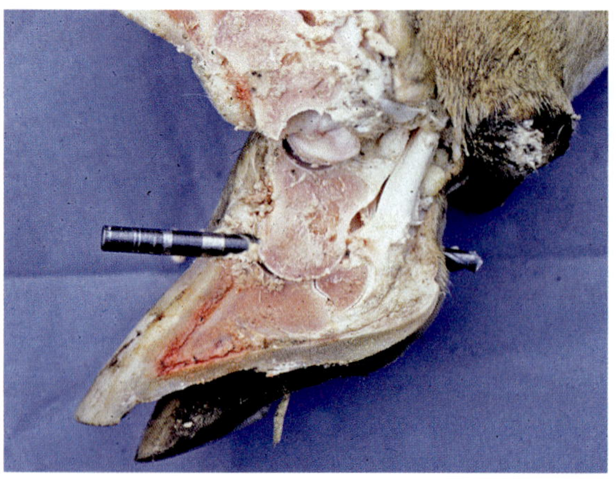

A new line is drilled across the joint to give better drainage.

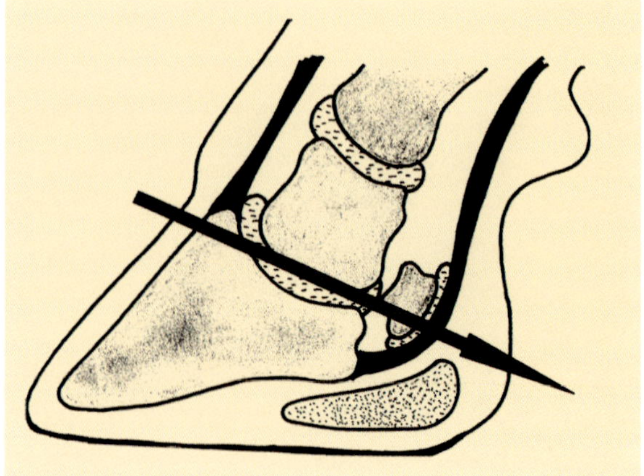

Sectional diagram through the foot to show the new line across the joint.

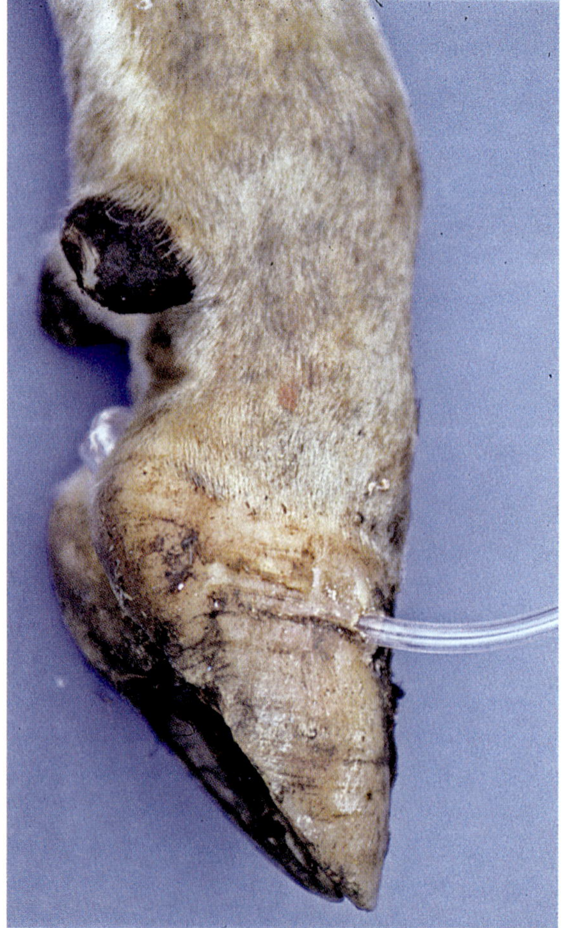

Tube in place through the new drilled hole.

the joint and establish a new drainage line. Thread the tube onto the trochar or through the cannula and position the drainage tube across the joint.

In both techniques the tube is sealed at one end, holes are cut in it along the length inside the joint, and it is strapped to the leg with bandage higher up the leg away from the foot to allow easy access for flushing. Flushing is simple and it is the physical flushing procedure that is the main objective, so the type of fluid used is not important. Simple homemade saline solutions are perfectly adequate. It will take several weeks to fully flush an abscess in the pedal joint so the drainage tube will need to be in place for some time.

Summary: It is quick and easy to perform, gives good access for flushing the joint and is relatively easy to maintain. It may leave a functional joint. There may be problems with removing thick clotted material and debris from the joint. However, in time these should break down and be flushed out.

Full open surgery – arthrodesis, arthrotomy: A large incision is made into the joint to fully evacuate the contents and remove all dead and infected material. The procedure requires general anaesthesia to obtain the best results. Arthrotomy implies that the incision is temporary, for removal and evacua-

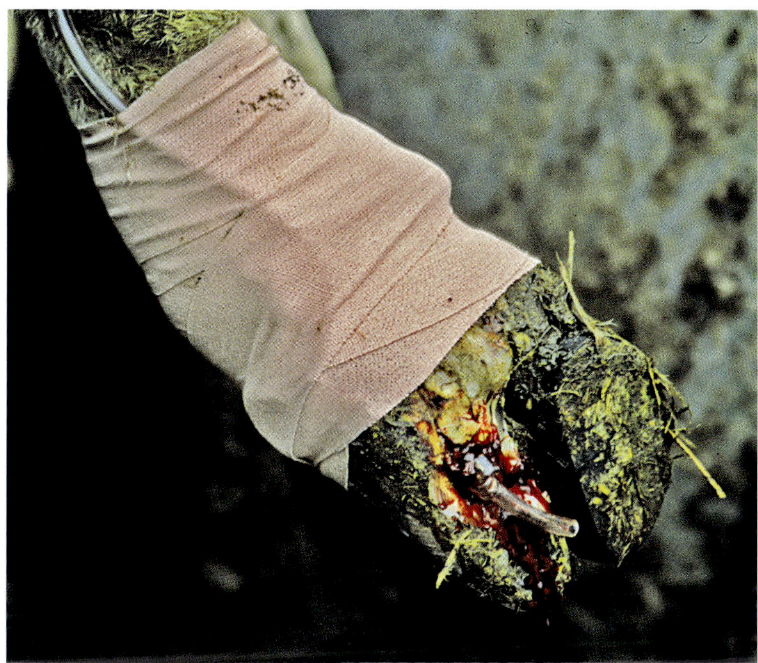

Drainage tube secured in place to allow easy access to flush the joint.

tion, while arthrodesis is aiming to produce a fusion of the joint.

Summary: It gives good access to the joint, good removal of infected and necrotic matter and good drainage after. However, aftercare is difficult and there may be problems if the tendons are cut when gaining access to the joint. Joint function will be completely lost with arthrodesis.

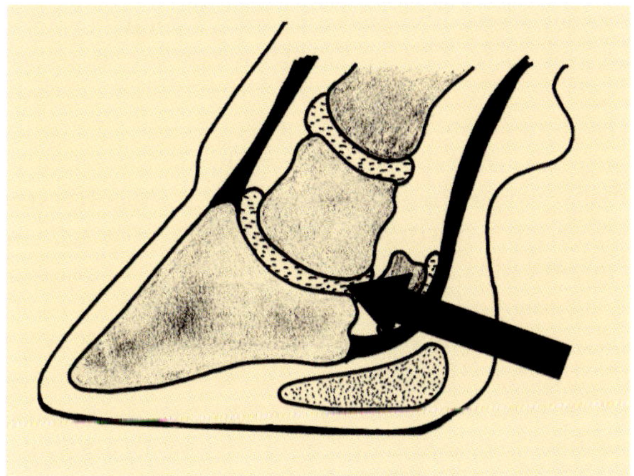

Approach to the infected joint if doing full surgery to open up and remove infection.

Amputation: This method completely drains the area by removing the entire digit with the infected joint and any other infected material. It is relatively easy to perform under regional anaesthesia; but it may not be very successful for the long-term future of the cow. Clinical studies indicate that cows with amputated digits are difficult to maintain post operatively and are not retained in the herd for very long.[14]

There will be failures and problems with all the above techniques. The most common are:

- Upturned toe – due to rupture or section of the flexor tendons. The superficial and deep flexor tendons pass behind and below the pedal joint through the retro bulbar area. If there is any infection in this area, or the pedal joint, these tendons are also affected and often end up rupturing as they become infected and rot away. If surgery to the joint is carried out, these tendons are often cut to gain access. Without these tendons the toe tends to lift up as the extensor tendons are still pulling from above and the weight of the animal is no longer being suspended

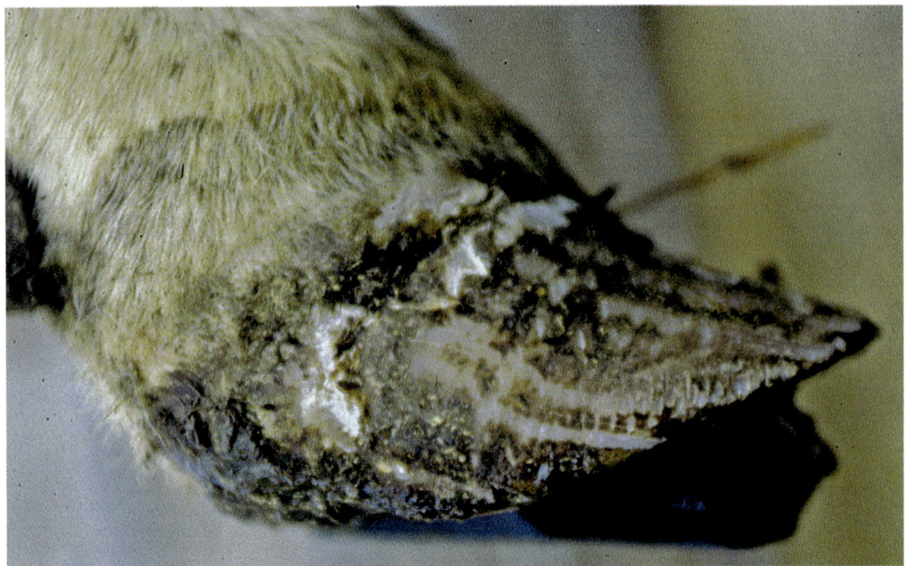

One common complication of infection in the joints or to the rear of the foot is that the flexor tendon breaks and an upturned toe is produced.

by the flexors. It is often worthwhile wiring the toes together to try and prevent this.

- Defective horn growth – due to damage to the coronary band. Drilling holes or establishing drainage could damage coronary band horn, which will then produce a defect that could affect the conformation of the foot.
- Enlarged joint – exostoses may limit movement.
- Chronic infective fistulas – usually temporary if drainage is effective.
- Ankylosis can be a problem in some joints. However, as most cases of joint disease involve the pedal joint, maintaining movement is not a problem.
- Infection tracking higher up the leg – tendons, tendon sheaths and bursae can all become infected and this can track up the leg to create a more extensive disease.

Conclusions

Without enthusiastic involvement of the farm staff and adequate farm facilities to cope with the problem there is little point in attempting any treatment of septic arthritis in the adult cow. But with co-operation and a skilled approach to the condition, especially early in the course of disease, the success rate is very good and there is an excellent prospect of the cow returning to normal production.

FRACTURE OF THE PEDAL BONE

It is tempting to say that this condition is rarely seen in practice, but it is also true that it is very difficult to diagnose and may be involved more than we think in some chronically lame cows. Diagnosis is based on the fact that there are no other obvious signs of a lameness lesion in the foot. The cow with a fractured pedal bone is usually affected in the inside claw of the front foot. The fracture is very painful and the cow tries to remove the damaged claw from weight bearing by crossing the affected leg when walking to transfer the pressure to the outside claw.

Treatment is by diagnosing the problem and putting a block on the sound claw. This sounds simple but there may well be some doubt as to which claw to block because there will be no lesion present in the lame cow to indicate which claw is affected. If you see the crossed-leg walking, you can be confident about which claw to block. Otherwise it may be worth 'speculating' as to the diagnosis and the claw involved by putting a temporary block on the foot to see if this helps the lameness symptoms. If it is successful, a more permanent block can be applied. If the wrong claw is blocked or the diagnosis is incorrect (e.g. it is a leg injury higher up), the lameness should worsen and the situation can be corrected.

STIFLE INJURIES

The stifle joint is one of the least stable joints in the whole hindlimb. There is no distinct encased joint where one bone locks into the other, as is the case with the hip and the hock. The stability of the joint is controlled purely by the ligaments holding it in place. The stifle joint is easily damaged when a cow falls or stumbles on concrete yards. The leg angle will tell you straight away whether there is ligament damage or not. Stifle injuries are seen as:

- A down cow with the stifle joint no longer in a straight line but angled outwards.
- A cow walking with rotation or twisting movement at the stifle.
- Severe lameness with an enlarged stifle joint.

As it is rarely possible to identify individual structures in it, the joint is difficult to examine. However, if you stand behind the cow and reach forward to clasp both stifle joints at the same time you can quickly appreciate if one of them is swollen and possibly damaged by comparing the feel of each one relative to the other.

LOCKING PATELLA

The kneecap or patella is the mechanism by which the extensor muscles exert their force past the knee joint to the lower limb; it works like a pulley arrangement. In cattle the patella is also part of the stay apparatus that helps the bovine remain on its feet for long periods of time for grazing and so on This stay mechanism is not as advanced as it is in the horse, where it is part of the weight support for the standing animal. However, the bovine still has the remnants of this system and the patella plays a key role.

When the leg is extended the patella will hook over a protuberance of bone on the end of the femur and the movement of the stifle joint is then locked up. The cow will appear lame, with the leg, fixed in extension, dragging behind it. The cow will walk a few strides with this awkward gait until the patella suddenly unhooks itself and it starts to walk normally again. Often both legs are affected, although one is usually worse than the other. There are surgical procedures to correct the problem if it is diagnosed correctly. The treatment involves cutting one of the patellar ligaments in order to prevent it hooking onto the bone and locking in extension.

DISLOCATED HIPS

The hip joint in cattle is very shallow and the absence of a large muscle mass (especially in the dairy cow) means that often a simple injury results in the femoral head becoming displaced from its normal position in the acetabulum on the hip to produce a dislocated hip.

Dislocations of the hip are not common, but cases do occur and many are not reported or are misdiagnosed, especially when you have a 'downer cow' situation. Cases in calves and youngstock are seen, but they need to be checked carefully because many are complicated by fracture of the femoral head.

Cows usually dislocate hips when in oestrus or involved in oestrous behaviour. The risks of it happening are higher during the winter housing period when management of the dairy cow usually involves access to areas of concrete.

A dislocated hip may seem a daunting prospect to attempt to correct due to the physical size of the problem involved. There are, however, logical and practical ways to approach

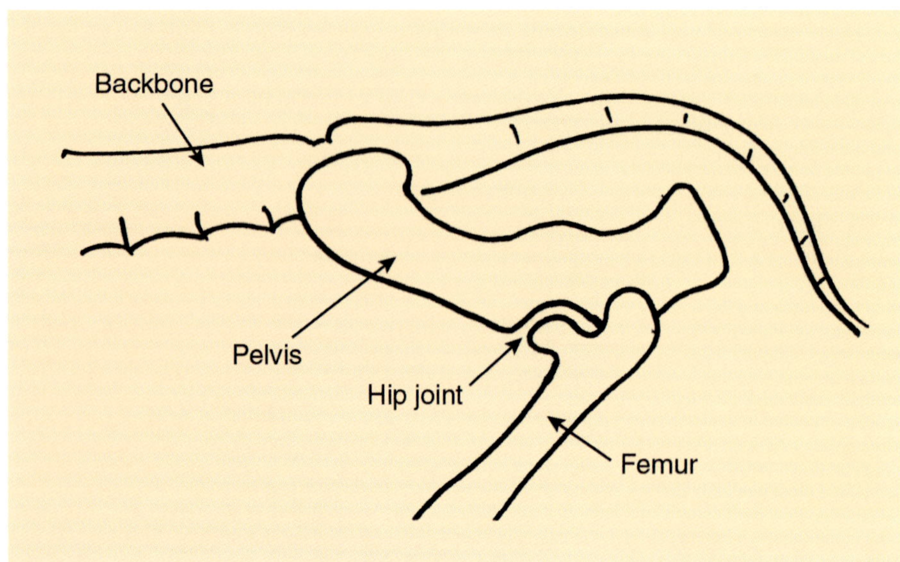

Side view of the bones of the hip joint.

this clinical problem. Dislocation of the hip should not present any more of a welfare decision than other causes of long-term lameness.

In practice, there are four stages involved in dealing with a dislocated hip:

1. Diagnosis.
2. Assessment.
3. Treatment.
4. Complications.

Diagnosis

Diagnosis can be difficult, especially if you cannot identify the structures of the hip joint. It is difficult to detect a dislocated hip in a fat cow down on the floor after falling. Often a lot of swelling is present after dislocation, which masks any attempt to accurately palpate the position of the hip. A severely lame cow will always alter the tilt of the pelvis as she walks, trying to take weight off the lame leg. This makes it difficult to determine if the hip is in place or whether another cause of lameness is producing the problem.

What are the likely presenting signs?

- The leg may be weight bearing or not. The degree of lameness varies enormously, with some cows adapting very well to the hip being out of place whilst others are profoundly lame.
- Comparing the relative positions of the points of the hocks on both hindlimbs may indicate one leg shorter than the other. This indicates whether one leg has the femoral head higher or lower than the other, i.e. they are not both in the same position in the hip joint.
- Rotated limb – stifle out, hock in. Dislocation of the hip allows much more rotational movement as the femoral head slides about on the pelvic bones. The stifle tends to rotate outwards.

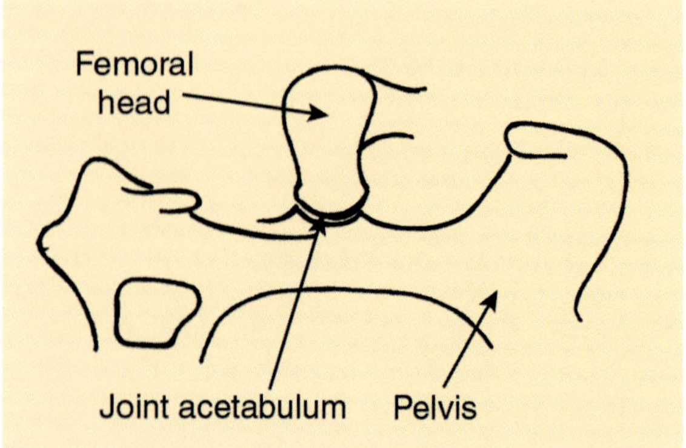

Dorsal view (from above) showing how shallow the acetabulum is.

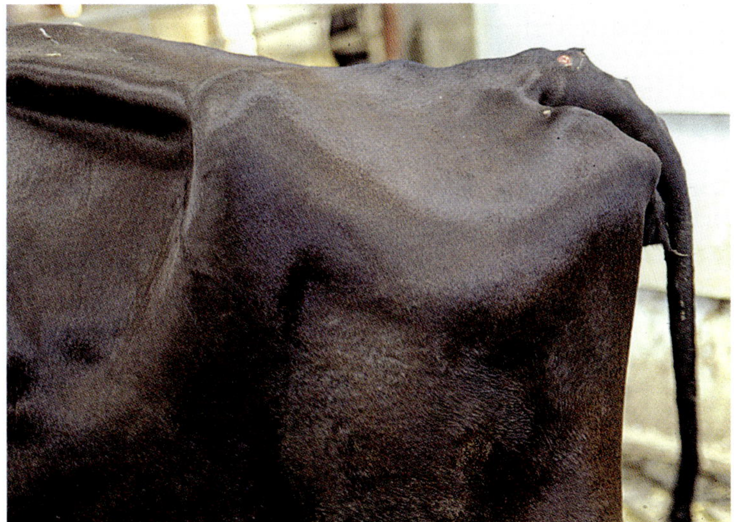

Normal hip – you can see the dip where the hip is in the joint.

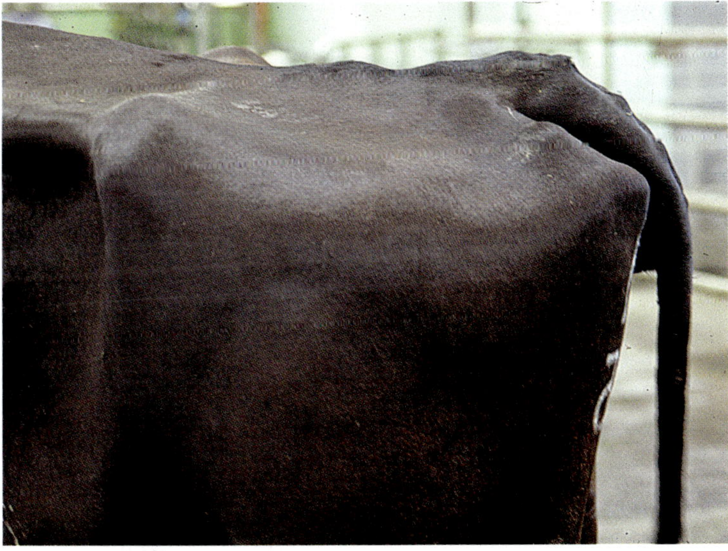

Dislocated hip (dorsal) – the line of bones has now straightened as the hip is out of the joint and moved uphill.

An examination of the cow should be carried out to confirm the diagnosis. It is important to check the following points:

- You may be able to feel where the head of the femur is. Can you feel the three key markers to check their relative alignment – the two pin bones and the head of the femur (tuber coxae, tuber ischii and greater trochanter)?
- Put your hand over the hip area during movement and feel for excessive movement of the trochanter up and down or a grating noise as the femur rubs on the pelvis and not in the joint.
- Be sure to check the stifle joint, as this is a common complication or misdiagnosis.

Assessment

Assess the likelihood of a successful outcome before attempting any treatment.

- Are there any other complications, such as stifle injuries or fractures?

- Are there enough facilities and help on the farm to do the job?
- Should the procedure be attempted in a downer cow?

The success rate for correction can be high for someone who has the skills and confidence and undertakes it early enough. However, the welfare of the animal is paramount so check on the age of the cow, its prospects as a productive animal and whether the farm is capable of dealing with the situation.

The femoral head, when dislocated from the acetabulum, can come to rest either above or below the pelvis and the hip joint. Dorsal dislocation (above) is the most common case seen in practice. In the dorsal position there are two possible options: the femur ends up either in front of or behind the hip joint – cranial or caudal dorsal dislocation to be fully accurate. The hip moving dorsally and caudally is the most usual dislocation seen. In ventral dislocation (below) the femoral head lies below the line of the pelvis and, although it is usually cranial to the hip joint, it can become lodged caudally in a large hole in the hipbone called the foramen magna. The hip may be felt internally, by a rectal palpation, protruding through this hole into the pelvic cavity.

Treatment

There are basically two approaches: non-surgical manipulation and open reduction by surgery. Obviously non-surgical reduction is going to be the treatment of choice if it can be achieved easily.

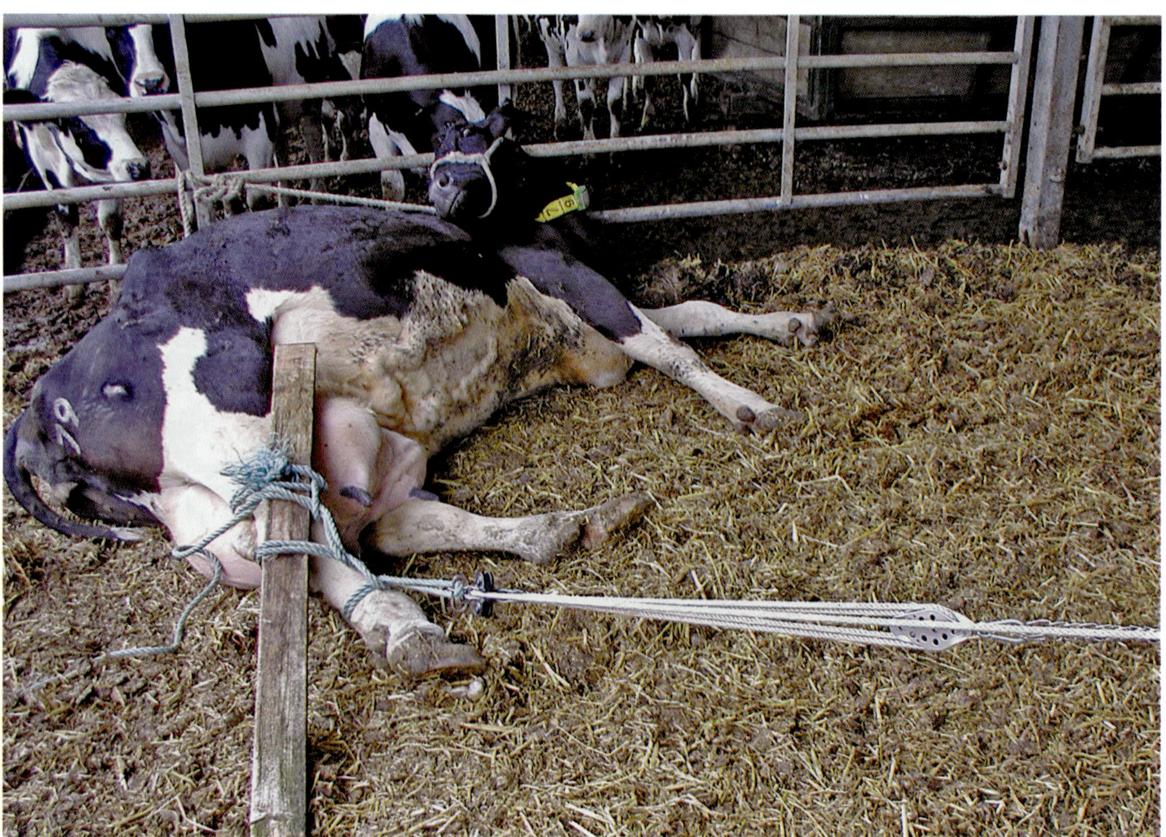

Pulleys can be attached to the dislocated limb to pull it back into the hip joint. It needs a lot of practice!

Non-Surgical Manipulation
The key to manipulating the hip back into place is to use both traction (and repulsion) as well as rotation. Rotation is not usually achieved, as without some experience it is difficult to accomplish. Rotation will reduce the resistance of the hip when it comes up against obstructions on the pelvic bones and help to lever it back into the cup of the acetabulum.

Heavy sedation is needed to achieve good muscle relaxation as well as controlling the cow. The cow is placed down on its side with the dislocated leg uppermost. It is then anchored to a fixed point with a rope around the abdomen between the back legs; this fixes the cow and allows traction on the affected leg from another fixed point using a set of pulleys. Getting a dislocated hip back in place is a skilful procedure and, unfortunately, even veterinarians will not get many cases to practice on. However, it is worthwhile considering this sort of manipulation.

Surgical Approach
It is possible and, in some people's view far easier, to relocate the hip by surgery because you can see what you are doing more clearly. A lateral approach through the large muscle mass of the leg is easier than it sounds and the hip can be grabbed with both hands and slipped back into the acetabulum whilst someone else manipulates the leg.

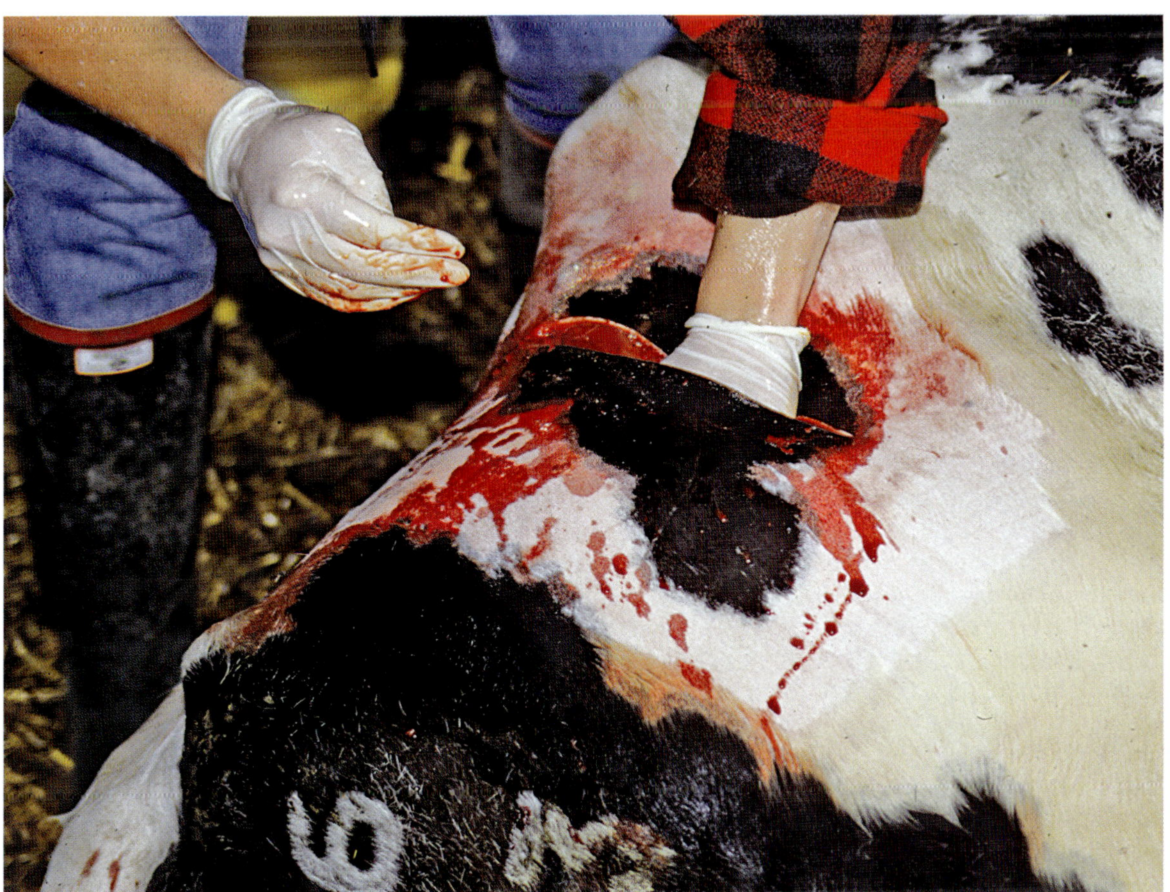

Surgically replacing a dislocated hip.

Complications

Fractures may occur, although they should be rare in adult animals as the anatomy of the cow's hip joint means it is far more likely to dislocate with an injury than it is to fracture. Fractures seem to be more common in calves, where the growth plate is more plastic. If the dislocation is left untreated, as long as there are no complications such as fractures, there are usually two outcomes to this condition. First, the cow is severely lame and remains so, which will mean she is culled after a short period of time because there may be an increased risk of falling and producing further damage. Some cows, however, do seem to settle down to form a 'false' hip joint and, although they walk awkwardly, they manage perfectly well with the dislocation.

Many cows have arthritic changes either later in life or soon after replacement, indicating that there has been other damage to the area affecting the femoral head and hip joint.

DISLOCATION OF THE PELVIS

Strictly speaking, the only articulation of the hip is with the hindlimbs through the hip joints at either side. There is, however, a 'potential' joint between the pelvis and the spinal column where the sacral part of the spine joins up with the wings of the pelvis (the tuber coxae). The joint is not quite solid and will normally, at calving, loosen so that the dimensions of the pelvis can enlarge for the calf to be delivered. This loosening can become more extensive in some cows at calving so that the bones move further apart and dislocate (it is usually more accurate to call it a subluxation as, most commonly, the relative movement apart is very small). The weight of the abdomen is carried from the spinal column, which pulls it downwards, and the weight passing up the hindlimbs tends to lift the pelvis. The structures drift away from each other, with the sacrum dropping into the pelvic canal.

Diagnosis is usually straightforward because the anatomy is clear to see; the line of the spinal column has visibly dropped between the wings of the pelvis.

The cow is not so much lame with this condition as unstable, tending to move with a staggering gait. Most cows cope with this dislocation very well and carry on being perfectly normal in the herd. However, they present a problem for future calving as the pelvic canal has been greatly reduced by the spinal column dropping into it and this will make it difficult, if not impossible, to deliver the calf. These cows will eventually be culled because there is no treatment for this condition.

FRACTURE OF THE HIP

The wings of the pelvis (tuber coxae) are very prominent in cattle and help support the huge weight of the rumen. They are easily damaged by protrusions around the farmyard buildings, especially when the cows are housed or have to go through confined gaps. Injuries to these wings may show as a mild temporary lameness, but the main purpose of discussing them here is to make sure that they can be recognized and are not confused with other abnormalities of the leg.

If the wing of the pelvis is damaged it usually fractures the tip, which then drops down below the hip due to the weight of the rumen pulling it down; the colloquial name for this injury is a 'knocked-down hip'. The fractured segment cannot be seen and, surprisingly, cannot be palpated through the abdominal muscle. However, these cases are very characteristic, appearing as a 'lop-sided' cow standing at the feed fence or in the crush.

Occasionally the injury can expose the fractured wing of the hip; it rubs through the overlying skin and pokes through as an exposed piece of bone. Fractured or exposed pelvic wings are a sign that the cow is damaging herself in the environment and there may be problems with the cubicles or the housing area. Check to make sure that this is not a symptom of more obvious problems in the herd.

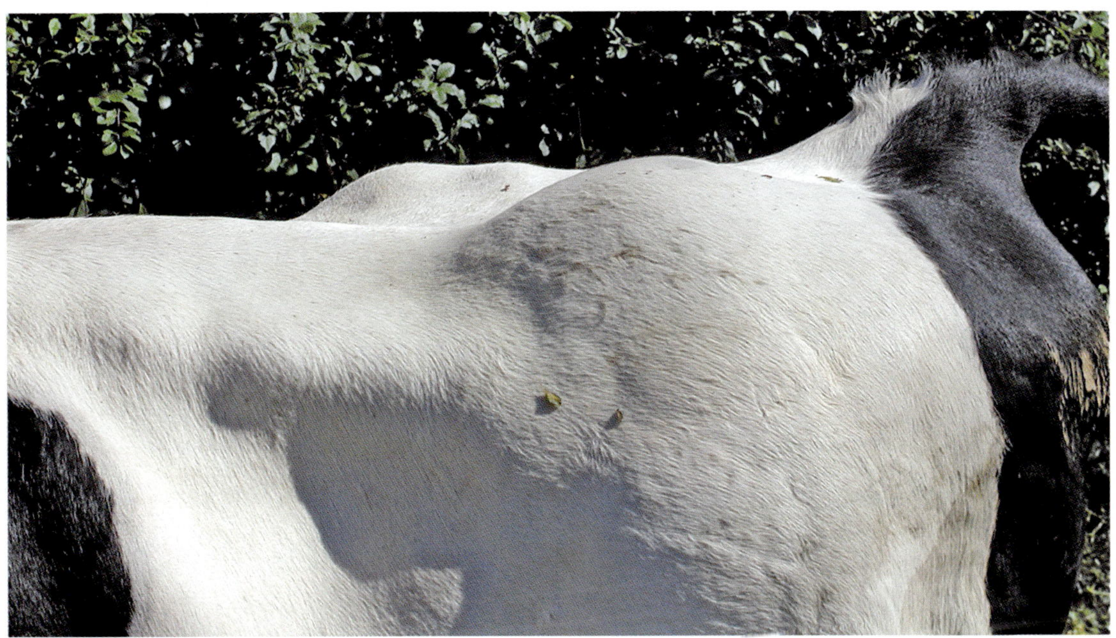

Subluxation of the pelvis – a distinct notch can be seen.

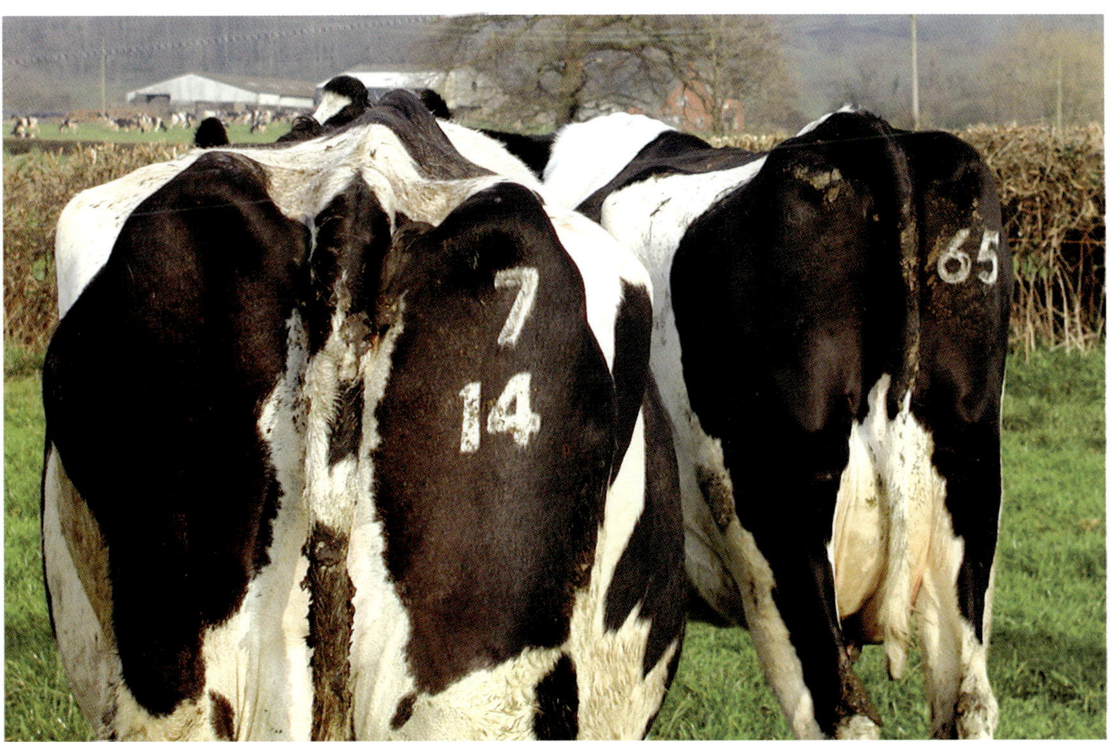

Subluxation of the pelvis. You can see the notch in the backbone where it has dropped. Compare with the normal cow next to it.

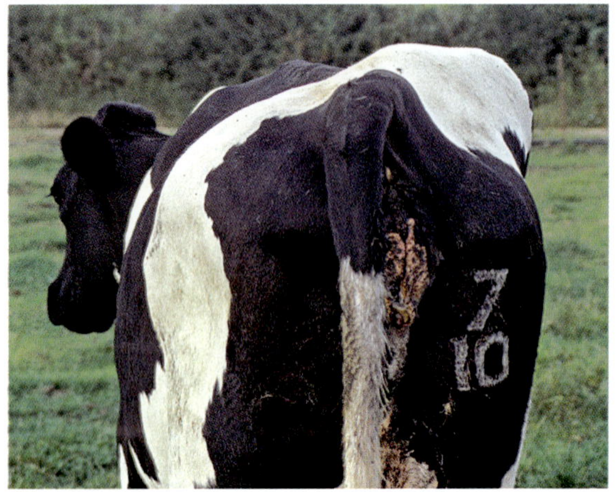

The wing of the pelvis has gone, indicating a knocked down hip.

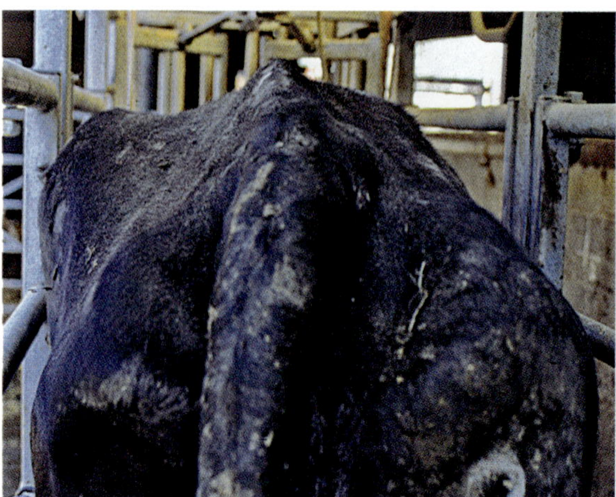

A cow with a knocked down hip at the routine fertility visit.

Treatment for a fractured pelvic wing is usually unnecessary because the acute signs of the damage – pain, swelling and tenderness of the area etc. – will resolve quickly. The cow may need some pain relief.

If the fractured pelvic wing pushes through the skin it will need topical antibiotic to prevent secondary infection. Both conditions will benefit from moving the cow into a straw yard whilst this recovery occurs. Here they will not continue to damage themselves and the wounds will have time to heal without being rubbed and further damaged by the cubicle housing.

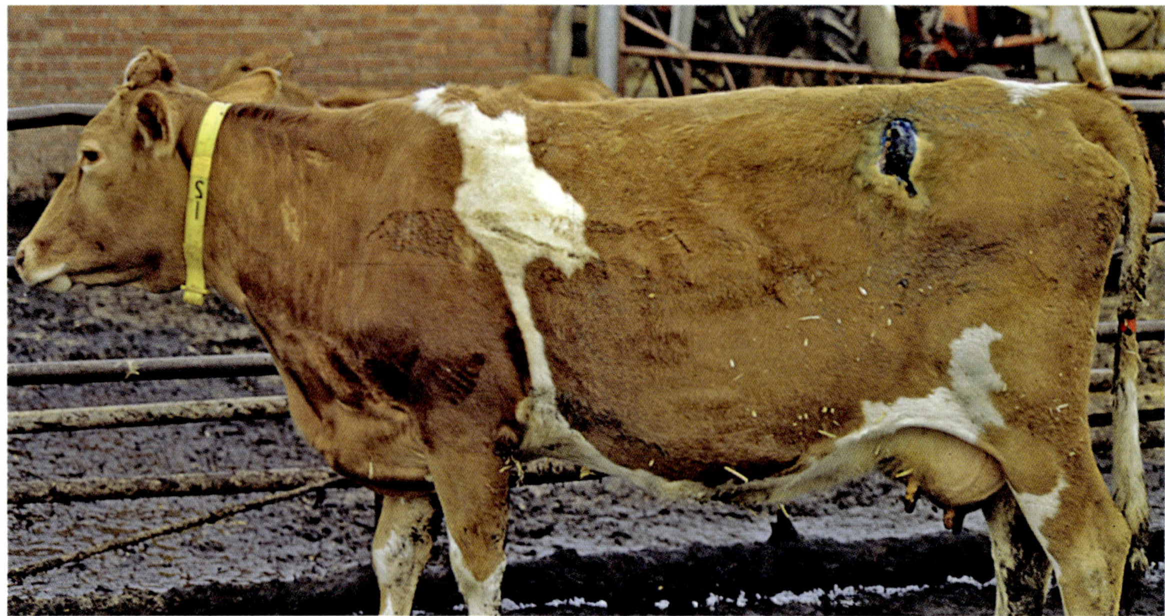

A fractured wing of the pelvis is sticking through the skin.

CHAPTER EIGHT

Miscellaneous Foot and Leg Conditions

The majority of lameness occurs when lesions affect the foot and this should be the starting point for any investigation of a lame animal. The DAISY survey in 1996 (Chapter 2) found that 96 per cent of all lameness could be allocated to lesions in the foot and only 2 per cent to defects in the leg. However, if no lesions are found in the foot, a thorough examination of the leg must be carried out despite the odds against this being the source of the lameness.

The leg itself can become involved in lameness through damage to various parts of it:

- Nerve damage. If nerves are affected, muscle control will be lost or become defective. This will alter the way the animal walks and produce apparent 'lameness'.
- Damage to muscles. This is rare, but if the large muscle masses are affected it can markedly alter the animals ability to move around.
- Tendons, tendon sheaths and bursae. The action of the muscles is through tendon attachments to the bones. These tendons frequently run through bony channels and across bony structures and they are protected and lubricated by sheaths and bursae. These can be affected by infection or inflammation.
- The joints and bones associated with the leg. This has been discussed in Chapter 7.

In most cases of leg lameness it is usually a combination of these structures that are damaged. When one part of the system becomes affected it soon puts increased stress on other parts of the leg and the damage is soon compounded.

HOCK DAMAGE

Hock injuries are predominantly associated with cubicle damage, especially chronic mechanical irritation due to:

- Rough cubicle surface with little or no bedding.
- Poor cubicle design that causes the cow to creep backwards when it needs to rise.
- Poor hygiene conditions in the cubicle.

In fact, the type of lesion to the hock and the incidence of it in the herd can be an indicator of cubicle problems and the likely prevalence of other types of lameness. If the cubicle design is producing hock injuries, it is also likely to be limiting cow comfort, and possibly producing other damage to the limb that may result in lameness. There is concern that the mattresses that are now the most common cubicle base used for cows in the UK are, without proper bedding down, causing this type of injury; this is covered in more detail in Chapter 10.

The initial damage is usually seen as a hairless area over the lateral aspect of the hock, especially over the protruding epicondyles. This will soon become reddened and sore if the damage continues, with the end result being the formation of what is known as a hygroma. A hygroma resulting from this sort of injury is usually lateral to the hock (on the outside), indicating contact injuries with the cubicle surface when the cow is lying down. However, occasionally the inside of the hock can be affected if the uppermost leg drapes behind the cow and catches on the lip of the cubicle, so injuring the inside face.

Description

A hygroma is diseased subcutaneous tissue, which is formed over the hock joint following a long period of chronic inflammation. Clinical signs start with a hairless area of skin on the outside of the hock, which soon progresses to a hyperkeratotic area – the skin becomes thickened as a direct response to the irritation. The subcutaneous tissue also thickens and a fluid-filled sac (bursa) develops in this area. When

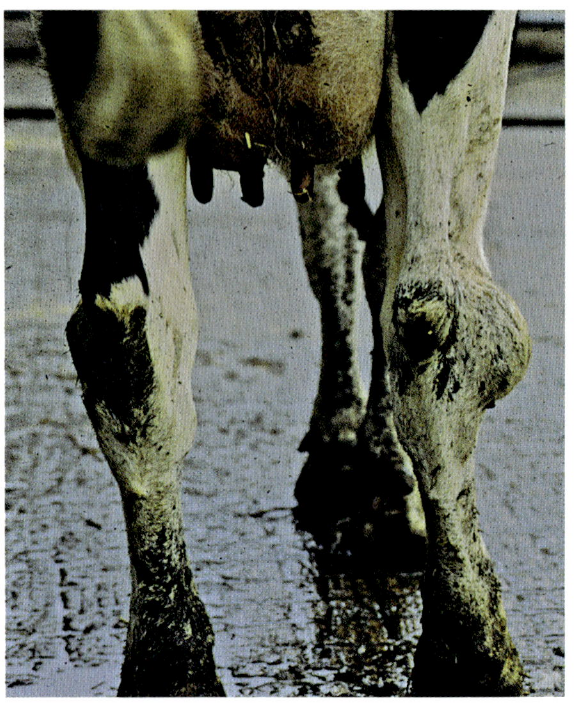

Swollen hock with typical hygroma on the lateral aspect.

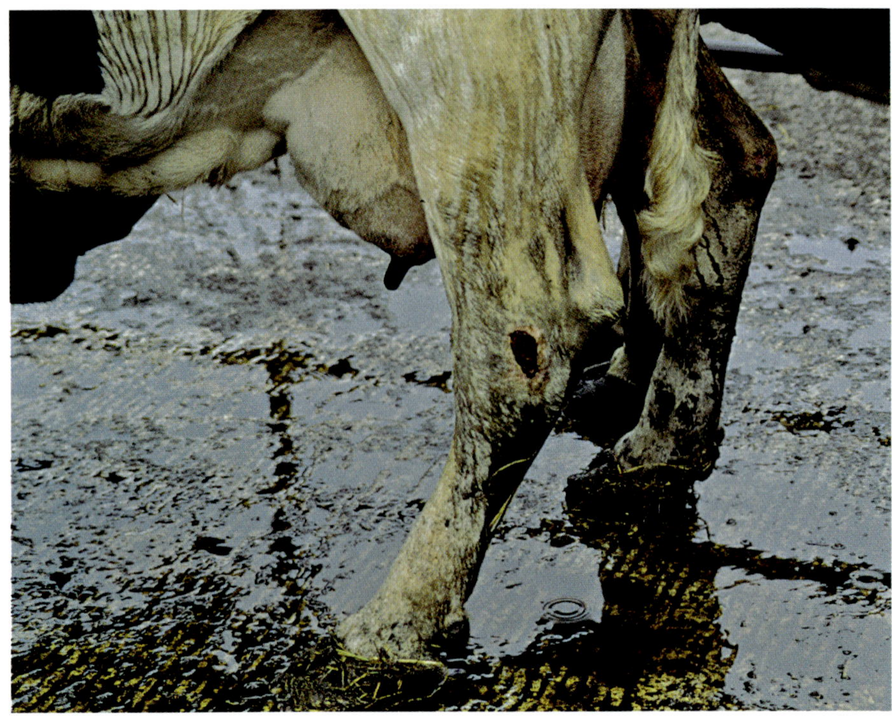

Hygromas start off as a hairless area where the skin has been rubbed on the outside of the hock.

116

the sac becomes inflamed (bursitis) it produces a painful condition and hence the cow shows lameness.

The underlying tissues of a hygroma at first consist of fibrotic tissue and blood clot formation, but they soon become infected and give rise to an abscess that usually bursts laterally and then resolves to give a fibrotic lump. The cycle of thickening and fluid formation followed by infection and abscessation continues if the original cause is not addressed. Both hocks are usually affected.

Another category of lesion affecting this area is the 'capped' hock, which is another type of bursitis. The bursa occurs on the point of the hock where ligaments run across the bony prominence of the tuber calcis of the fibular tarsal bone. In dairy cows housed in cubicles this lesion is usually associated with sand cubicles where the curb of the cubicle has become exposed due to poor management of the bedding. If not replenished and 'groomed' regularly, the sand hollows out on the cubicle base and exposes the point of the hock to damage through rubbing on the curb lip. If this is a concrete curb, the damage can be quite marked; wooden curbs will produce less damage. This rubbing or knocking to the

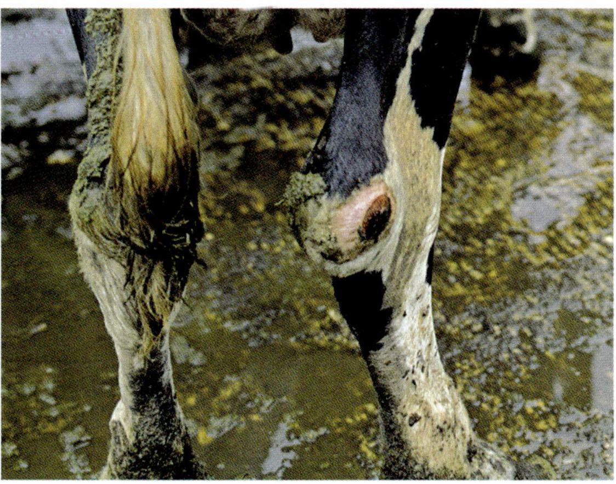

Capped hock – the lesion is on the tip of the hock and if the bursa becomes infected it can be very serious.

point of the hock produces the same sequence of damage as in the lateral aspect of the hock with hygroma formation. Both hocks are usually affected. The initial lameness may not be marked, but the lesion becomes extremely serious if secondary infection becomes established. This type of infection is difficult to deal with and the cow usually becomes critically lame and is culled from the herd.

Septic arthritis of the hock joint is rare, but it can occur from direct extension of infective processes from a hygroma or a capped hock lesion. Sepsis in the hock joint is difficult to treat because movement is essential in this joint for normal gait; any attempt at drainage and immobilization will be difficult to manage in practice.

Treatment

The cow is best moved out of the cubicles onto a straw bedded area; this will remove the constant injury element from the cycle of events and allow the wound to settle down.

If the irritation has formed a bursa or abscess, it will probably need to be drained surgically at some point. Although this sounds simple, the infected area has a thickened capsule wall and is often 'multilocular', i.e. there are many different compartments, which makes it difficult to drain. The aim is to drain the area ventrally to encourage fluid to run out, but the thick capsule and compartmental structure means that this is often unsuccessful. It may be worth putting a drainage tube through the wound to remove fluid and necrotic tissue from the area; this will keep the exit hole open and enable the wound to be flushed out with fluid. This treatment requires time and effort, often over a long period of time.

Prevention

Hock injuries are in direct response to the design and physical nature of the cubicle. They are a sensitive monitor to the success or otherwise of this aspect of cattle housing and can be used to investigate lameness.

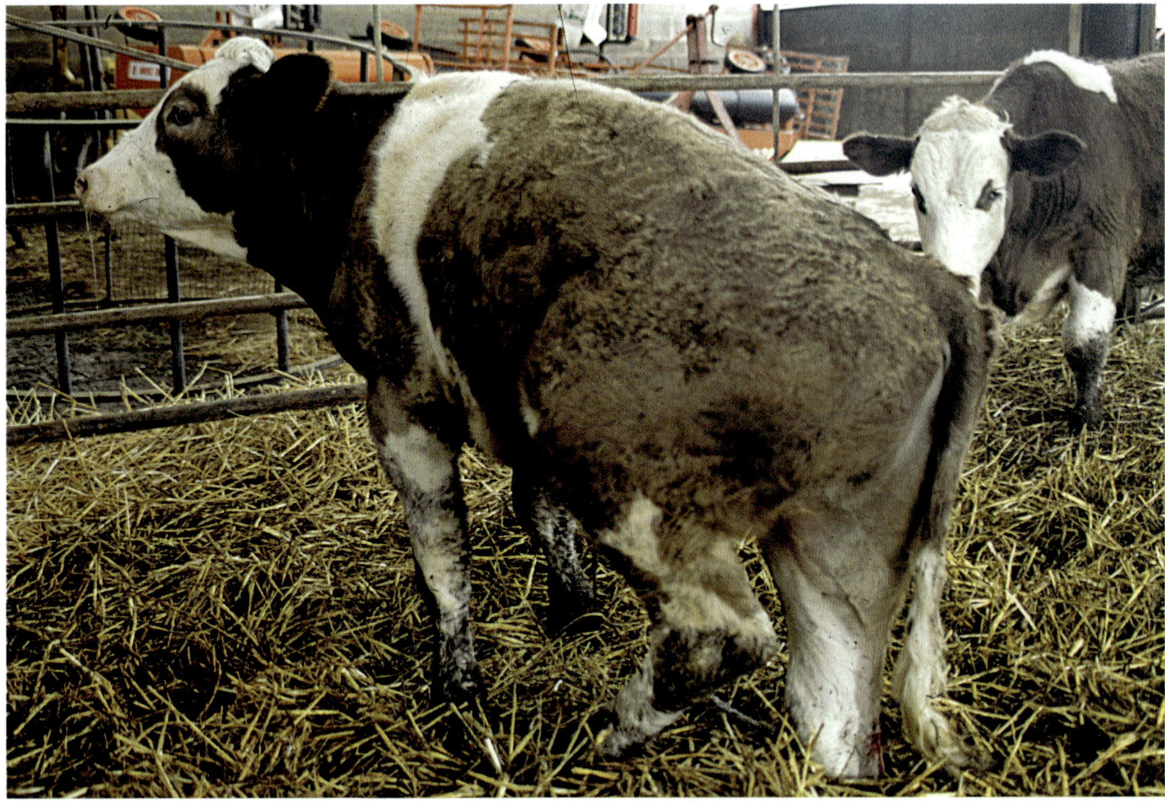

Collapsed yearling due to the gastrocnemius tendon snapping with muscle damage.

WHITE MUSCLE DISEASE

Selenium and vitamin E act in combination to protect the cell membrane and keep it functioning properly when constantly threatened by toxic radicals in the animal's system. If there is a deficiency in either selenium or vitamin E, cell walls can be seriously damaged, which will damage the cellular structure of the organs involved. Muscle is the main cellular structure damaged and this is often seen as an acute lameness or recumbency. This condition can occur when housed cattle are turned out onto grazing for the first time in the season; several of the herd may collapse or become acutely lame. The damage may be so severe as to produce rupture of whole muscle masses, typically seen as ruptured gastrocnemius muscle, which causes the hock to collapse to the floor; the animal will try to walk on the flat aspect of the lower tarsal limb. Diets low in selenium or the presence of toxic elements that are depleting vitamin E are the usual scenario.

CRUSHED TAIL HEAD SYNDROME

Crushed tail head syndrome has been reported in the USA as occurring commonly in Holstein dairy cattle.[15] Some cattle veterinarians in the UK have also reported the condition, especially in high genetic merit Holsteins. An outbreak was described in Somerset in 1997, which, although not presenting the same disease profile, was similar and affected young Holstein cows.[16] The apparent incidence of this disease reported in the last few years suggests that it has become more common and

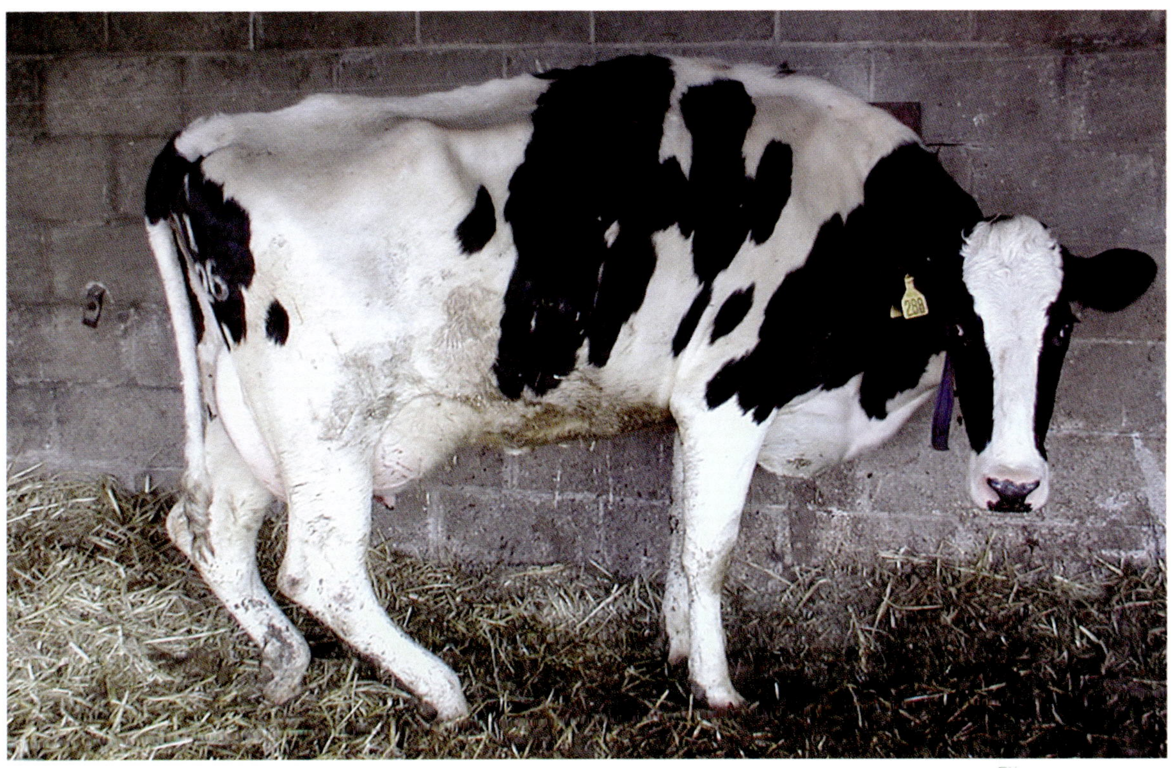

What looks like a peroneal nerve damage but it is affecting both legs and the back is dropping, indicating crushed tail head.

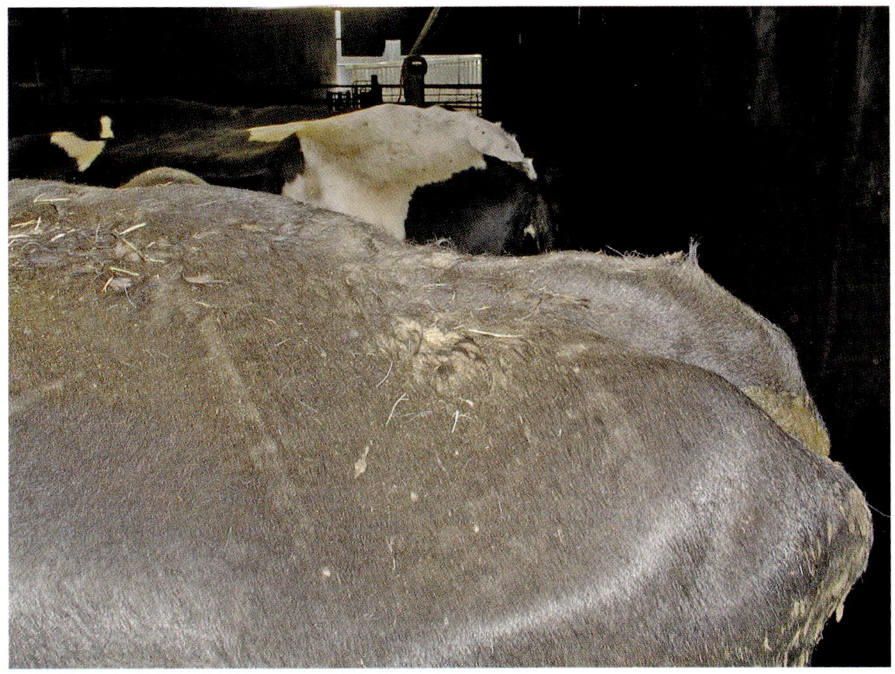

The sacral section of the spinal cord has dropped and this may have trapped the nerves, producing a crushed tail head paralysis.

may be increasing in frequency. It should now be an important differential consideration in any recumbent cow, but these animals are frequently initially presented as lame cows.

Clinical Signs

A typical case history would be an initial observation of lameness in one of the hindlimbs, usually presenting as a knuckling of the fetlock area. The cow will often be trembling and nervous. Although one leg is affected at first, the other hindlimb starts to show the same symptoms. The cow can become recumbent if these initial signs are not seen or if a thorough examination is not carried out. Hindlimb weakness with a lowered posture on the hindlimbs is a common sign of this paralysis and the tail may be affected with either spasm and stiffness or flaccid paralysis. Sometimes the sacrum can be seen to be out of alignment with the lumbar vertebrae or there may be movement of the vertebral column in the sacro-lumbar area.

These cows are not usually freshly calved, which distinguishes the condition from other nerve injuries that normally occur due to, or around, calving, for example peroneal nerve paralysis. There may be a history of a breeding bull being used in the herd or the animal having been in oestrus in the last day or so, which may indicate a physical element to the damage caused.

Damage Caused

The initial site of the injury is the spinal cord in the lumbar-sacral area. Indications of the disease are:

- Haemorrhage and blood clot formation is evident in the roof of the spinal canal at the level of the lumbar sacral junction.
- There is often some joint 'looseness' in the region of sacral vertebrae numbers one and two. They can be moved easily by handling the tail.

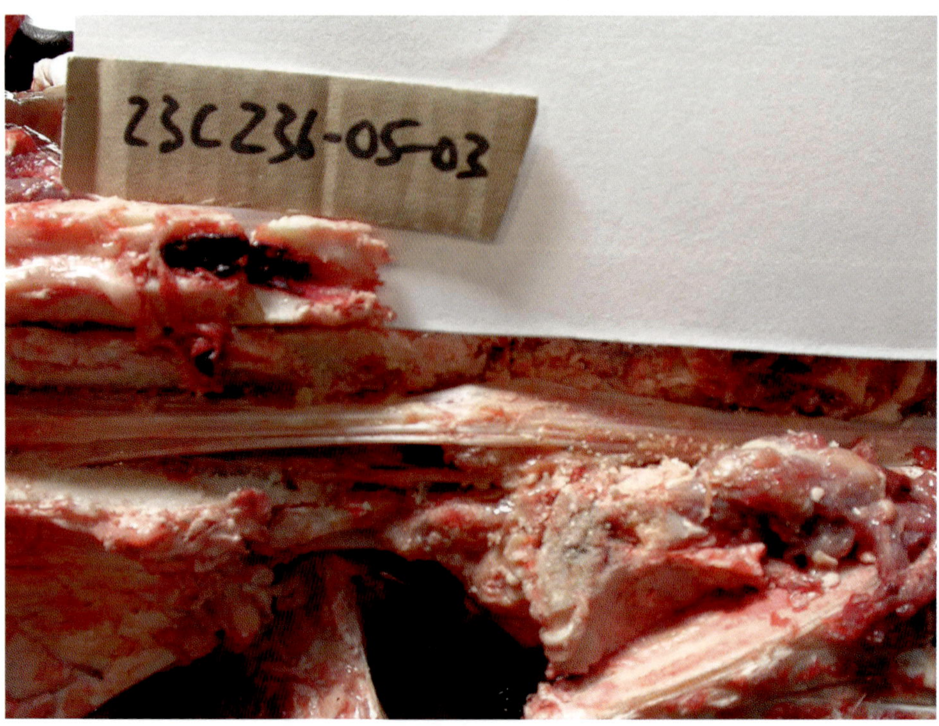

A section through the spinal cord in a crushed tail head cow. The bleeding is due to bone damage pressing on the cord and causing paralysis.

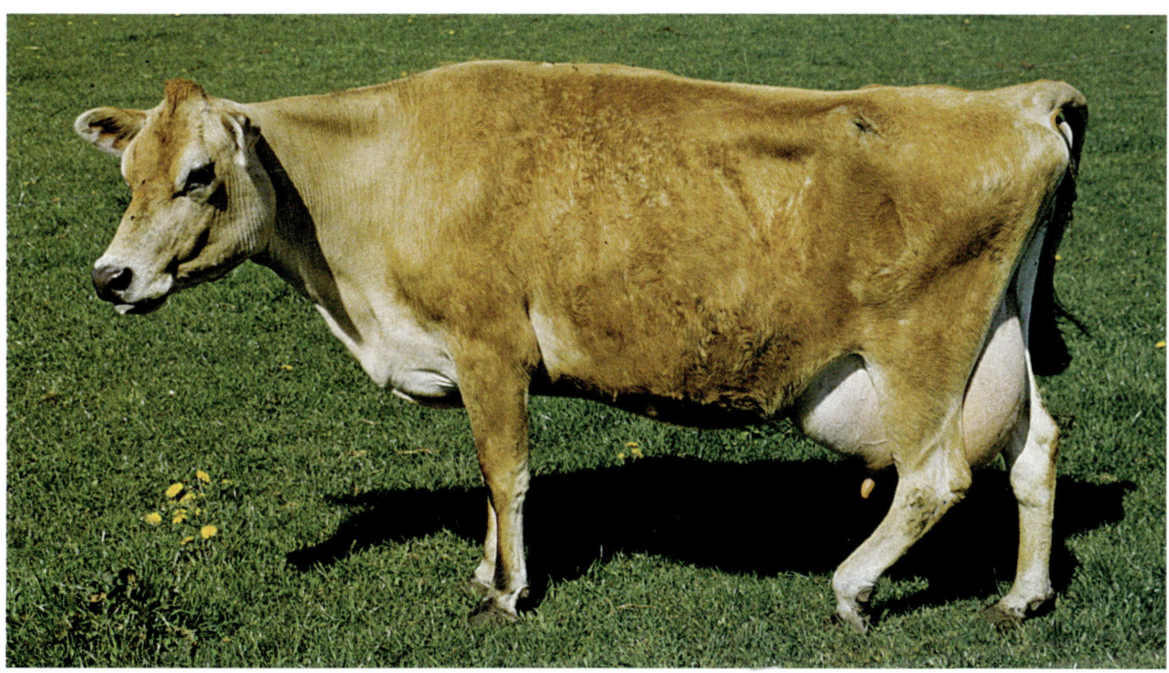

Peroneal nerve paralysis. It is usually one-sided and occurs soon after calving.

- The cut surfaces of the bone in this area are discoloured and may show haemorrhage involving the outer periosteal covering.

The pathology indicates that, due to movement of the sacrum, there is damage to the spinal nerves as they exit the vertebral column in this area. This nerve damage produces the clinical signs seen in typical cases.

It is possible that this condition is becoming more common due to some weakness or susceptibility in the sacral area of the vertebral column and its attachment to the pelvis. As this condition is usually seen in the higher yielding cows, it may be associated with extreme demineralization of the bone occurring with higher milk yields. Or it may be a hormonal effect loosening the attachments of the sacrum to the pelvis and allowing it to become damaged and to dislocate more easily. At present it is not known what the underlying problem may be.

Treatment

Treatment has been applied with varying degrees of success. Long-acting corticosteroid or similar drugs have been used. The age of the cow often determines the likely outcome, with older cows being less able to cope with the situation whilst the sacrum stabilizes and the nerve damage repairs. It would appear from limited field experience with this disease that the outcome of treatment may be more related to the severity of the symptoms displayed and not a reflection of any treatment protocol.

PERONEAL NERVE PARALYSIS

A common condition seen at or soon after calving is peroneal nerve paralysis. The reason for including it in this chapter is that these cows appear lame and are often referred for veterinary treatment. The cow is not strictly lame, but it cannot move the leg correctly due to nerve paralysis. It can be difficult sorting out precisely which nerve is damaged in this condition, but most textbooks refer to it as peroneal nerve damage.

The peroneal and the tibial nerve both run across the outer aspect of the stifle joint. The peroneal nerve, in particular, is very superficial and can be damaged by compression. This can easily occur in a cow that has been recumbent. This recumbency can be caused by a prolonged calving on an unsuitable surface or is more commonly due to post-parturient hypocalcaemia (milk fever).

Description

The cows have a typically flexed fetlock joint as the nerve paralysis prevents them from using muscles to fully extend the joint into a straight line. This flexion causes the cow to drop on the affected leg, especially when it walks, and thus appear to be lame. The fetlock joint is often the most obvious feature seen. As it is unable to extend properly, the joint bends forward and causes the characteristic 'knuckling' seen in these cows. Sometimes there may be damage to the ligaments of the fetlock joint, which allows the bones to move abnormally out of line. This can be seen when the cow walks: the upper metatarsus bone slides forward over the lower phalangeal bone (the bones of the fetlock joint) with an audible 'click' as the bones move over the cartilage joint surfaces. This damage may produce a permanent fetlock weakness with persistent knuckling and lameness. In rare cases the flexion is severe enough to cause the whole fetlock joint to bend over forwards and come in contact with the floor surface. This soon damages the skin and infection enters the joint.

Treatment

The condition does not usually need treatment as most cases recover with time; only in persistent cases or where excessive knuckling is damaging the fetlock is any treatment needed. Sometimes the lower leg can be placed in a cast to set the leg position in as near normal extension as possible. It is also possible to put

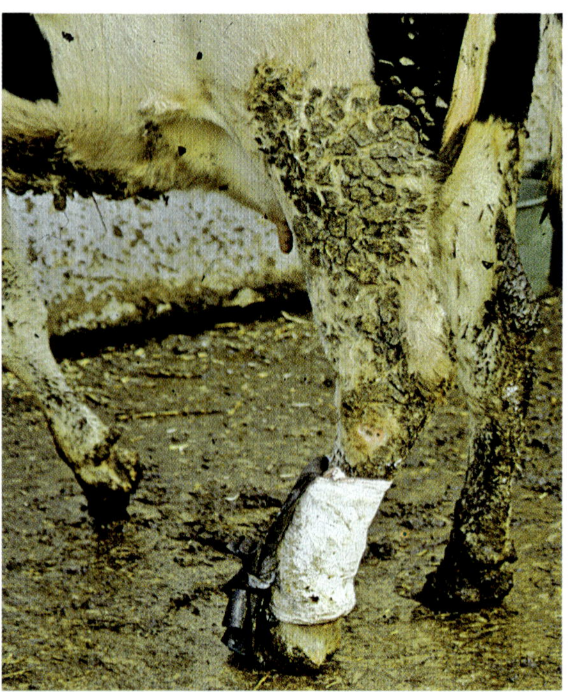

A plaster cast has been put on the leg and a false tendon constructed with an inner tube tightened up onto the claws.

in place an external false tendon made from a rubber inner tube. This acts as a flexor for the fetlock joint, forcing it to 'spring open'. Advice on housing these animals is difficult because the natural tendency is to prevent any further damage to the joint by taking the cow off concrete and out of the cubicles. However, a soft surface such as a straw yard enables the toe to dig in and the foot to stay flexed at the fetlock as the animal bears weight. Keeping the cow on concrete may speed recovery. On a hard surface the foot is forced to extend as the weight transfers to the affected limb; as the toe comes into contact with the solid surface it levers the joint open.

Prevention involves attention to the care and housing of the calving cow and avoiding diseases such as milk fever that will cause recumbency at calving.

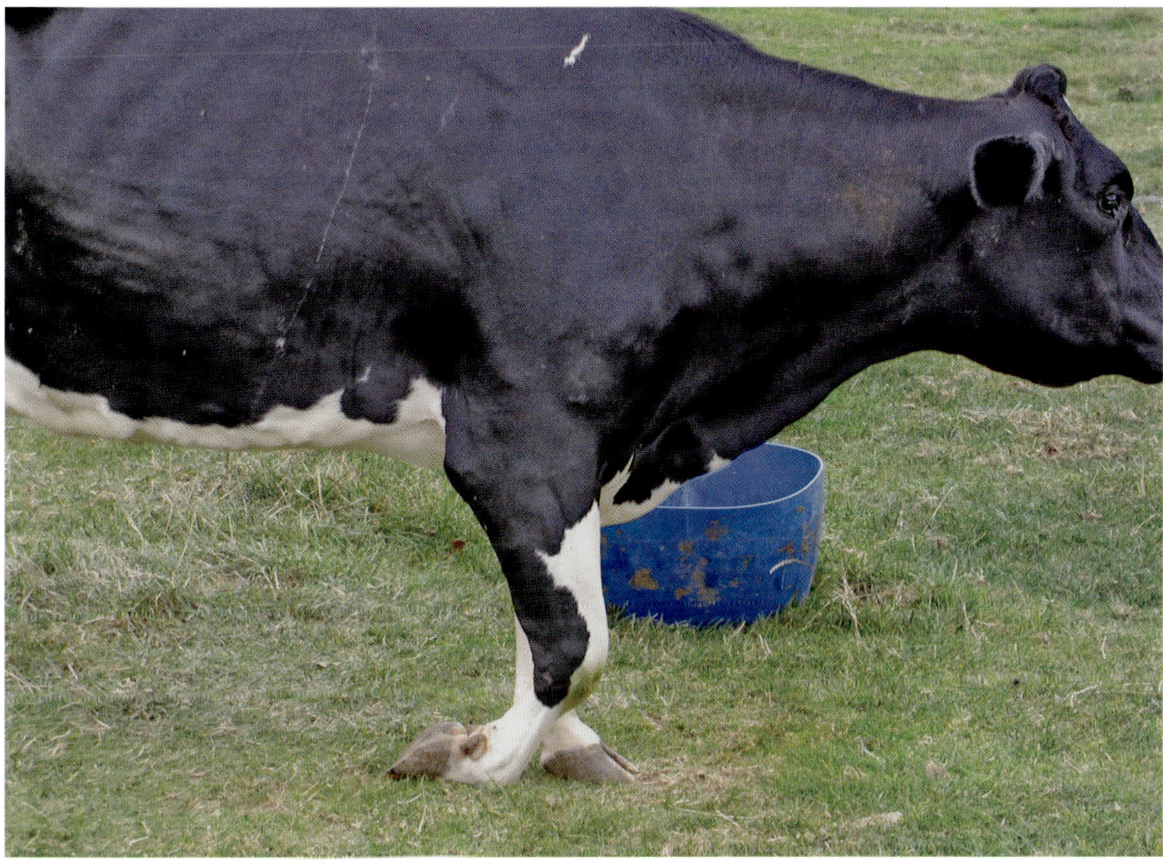

Radial nerve paralysis. This cow has just calved on a very hard dry paddock.

RADIAL NERVE PARALYSIS

The radial nerve in the forelimb runs laterally in a groove in the humerus and, like the peroneal nerve in the hindlimb, is prone to damage and paralysis. It can occur at calving due to recumbency, but it can also be associated with normal everyday trauma around the cubicle during winter housing. It is rare compared with peroneal paralysis. The symptoms are similar except that it is the forelimb that is affected. The fetlock is held flexed and the limb appears to be dropped with the elbow loose. The limb is often dragged across the floor, which can easily cause abrasion and secondary problems with the fetlock joint. The cow appears to be lame, but the limb is incapable of being extended forward as the cow moves. There is no specific treatment except to prevent secondary damage by ensuring the cow is housed on deep straw. They usually recover within a short period.

SPASTIC PARESIS

This condition is usually regarded as being genetic in origin, although there has been little work done to be certain. The primary defect appears to be a muscular abnormality that produces excessive straightening of the hindlimb above the hock. In fact the term spastic paresis is a poor description and there is no evidence of nerve damage centrally or peripherally. It is likely to be associated with over-activity of muscle reflexes causing the muscles to exaggerate normal postural and movement reflexes. The limb is over-extended, with the hock almost straight, and affected animals are lame due to a very stiff gait. The condition can affect both hindlimbs, but usually one leg is worse than the other. In the later stages of the condition the over-extension often makes it impossible for the other 'unaffected' limb to reach the floor because the extended limb lifts the hindquarters off the floor. The condition is usually seen in young animals, although heifer replacements can be affected up to a year in age.

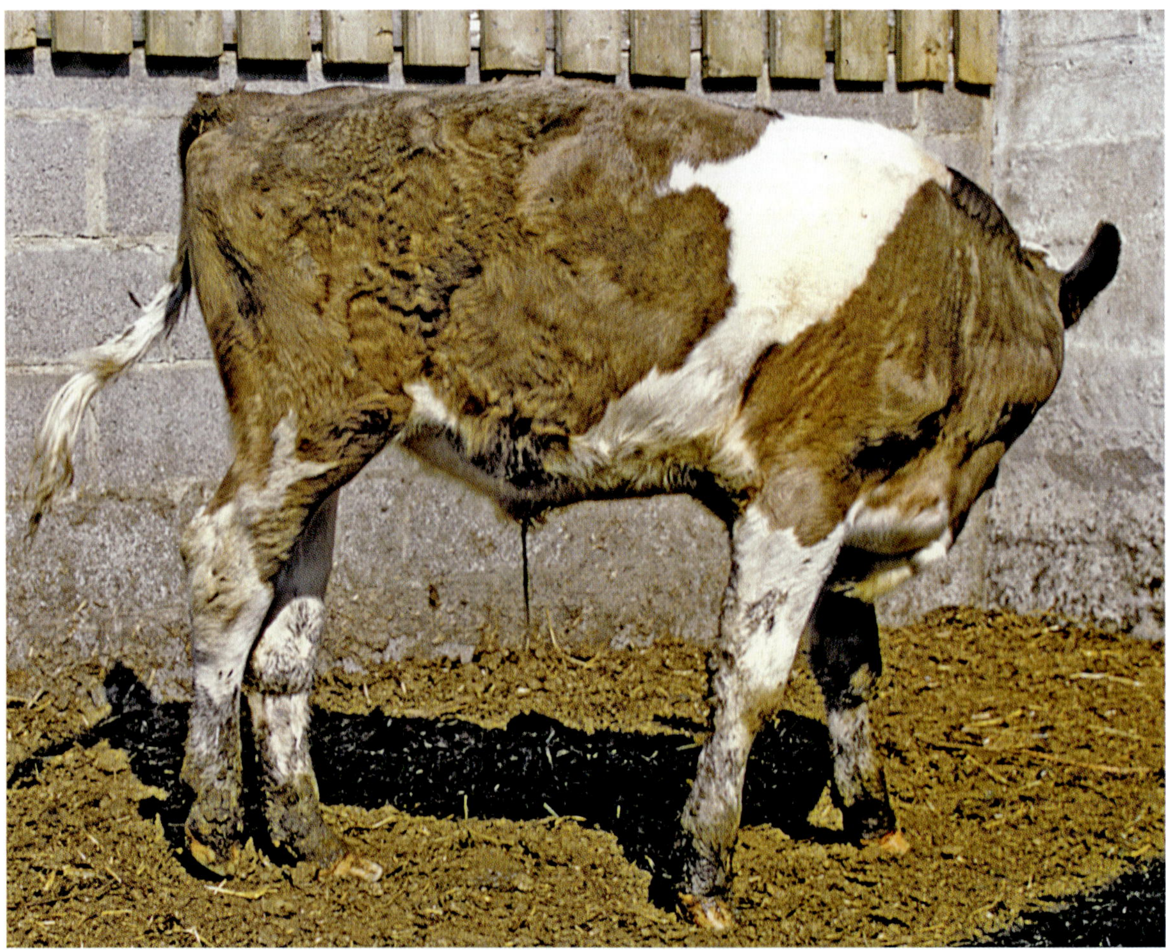

Spastic paresis. Note how straight the back legs are. One leg cannot touch the floor.

CHAPTER NINE

Preventing Lameness

Prevention must be the long-term aim in tackling any disease process; relying on treatment alone will always create economic losses and put the welfare of the animal at risk. Lameness must be viewed in this way because the aim is to prevent disease and not rely on treatments to overcome the problem, no matter how effective they are. Prevention is about understanding the underlying disease process and identifying the critical points that predispose or precipitate lameness in the animal. The aim is to avoid or minimize these critical areas and reduce the level of lameness. There may be active measures that can be taken to minimize risk factors and to modify the predisposing causes. Trimming the foot should be included in this list, but as this subject has already been dealt with in Chapter 4 we now look at other aspects of lameness prevention.

Predisposing factors for lameness are thought to include:

- Physiological and hormonal changes associated with calving.
- Nutrition.
- Housing, environment and the way cows are managed.
- The stresses of social interactions – cow behaviour.
- Genetics – can we breed for less lameness?

It is difficult to separate out the possible effects of lameness on nutrition, genetics, environment and management because they all interact. For example, a farm that feeds wet silage may also have poor slurry conditions underfoot and be feeding excessive quantities of concentrates to make up for poor silage. So many factors start to link together and become interrelated that it is impossible to prioritize any single one.

Despite much research, there is also little definitive evidence to substantiate many of these relationships. There is too much anecdotal evidence and very little hard fact to show how these factors affect changes in the foot or even what these changes are. How is the physiology, pathology or biochemistry within the foot affected by these influences?

Although it is difficult to rank the involvement of any one factor, the basic concept is that the process of calving and early lactation allows changes in the hoof to occur that create 'disruption' (coriosis – *see* Chapter 1), with the consequent loss of support for the pedal bone and possible impairment to horn growth and horn quality. These underlying changes make the foot more susceptible to further damage from the external influences associated with housing, feeding, management, and most importantly, the behavioural responses of the cow.

Work has shown that these lesions occur at or around calving regardless of the environmental issues present for the animals. They are an inherent problem of parturition and are due to basic physiological systems and changes that occur at this time. These lesions become exacerbated in response to adverse conditions at or around calving, which indicates that there is an underlying problem that is then acted on by outside stimuli to produce the effect – lameness.

As mentioned earlier in Chapter 1, there are regular growth patterns in the horn of the foot. The growth rate in summer is higher than that in winter, which means that calving cows on concrete surfaces in the winter are automatically at a disadvantage in defending the foot against injury. The foot attempts to counteract this trauma by increasing horn growth after calving in response to the harsher winter environment, but this may not succeed in stopping lesions forming. To minimize foot problems, some herds may consider summer calving as the best time to bring cows into milk. This is unlikely to be a useful option for most UK dairy herds because the trend towards all year round milk supply is the standard required by most milk buyers.

NUTRITION

It is not clear what impact nutrition has on the claw and its association with lameness. Therefore we need to look at the acknowledged areas of nutrition likely to be involved in lameness and try and assess their importance. The issue becomes even more difficult when we have to balance the nutrition of the animal in preserving its own well-being with the demands that the industry places on it for production. The true answer as to what degree nutrition is associated with lameness is likely to be a compromise. Nutrition can, with other factors, influence the severity and type of lameness and we must address it in producing schemes to reduce lameness or prevent it. However, it is likely that environmental issues will have more impact on the incidence of lameness and that nutrition will be only a small part of the risk assessment.

Good nutrition is likely to have an overall benefit on the dairy cow in trying to achieve good levels of milk production without compromising health. The health of the fresh calved cow is essential for many reasons, and preventing diseases such as metabolic disease, mastitis and so on will have a positive effect on the feet and the level of lameness found.

Nutrition can affect the health of the foot in two ways:

1. The release of metabolites or endotoxins during the peripartum period as the cow adapts to changing diets. These compounds may damage and disrupt horn growth along with the attachment of the claw inside the horn capsule. This is the basis of the endotoxin theory outlined in Chapter 1.
2. Inadequate nutrients impair the ability of the cow to form good-quality horn and preserve the integrity of the foot, and ultimately impair the cow's ability to withstand environmental pressures. This inadequate nutrition could be from absolute deficiency or more usually because the pressures of production force the nutrients to be partitioned in favour of milk and not health.

Low Rumen pH – Ruminal Acidosis

Excessive starchy concentrates (starches that break down readily in the rumen), or poor adaptation to them as rations are changed at calving, can cause rumen overload. This will precipitate a fall in rumen pH and the release of high levels of volatile fatty acids such as proprionic acid. It has been suggested that rumen acidosis also releases endotoxins and what are known as vasoactive substances (acting on the circulation), such as histamine.

The expression 'laminitis' is frequently used when referring to the effect of rumen acidosis on the feet of the cow. As outlined in Chapter 1, reference to laminitis and even subclinical laminitis is not the way forward because these terms do not describe what is occurring in the foot.

The laminitis theory cannot be supported by trial work. Giving cows endotoxins and histamine fails to produce claw horn disease and there are no signs of an acute inflammatory response being present in the laminae. In

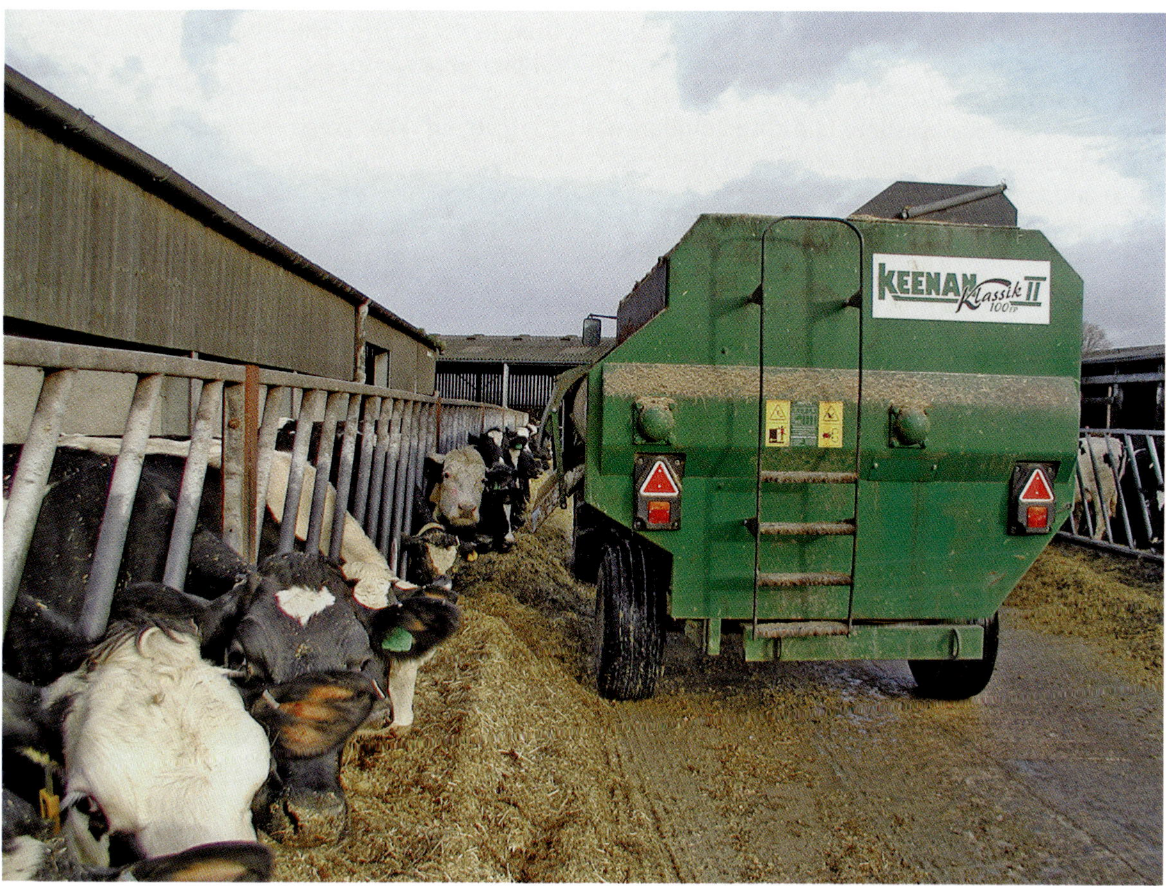

Total mixed rations removes the extremes of nutritional stress on feet.

fact, as indicated earlier, the primary insult in the foot is on the corium and not the laminae, therefore the correct term should be 'coriosis' and not laminitis, which produces a 'disruption' or 'insult' to the foot.

A diet with high starch content, with less than 40 per cent of the dry matter from forage, fed without being part of a total mixed ration (TMR), will increase the level of solar haemorrhages and claw horn disease such as solar ulceration. This is likely to be associated with a high level of rumen acidosis. If the same ration mixture is fed as a TMR, the effects will be less clear and the complication of the environment the cows are kept in becomes a more important issue. In fact, few of the foot lesions seen can be attributed to the effect of diet. It is likely that extreme diets fed as separate components could create enough of a change in the rumen to disrupt the foot.

Lower rumen pH can also affect the way the rumen manufactures other metabolites such as the B vitamins. Although biotin deficiency is not usual in cattle, as they synthesize their own in the rumen, low pH values can reduce production and create what is known as a 'relative deficiency', i.e. the rumen changes have created a lower output in a situation where the animal requires more.

Recent studies have outlined the possibility that instead of outright ruminal acidosis occurring with modern TMR feeding there is more likelihood of subacute ruminal acidosis (SARA) occurring.[17] This condition is more common in the USA and is a sign of poor ration formulation and feeding practices (e.g.

mixing the ration so much that it destroys the physical nature of the fibre). It is associated with poor cow health and increased levels of lameness. At present there is limited evidence that UK feeding practices are likely to create this condition.

Adaptation to Diets

The way a cow adapts to or is introduced to a diet may affect the way the rumen responds, with acidosis and excess volatile fatty acids being produced in some cases. This adaptation to the milking ration is an area of debate. The commonly held view is that the rumen should be adapted to the milking ration pre-partum in order to develop the rumen papillae sufficiently to cope with large levels of concentrates and absorb the nutrients created. However, there is much anecdotal evidence that this is not necessary and could be counterproductive to the cow's health and especially to the well-being of the feet after calving. Many farms now introduce the milking ration after calving. There are several methods of doing this, but they are usually based on one of the following procedures:

- Putting the fresh calved cows into the lower yielding group, so that they get less concentrate and more forage for the first week or so after calving, before moving them to the main fresh calved group.
- Do nothing. Some workers think that because the cow's feed intake is still quite low immediately after calving and takes some time to recover, the cow will control its own intake of high-concentrate fresh cow feed and adapt itself.[18]
- Shorten the dry period. If the cow is not allowed to go dry for long it can be kept more 'metabolically active' so that it never becomes 'unadapted' to the milking ration. There is no transitional feeding.

When concentrates are fed they should ideally be incorporated into a TMR because this avoids the 'slug' effect of large amounts entering the rumen at any one time. Even with TMR it is

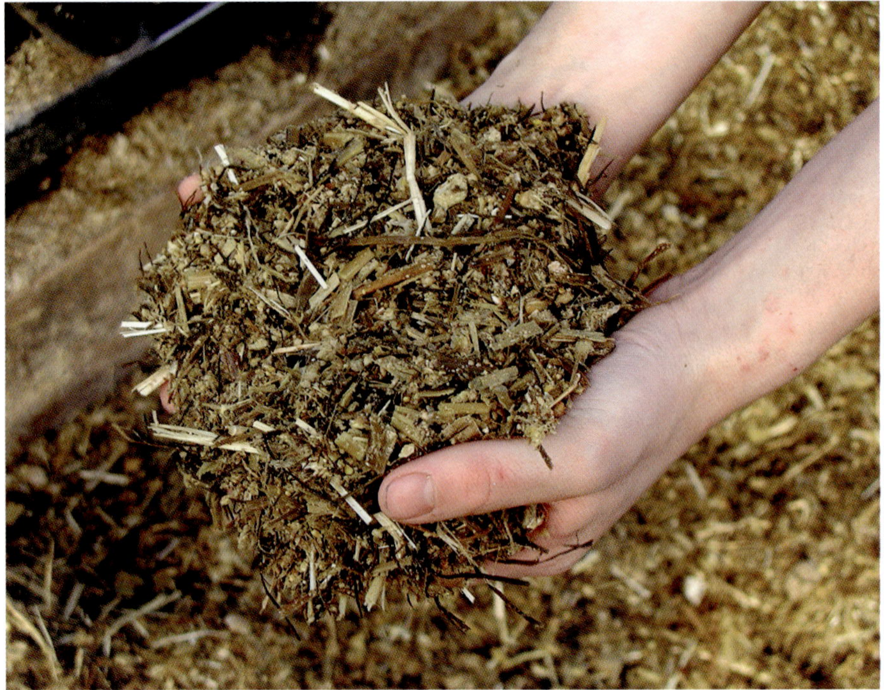

Quickly check the effective fibre and moisture in the diet by looking and feeling.

still possible to see a marked diurnal change in rumen pH associated with feeding times.

Protein

It has long been thought that the protein level of the diet can affect lameness, although again there is no real evidence to support this. Protein may affect the feet in the following ways:

- By producing high levels of urea in the blood as it is broken down to metabolize energy in fresh calved cows.
- Histamine production in the rumen – this is a powerful stimulant associated with inflammatory processes.
- Toxins are created from protein digestion.

Some workers have seen levels of lameness rise when diets have been increased to 20 per cent crude protein (CP) concentration;[19] this is associated with high levels of rumen degradable protein. Other workers have shown that increasing undegradable protein in diets produced no lameness problem. The effect here may indeed be due to urea.

Recent changes to dairy cow nutrition include the introduction of the new 'feed into milk' (FIM) strategy from the Milk Development Council (MDC), which has adopted a much lower recommendation for protein levels in cow diets. This may have benefits in other areas, but the effect on lameness remains possible but at present circumstantial.

Imbalance of Amino Acids

There is much talk about using specific proteins to increase the amount of sulphur-containing amino acids in the diet. Sulphur bonds are important in giving keratin its strength when it is formed in the hoof, so, if sulphur amino acids are limiting, it may improve horn quality by supplementing them. Methionine was widely quoted as having some beneficial effect, although the results of feeding trials failed to find any effect. It is possible that the type of protein and thus the type of amino acid released when it is broken down could have an

outcome on horn quality. More work needs to be done in this area to provide convincing evidence that this sort of supplementation is worth adopting in practice.

Dry Matter of the Diet

A study prepared for the MDC showed clearly that diets that were higher in dry matter (more than 60 per cent) were associated with less lameness due to claw diseases when fed to dairy heifers, both before and after their first calving, than diets with a lower dry matter content.[20] We know from previous studies that cows that suffer lameness in their first lactation are three times as likely to have lameness in subsequent lactations. Therefore, the feeding of a high dry matter diet affects lameness during most of the animal's life in the herd; this makes it even more important to address lameness issues in the young animal.

Several other studies have shown that feeding high dry matter feeds has beneficial effects on the feet of dairy cows;[21] however, the evidence is complicated by the fact that the relationship is not straightforward. The effects of these diets may come from indirect benefits:

- High dry matter diets reduce milk yield, so the effect may be one of yield depression rather than a direct effect on the feet.
- The main effect of high dry matter diets is that the animals have much firmer faeces. Therefore the environment is drier and there is less slurry, so the feet are less likely to be wet and covered in manure.
- The cattle on a high dry matter diet spent less time standing and feeding, and more time lying down.

The problem with high dry matter diets is that they are more expensive and may reduce lactation performance, and thus be at odds with the economic aims of the herd. However, a reasonable compromise to aim for is:

- Youngstock rations should achieve 55 per cent dry matter during the rearing period.

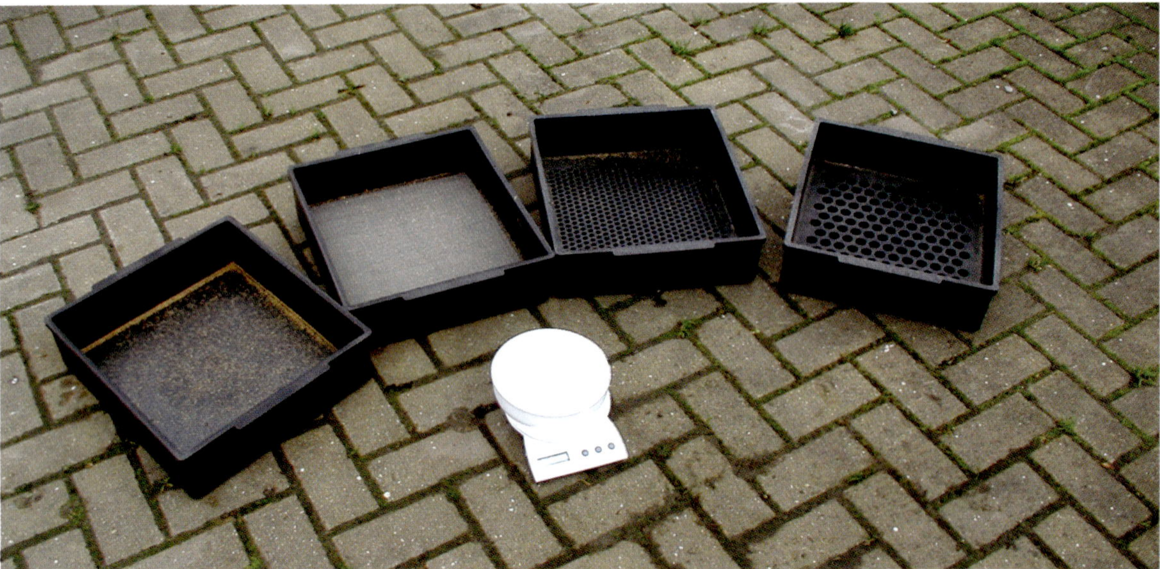

Penn State separators are a precise way of looking at particle (fibre) size in the ration.

- The first lactation ration should aim to be about 40–50 per cent dry matter.

Fats in the Diet

In general, use no more than 5 per cent fats in the diet unless you know that protected fats will bypass the rumen. Oils in the diet primarily come from grass, but adding fats or oils to the diet will have beneficial effects up to about 5 per cent of the total dry matter. Above this level the fat in the diet will interfere with rumen metabolism by coating the fibres in the rumen and making them less readily digested by microbes. This reduces the fibre element of the ration, which will increase the starch effect. To increase the fats in the diet above 5.5 per cent you need to use protected fats. Protected fats can pass through the rumen unchanged and be digested lower down the gut. A further 1.5 per cent of fully protected fat can be used in the diet.

Vitamins, Minerals and Microelements of the Diet

As with most of the vitamins and minerals, biotin affects the various metabolic pathways that are needed for normal health and function. Biotin is involved with gluconeogenesis (the production of glucose), fatty acid synthesis and protein synthesis. It has been shown to be necessary for the production and keratinization of hoof horn tissue. The microstructure of the horn is seen to improve with biotin supplementation; there are less microscopic cracks and the tubules are better formed with smaller intracellular spaces and lower water content. These changes represent a more clearly defined and stronger structure to the horn, with wear-resistant characteristics greatly improved. Many investigations have reported an advantage to horn health and healing by using biotin supplementation in a wide variety of species of animals.[5]

The bovine gets nearly all of its supply of B vitamins from microbes in the rumen. The microbes are themselves digested and absorbed lower in the gut. Thus ruminants should not become deficient unless the rumen flora is disturbed sufficiently to reduce the amount of B vitamins produced. This can happen when biotin and several of the other B vitamins are affected by acid conditions in the rumen, which reduces microbial production. This is classically seen in starch overload when cattle have eaten too much high-starch food. It may also be present to a lesser degree with modern dairy cow diets, especially the high-yielding cow in early lactation, which could encourage some degree of acidosis in the rumen on a regular basis. It has been proposed that many dairy cows are biotin deficient to some extent and that this could be producing poorer quality horn and increasing their susceptibility to lameness.

An intervention study in 1998–99 carried out on five Gloucestershire dairy herds showed that supplementing dairy cows with 20mg per day of biotin resulted in a significant reduction in the incidence of white line disease.[5] The effect started to appear after the cows had been supplemented for around 130 days. This is in line with the length of time it takes for solar horn to completely grow out and renew. After 130 days the horn growth at the start of the supplementation period would have become exposed to the surface and the effect of environmental wear and so on. It is interesting that the supplementation only improved white line disease, which implies that horn structure improvement is not enough in itself to prevent other forms of horn lameness, for example solar ulcers. However, the origin of white line disease may be more reliant on the quality of horn, especially at the white line junction. It is most likely true that pedal bone movement also has some role to play in worsening the condition but that the horn structure is the key element in producing this disease.

There are other specific trace elements that are thought to increase the strength of horn. Adding 3g per day of zinc oxide to dairy cow rations has been suggested as being beneficial to horn structure, resulting in decreased water content and thus harder and more wear-resistant horn. Sulphur has also been suggested as being important in protein synthesis to provide strong molecular bonds that improve the quality of the keratin in horn. The evidence for this is poor and there is a danger that too much sulphur in the diet could interfere with copper absorption and lead to an indirect copper deficiency.

In conclusion, unless the diet is very extreme, nutrition is unlikely to play a significant role in the development of horn lesions in cattle. High-starch diets fed without a TMR can encourage rumen acidosis and this has been shown to increase the level of horn lesions. However, environmental factors are likely to be more important. The exceptions to this may be the role of biotin in the formation of white line disease and to some extent the dry matter of the diet, although this may be acting through changes to the environment and the behaviour of the cow (see above). More work is needed on the possibility of less dramatic rumen pH fluctuations affecting cow health in conditions such as SARA.

ENVIRONMENTAL FACTORS

If we accept the basic principle that some underlying damage will occur in the claw at or around calving, the aim must be to prevent environmental factors adding to this forming claw lesions in the foot and producing lameness. Therefore, we must prevent stage three of the sequence outlined in Chapter 1 (the formation of lesions) occurring and forming a basis for horn disease.

Environmental damage to the hoof can be minimized by:

- Ensuring aspects of the housing do not damage feet.
- Management of water and slurry exposure to keep the cows clean.
- Having good cow comfort reflected by long periods of lying time.

When investigating lameness problems we can use each of the following to measure what is happening and put figures to them to help assess their adequacy (*see* Chapter 10):

- Inspect for hock and leg injuries and assess the type and severity.
- Inspect the animal for cleanliness as an indicator of housing hygiene.

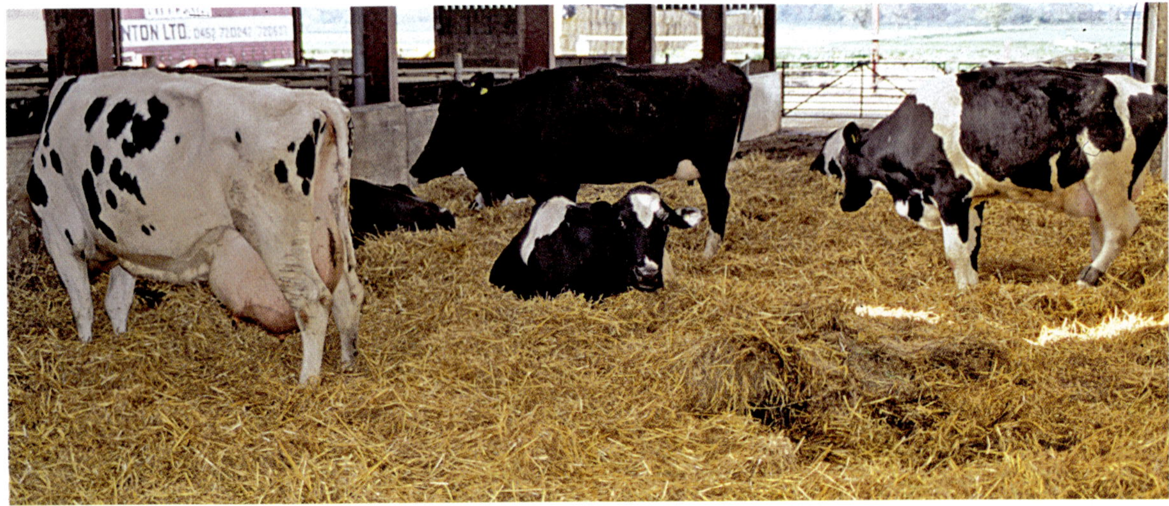

Straw yards are essential in combination with cubicle systems.

- Measure cow comfort by observation of lying times and standing behaviour.

The overall aim of winter housing is to protect the animal from adverse conditions at pasture and protect the grazing area from damage. This requirement has changed somewhat in recent years, with many cows being housed for longer periods of time to maximize the feeding and management aspects in many production units. Any housing system must supply all the freedoms necessary for the cow's best health and welfare. The most important consideration is the actual resting bed for the cow, in either straw yard or cubicle.

Straw Yards

Straw yards are still important and especially so immediately after calving. As mentioned previously, work carried out by Bristol University has shown that the actual event of calving encourages changes in the foot, which can be reduced but not prevented.[21] The process of minimizing the effects of these changes is based on producing good lying times and as little environmental damage to the feet as possible. The use of straw yards at calving has been shown to have huge benefits for claw health. Bristol University showed that housing heifers on straw yards for 4 weeks before and up to 8 weeks after calving significantly reduced the level of overall claw horn lameness, mainly solar ulceration and haemorrhages (but not white line disease). This regime lessened the environmental effects on the calving disruption to the hoof. In practice, many herds find that housing freshly calved cows in a straw yard for as little as 7–10 days after calving is enough to reduce environmental damage and give the cows a good start.

The benefits of straw yards are:

- Less impact on the feet due to softer, less resistant bedding.
- Increased lying times due to increased comfort.
- Less problems with slurry and wet surfaces on the feet.

However, they often carry an increased risk of environmental mastitis and because of this and the high straw prices many units are now seeking to restrict the use of straw yards to essential areas and groups of cows.

Despite popular opinion, straw yards are not easy to maintain. They require detailed planning in their layout and maintenance. For instance, the moisture content of straw used as bedding should always be less than 15 per cent; any higher than this will create a wet bed that will heat up and increase the risk of mastitis. The area allocated for the cows should be in line with the guidelines in Table 10. Care needs to be taken that all water troughs are placed at the front of the straw yard away from the bedded area and, in large units, some means of stopping the cows charging round the bedded area by using partitions to form smaller 'cells' in the yard is advisable. Ideally straw yards need to be bedded down twice a day and will need completely cleaning out every 4–6 weeks. As a rough guide, 10kg of straw per animal per day is needed.

Cubicles

Cubicles, or 'free stalls' as they are usually referred to abroad, have many benefits over the straw-yard system for housing cattle. The cubicle is a very efficient means of housing the cow. It is cheap on materials because it requires far less bedding and it can be cleaned out and re-bedded by mechanical means quickly and efficiently on a regular basis. However, it can create problems with slurry disposal as it accu-

Cow management group	Space required	
	ft²	m²
Freshly calved	70	6.5
Mid–late lactation	60	5.6
Dry cows	50	4.6

Table 10 Space requirements for milking cows in straw yards

mulates in the various concrete passageways associated with the cubicles, which increases the risk of digital dermatitis. It is important in new designs for cubicles to make allowances for this (see below under 'slurry handling').

The design of the cubicle is crucial. A fixed area is allocated to each cow and this area must supply all her needs. The cubicle requirements should be considered in general design terms before actually specifying details and measurements. This approach is essential. In Chapter 10, on investigating lameness, we introduce the cow as the final arbiter of the cubicle – in other words it does not matter

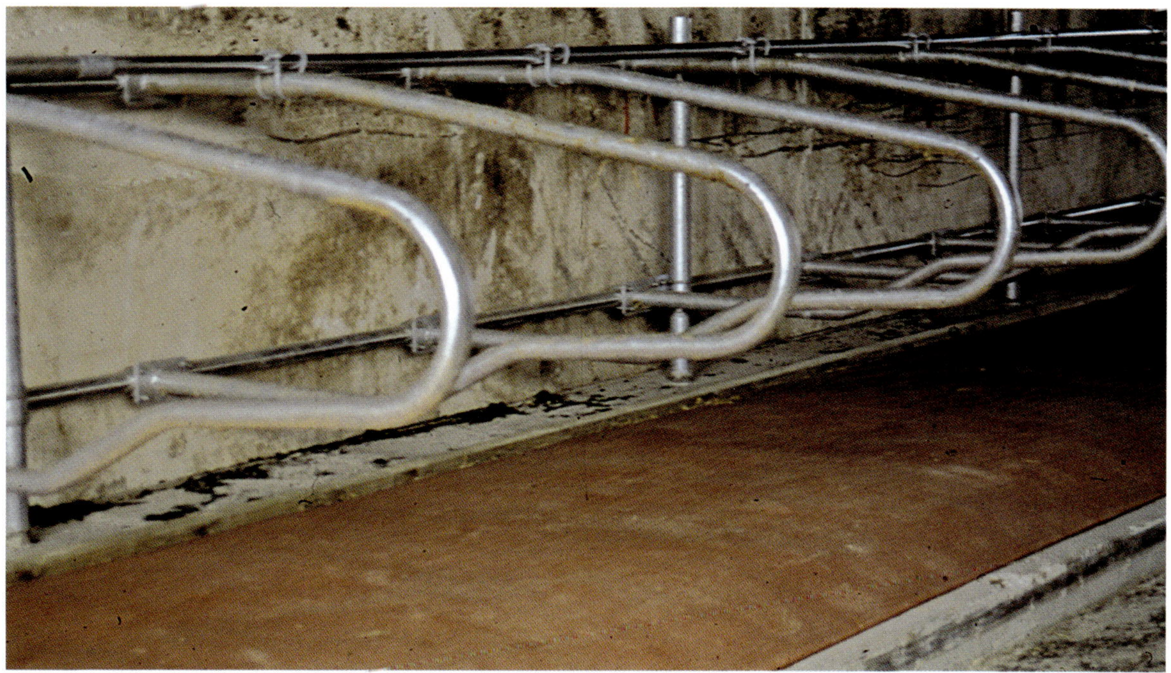

Most cubicle systems in the UK are based on mattress surfaces.

what we think about the dimensions of the cubicle, it is what the cow does with it that is important.

However, we need to start with some sound principles about design features and actual measurements. These can be considered under the following headings:

- Surface cushion and bedding.
- Actual lying area.
- Ability to rise and lie down.
- Positioning of the cow on the cubicle bed.
- Kerb height and general features.

Surface

The surface material of the cubicle affects the pressure on the lying cow and the surface grip when it stands up or lies down. A combination of the surface material and the bedding used on it creates an overall cushion effect and gives the surface the qualities we need. The ability of the surface to 'meld' – to conform to the shape of the foot and provide a greater contact with the whole foot – is important. As a result, pressure is distributed more evenly and grip

for the foot is increased when the cow either lies down or rises from the cubicle surface.

The aim of the surface material must be to:

- Provide support and cushion the animal's weight so that it is distributed evenly over the cubicle bed. The bed will then be comfortable enough for the cow to lie in for long periods of time and injuries to the legs will be prevented.
- Provide grip when standing up or lying down. The cow needs to be confident that the surface will enable her to both physically lie down and get back up again without causing any pain or injury. These requirements may be different for the lame cow as opposed to the sound animal.
- Soak up water, faeces and milk to prevent contamination of the cubicle and keep the cow clean.

It is not surprising that studies have shown that cows consistently prefer a soft bedding in the cubicle to lie on. This is usually determined by two separate components of the cubicle

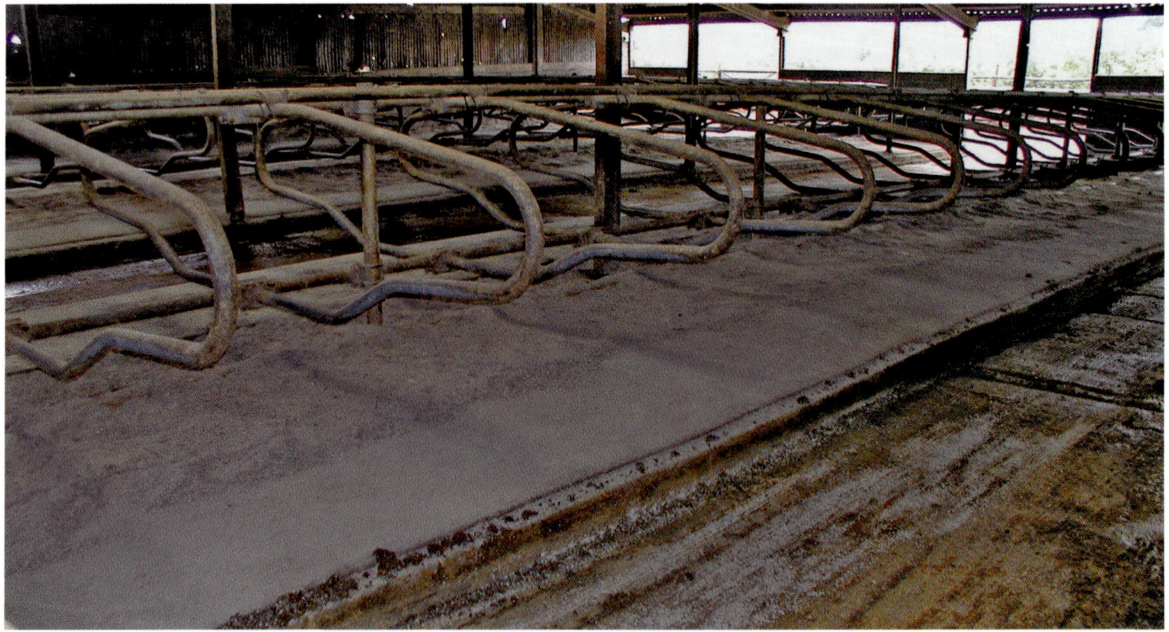

Mattresses are not enough by themselves – they still need bedding down. Waste paper is being used here.

surface – the surface material itself and the bedding used on top of it. Sand is, however, a complete bedding, being both the soft surface and the bedding material.

Most cubicle systems in the UK use mattresses filled with a variety of material but usually rubber or foam material. The surface must allow the animal to lie comfortably for long periods and it must not cause damage to the leg through abrasions to the hocks or pressure sores higher on the leg. This may be an inherent problem of many mattress systems and great care needs to be given to bedding these cubicles with adequate quantities of the right material. The cubicle surface must be hygienic because it is an integral part of udder hygiene for clean milk production and mastitis prevention. A study carried out in Wisconsin, USA showed the effect of using different bases for cubicles (Table 11).[22]

It was concluded that the cubicle surface used could significantly affect the level of lameness seen and the incidence of hock lesions observed. The study does not, however, show that sand is superior to all other bedding materials; this depends on how the materials are used and in what quantity.

| | Lameness prevalence (%) on: | |
	Sand base	Non-sand base
Summer	18.4	26.8
Winter	21.2	33.7
Hock lesions	5.4	38.8

Table 11 Lameness prevalence in twenty-six cubicle-housed herds studied in Wisconsin, USA

Sand is usually quoted as being the gold standard against which all other materials are judged, especially when you look at the work on cubicles and lameness carried out in the USA. It is a very good material, but it has some serious drawbacks. Sand, as a bedding material in the UK, is expensive and can cause problems for handling because it has an abrasive effect on slurry handling equipment.

If sand is used it must be washed, screened and graded to make sure that there is very little soil contamination, which would impede drainage and make it wet and difficult to handle. Also there should be no large particles present that could injure the cow. The sand must be added weekly to provide a depth of 150mm over the cubicle bed. It needs cleaning off the heel stone and levelling or 'dressing'

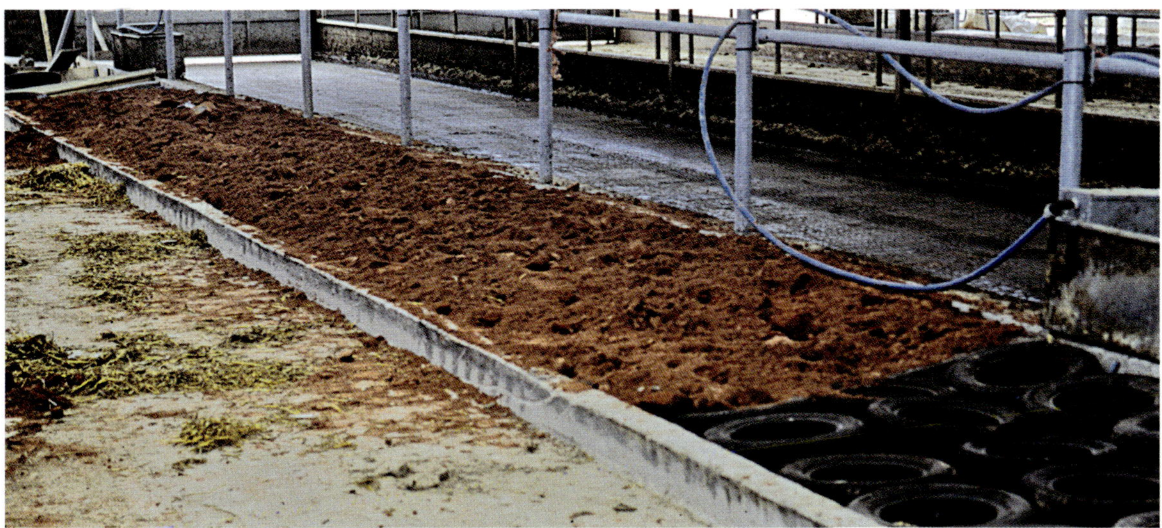

Using tyres under a sand bed seemed a good idea at the time until the cows dug them all out!

daily to distribute it evenly over the whole bed and maintain the required depth. Despite appearances, it needs a lot of work and effort to keep it 'adjusted' on the bed; there are specific machines for 'dressing' the sand cubicle. If sand is neglected, parts of the cubicle may become exposed and cause damage to the cows hocks (*see* Chapter 8). The quantity of sand required is usually quoted as being about 32–45kg per cow per day, although some of the best units can reduce this to about 22kg per cow per day.

Even a rubber- or foam-filled mattress needs some bedding material on the surface. A variety of materials – dried paper waste, sawdust, shavings and chopped straw – are available in the UK. Sand can also be used on this surface. When choosing bedding, certain factors must be taken into consideration, for example whether softwood sawdust should be used – it is more adsorbent than hardwood; also chopped straw keeps cows cleaner than long straw because there are more particles to stick to the manure and stop it sticking to the cows. The cubicle needs daily attention to remove faecal-contaminated bedding and to redistribute new bedding over the mattress. This will determine how often new bedding is introduced into the cubicles – daily or less often. There are few guidelines for the amount of bedding required, but as a rule it should provide a decent cover for the lying area to prevent hock and leg damage. Some suggested quantities for chopped straw are 2.5kg per cow per day for a plain concrete surface and 1–1.5kg per cow per day on mats or mattresses. Several studies have shown improved lying times and less hock injuries by increasing the amount of bedding material on the mattress.[23]

The current design of mattresses on a concrete base may make it difficult to retain enough bedding over the mattress, which is higher than the base. Some herds are using a raised heel retainer to hold more bedding over the mattress. This is very effective, but the heel retains fluid and faeces and may require more attention. Great care needs to be taken to ensure that the heel retainer does not become exposed and damage the cows' hocks, or raise the kerb height too much.

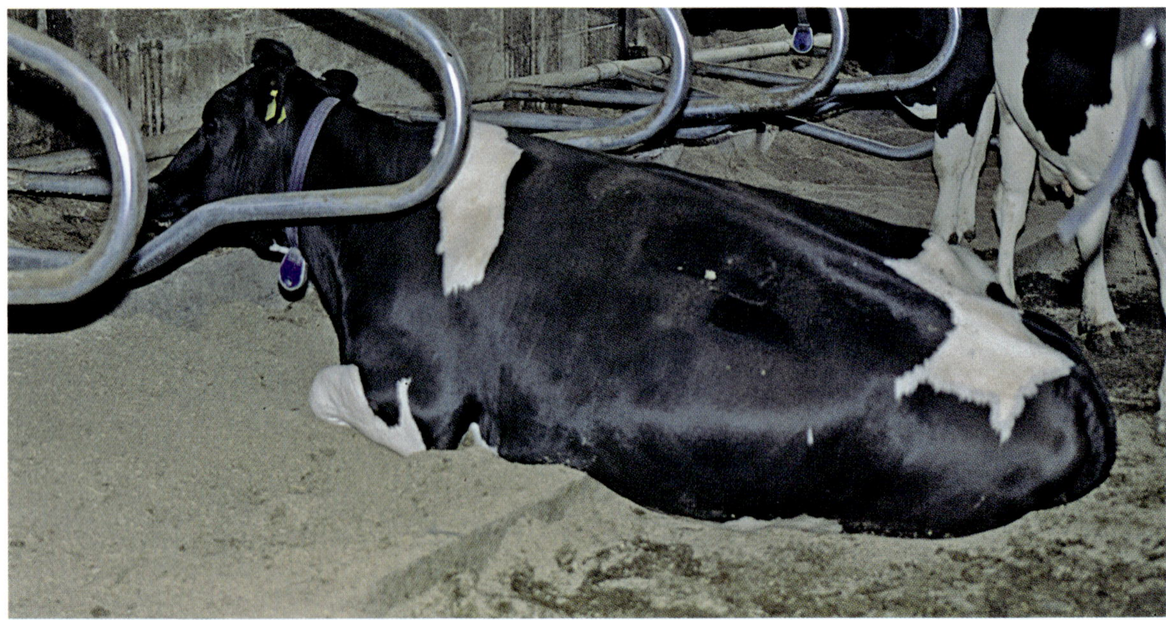

No matter what we think of the cubicle design or size, it is the cow who makes the final judgement.

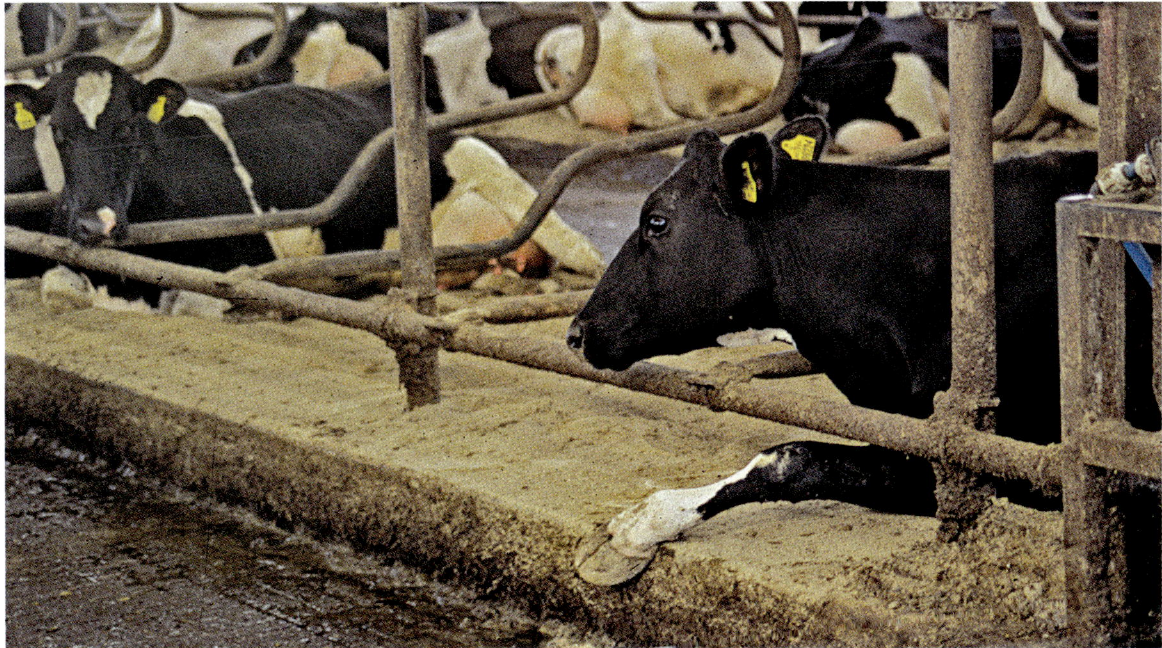

Cows lying comfortably often throw their front feet forward.

The requirements of the lame cow may make the choice of cubicle surface quality even more important. It has been shown that lame cows can lose their confidence on mattresses and thus spend longer standing than they do on sand surfaces. This does not mean that we ought to use sand, but with lame cows we may have to use different bedded areas to improve healing and avoid further complications of the lameness.

Actual Lying Area

If you study the imprint of a recumbent cow in the field, you will see that the impression left in the grass has the following measurements: the length is about 1.8m from tail to brisket, with an overall length of 2.4m if you allow for the neck and head forward of this; the width is about 1.2m. The actual lying area required in a cubicle should reflect this basic pattern, but, because the actual lying space needed varies according to the weight of the cow, we can make the calculation more accurate (Table 12).

Weight of cow (kg)	Width of stall		Total length of stall	
	m	in	m	in
600	1.17	46	2.39	94
650	1.22	48	2.51	99
700	1.27	50	2.62	103
750	1.32	52	2.74	108
800	1.37	54	2.84	112

Table 12 Average cubicle size for various weights of cow

The cubicles should be based on the dimensions needed for the largest quarter of the herd. This inevitably means that it may be necessary to consider housing first lactation cows or heifers in separate cubicles more accurately sized for them.

Cows like to lie facing uphill as it doubtless takes the weight of the rumen off the diaphragm, so making lying more comfortable. The cubicle surface should be sloped to allow for this: 100–130mm fall overall from front to back.

Ability to Lie Down and Rise

The ability of the cow to lie down and, perhaps more importantly, rise from the cubicle bed depends on several features. The overall size of the cubicle and the presence or absence of obstacles in the design determines, first, the lying position of the cow and, second, the movements involved in rising up from, and lying down on, the cubicle surface.

Detailed study of the way a cow stands up will show that there are over 30 separate movements involved, but these can be reduced to three key stages:

1. The front legs lift the cow up slightly and the head extends forward.
2. A slight lift in the front legs acts as a fulcrum to allow the cows weight to move forward so that the hindlimbs take less weight, allowing them to move and align themselves. The hind end of the cow then starts to come up. The whole action causes the head to lunge forward and drop down to the cubicle surface – commonly referred to as the 'lunge and bob' movement.
3. The hindlimbs straighten and take the majority of the weight, allowing the head to come up, followed by the front legs fully straightening. The forelimbs may extend forward over the brisket board in the final stage before taking weight fully on the hindlimbs.

The design of the cubicle must allow for a 'lunge and bob' movement. A free zone is necessary for forward movement, to allow the lunge and to make sure that there are no obstructions that could cause the cow to hit her head as it bobs. The cow would naturally prefer to lunge straight ahead and a free zone would persuade her to lie straight in the cubicle. This should always be the preferable option in cubicle design; however, there is the option to 'borrow' space either from the cubicle in front, if it is based on a head-to-head design, or from

the side by allowing movement through the divider into the space of the next-door cubicle. If the cubicles are up against a solid wall there is no forward space to borrow, so it has to be allowed for in the length of the cubicle design or borrowed from the side space of the adjacent cubicle.

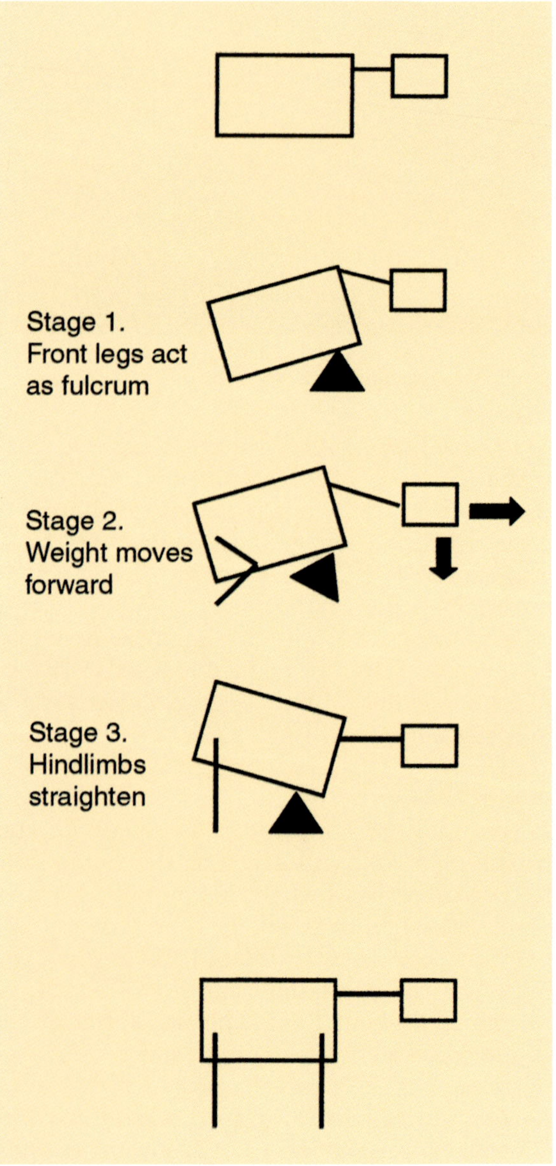

The essential stages in how a cow gets up.

Cubicle design feature	Measurement
Length of cubicle against a solid wall	2.9–3.05m (114–120in)
Length of cubicle in a head-to-head cubicle	2.74m (108in)
Overall length of a double head-to-head unit	5.5m or 2 × 2.74m (218in or 2 × 108in)
Lunge zone in front	No obstruction from the cubicle surface to a height of 1.02m (40in)
Bob zone	Nothing in the lunge zone higher than the surface of the cubicle
Side lunging	Cubicle divider should be no higher than 280mm (11in) above the cubicle surface so that the cow can bob and lunge to the side easily
Safety	Not less than 130mm (5in) between the brisket board and the lower divider arm so that the feet do not get trapped underneath it
The brisket board	Should not be so high as to prevent the cow placing a foot forward when lying or when taking weight in rising – 100mm (4in) maximum above the cubicle surface

Table 13 *The various measurements and design limitations for cubicles.* *Note that widths of the cubicles and variations for the size of the cow are shown in Table 12*

Cubicle Space Requirements
The various design features of the cubicle are summarized in Table 13 above.

These measurements and design specifications involve several aspects of cubicle construction:

- Cubicle dividers will need to be supported from vertical posts or be attached to a transverse connecting rail running below or at the cubicle surface level on which vertical fixing brackets are used to hold the lower arm of the divider, preventing an obstruction in the lunge and bob zone.
- The divider loop should be at least 890mm (35in) wide to allow the neck rail to be fitted at the correct height; again, vertical fixing brackets may need to be used.
- A deterrent strap may be needed at the front at a height of 1.02m (40in) to prevent cows going straight through the front of the cubicle and becoming trapped or damaging themselves. A simple plastic-coated wire suspended at this height should be adequate.

Remember that the lame cow may behave differently. Its inability to lie down or get up easily on some surfaces indicates that the surface material, as well as the cubicle design, is an important feature in the time taken to recover from lameness.

Position on the Cubicle Bed
How a cow lies in a cubicle is important because it not only affects the way she lunges when rising, but it is also an integral part of keeping the cubicle surface clean to prevent udder contamination or contamination of the feet. Some aspects of design affect how the cow stands in the cubicle, which, although we would prefer to minimize this activity, does occur for a period in the cow's daily schedule. Standing with all four feet in the cubicle is preferable, as standing with the hind feet in the passageway has been associated with higher levels of lameness due to more stresses being put on them.

The criteria that define where a cow lies down, and how it does so, are dictated by:

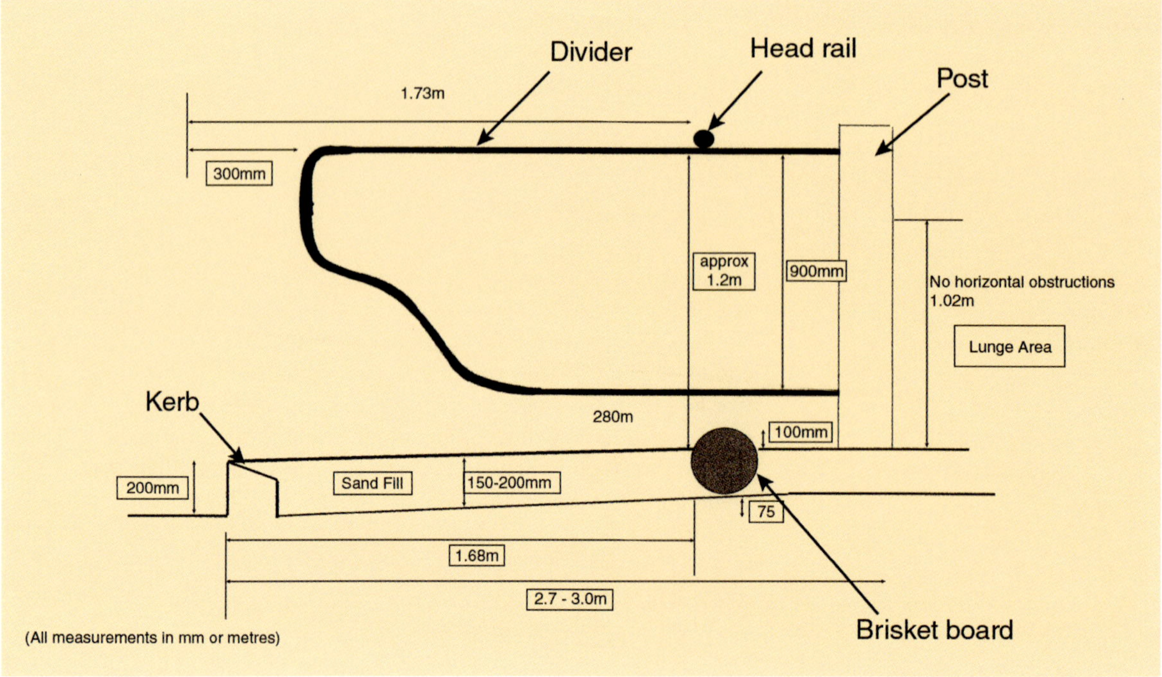

Cubicle dimensions and design – an outline of the principles involved.

- Stall width.
- Stall length.
- Neck rail.
- Brisket board.

As well as the size of the stall, we need to look at the other factors that dictate how a cow lies within the space allowed.

The brisket board is a means of stopping the cow lying too far forward in the stall. It should be placed carefully and, again, the distance is going to depend on the size of the cow (*see* Table 14). The distance should be such as to prevent the cow going too far forward and mucking in the cubicle but not so far back that the hindlimbs (or tail?) hang into the dung passage. The board or divider itself should be no higher than 100mm above the surface of the cubicle bedding and of a construction that will not damage the legs if they are pushed forward over it. A wooden board is often used, but round plastic drainage pipes, which are easily fitted and

Weight of cow (kg)	Length to briskest board		Height of neck rail	
	m	in	m	in
600	1.63	64	1.12	44
650	1.68	66	1.17	46
700	1.75	69	1.19	47
750	1.8	71	1.24	49
800	1.88	74	1.27	50

Table 14 The positioning of the brisket board and the neck rail for different sizes of cow

are very effective without harming the cow, have been used.

The next most important feature that determines the lying position is the neck rail. Again, the measurements associated with this are dependent on cow size (Table 14). The neck rail helps determine the position of the cow when she is lying in the cubicle. If the neck rail is too near the rear of the cubicle, the cow may take a diagonal line when standing and a more

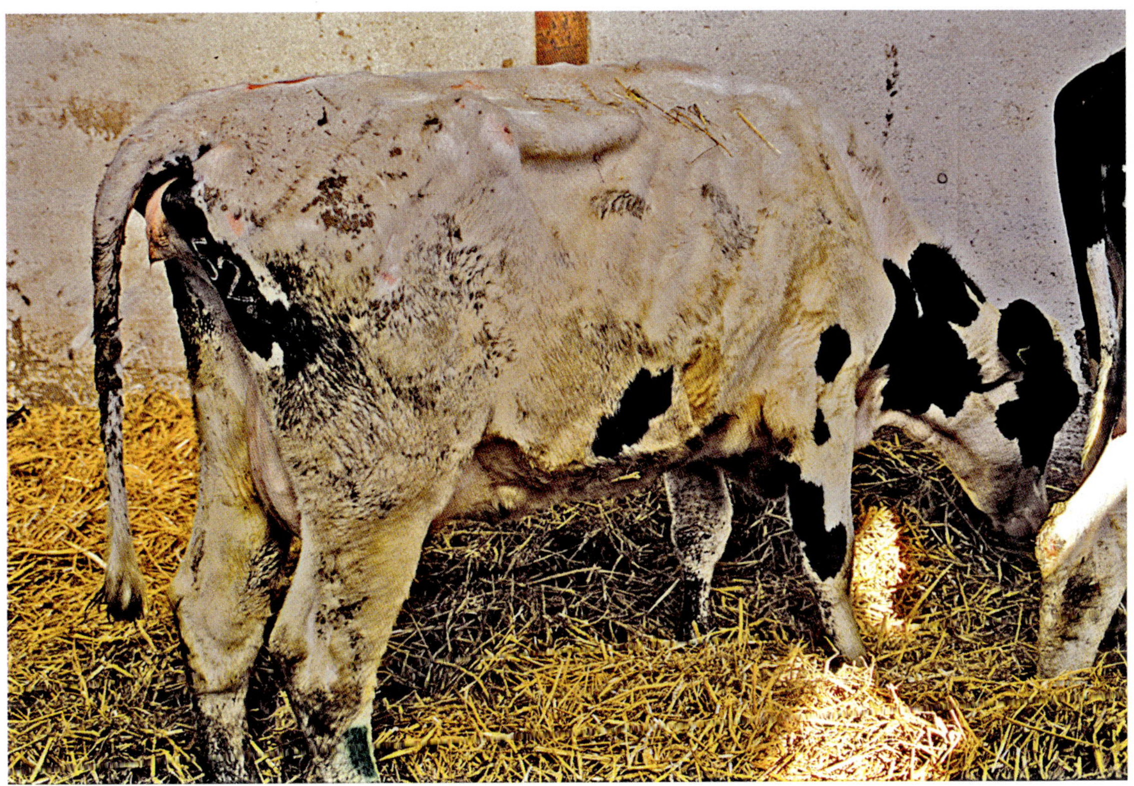

This heifer has many self-inflicted injuries from getting stuck under the divider. The cubicles must be designed for the largest quarter of the herd. Therefore, small heifers will need a separate housing.

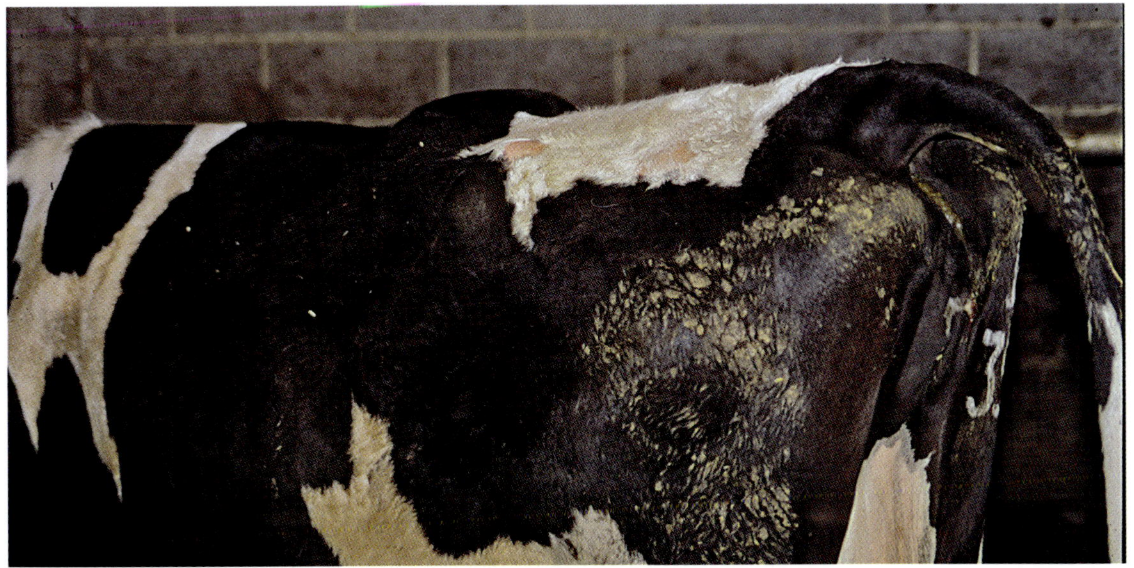

This heifer has a large bruise on the back from going through the head of the cubicle. A deterrent strap is needed.

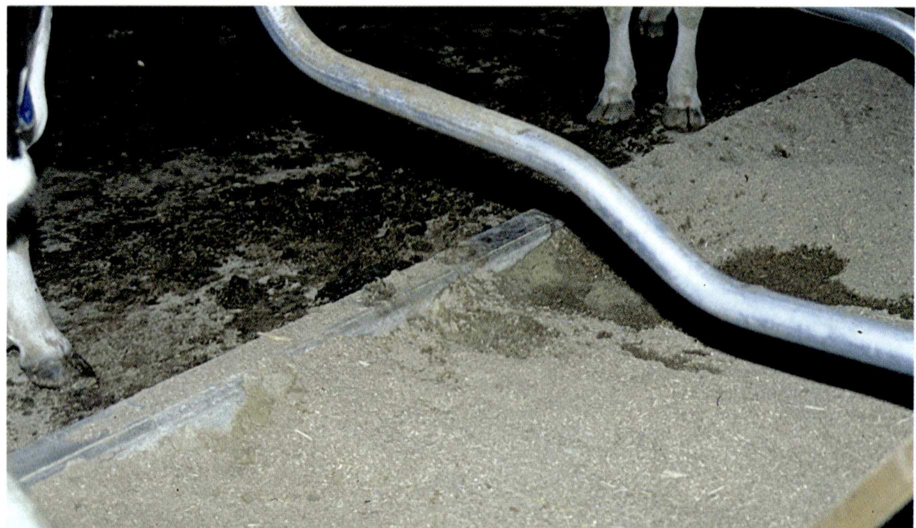

Sand cubicles where the kerb has become exposed and could damage hocks or alter standing behaviour.

diagonal line when lying down. The function of the neck rail is to prevent the cow standing too far forward in the cubicle. By placing the cow in a set position, it will also determine how the cow lies down and stands up, and will form an obstacle when the cow moves into position. If the position of the neck rail is wrong, the cow will stand too far back and the hindlimbs will be in the dung passage, which can affect lameness. As a rule, the neck rail in mattress cubicles should be positioned roughly over the brisket board to encourage the cow to stand in the cubicle with all four feet. In sand cubicles, however, the kerb that keeps the sand in the cubicle can be prominent and uncomfortable to stand on and many people feel that the best option is to persuade the cow to stand with the back feet in the dung passage rather than

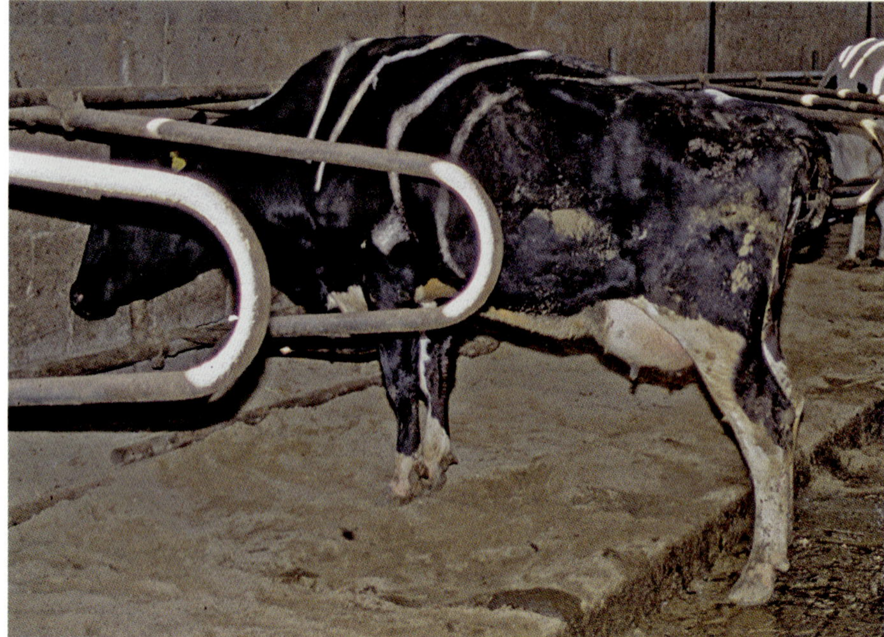

It may be an acceptable compromise to allow cows in sand cubicles to stand with the hind feet in the passage.

too far forward. In other words, the disadvantages of having the cow forward of the kerb and defaecating in the cubicle outweigh the disadvantages of the hindlimbs standing in the dung passage.

Lying Diagonally – Problems With Cubicle Position
Cows that lie diagonally are prone to two major problems:

1. They muck onto the cubicle bed and contaminate the lying area.
2. They are more likely to rise using side lunging in order to get the space required, which is more likely to harm the cow than straight lunging.

The problem of a cow lying diagonally brings together all the topics about the cubicle that we have discussed – position of fixed points such as the neck rail, measurements such as the cubicle size, and the behaviour of the cow in wanting to lunge and bob into a certain area. The lying position may be dictated by the social status of the cow in the herd. If a dominant cow is lying opposite, the diagonal lying pattern avoids contact and enables the subordinate cow to lunge away without risking a social confrontation. Diagonal lying is thus a complex issue. It is an indicator of how successful the cubicle design is and of the social mixing within the herd.

Kerb Height
Work by Liverpool University in the 1990s showed that there is clear relationship between lameness incidence and the height of the cubicle kerb.[24] This is likely due to increased stresses and weight imposed on the hindlimbs if the kerb is too high and the cow stands with the hind feet in the cubicle passage. If the cubicle promotes a longer lying time, standing in the muck passage may not be a problem. If the mattress-type cubicles are associated with more lameness, the issue becomes more important. As a rule, the kerb height should be no greater than 150–200mm (6–8in). If it

is lower than this, there could be problems in scraping out the muck passages because the 'bow wave' of slurry being scraped may overflow onto the cubicle bed. Solving one problem could create another.

Dry Cow Housing
Housing the milking cow is fairly straightforward in cubicles. The dry cow should be just as easy to manage provided allowance is made for the increased abdominal size of the heavily pregnant cow and a more inert bedding material is used. Sand is a good option for dry cows due to hygiene considerations to prevent mastitis organisms building up and getting in to the udder. Sand cubicles can be made very comfortable for the lame cow, especially if she has difficulties rising or lying down due to heavy pregnancy. In the cubicle environment the dry cow is kept on concrete, helping to stimulate the horn growth that will be needed when she calves.

Summary
Any discussion about the housing of dairy cows should not revolve round whether to use a cubicle or a straw yard because they are both essential to the well-being of the cow and minimize lameness problems. We should consider the use of a combination of cubicles and straw yards after calving. Cubicles have advantages because of hygiene. We can make them just as comfortable as the straw yard, yet they are much easier to maintain. Similarly, discussions should not be about whether we use sand or other types of bedding on the cubicles; there is a place for using both. Straw yards used immediately at and after calving have the advantage of minimizing damage and encourage increased lying times, as well as preventing moisture and muck damage to the skin, which encourages digital dermatitis infection.

Several investigations have looked at the differences between straw yards and cubicles and the conclusion has always been that, provided the housing system is well designed and maintained, there are essentially no overall differences between the two systems.[23, 24] However, each has its place and the combined use of both has great potential for the health of the animal, and lameness in particular.

Slurry Handling

Slurry presents a hygiene problem for the cow. Too much slurry could cause the following problems if the cow spends long periods of time standing in it:

- Water is retained, causing the horn to soften.
- The slurry could be toxic and erode horn and skin.
- Skin lesions, for example digital dermatitis, can be formed by close contact with water and slurry.

It is important to ensure that slurry is removed as often as is practicable and without producing problems, such as pooling, in collection areas before being finally removed.

Automatic scrapers make removal a regular and efficient process. Many units use automatic scrapers to collect large pools of slurry over slats or at the passage ends. However, this means that the cows have to walk through areas of deep slurry on their way to the feed fence for example.

The width of the housing passageways should be sufficient to allow slurry levels not to get too high – 3m (10ft) for a movement passage and 4.6m (15ft) for a feeding passage.

Floor and Track Surfaces

Concrete is, by necessity, the most common material for flooring in winter housing for cows. It is tough and cleaned easily, although it should be 'finished' correctly to make sure it is suitable for cattle housing environments. Damaged, old concrete can cause problems by

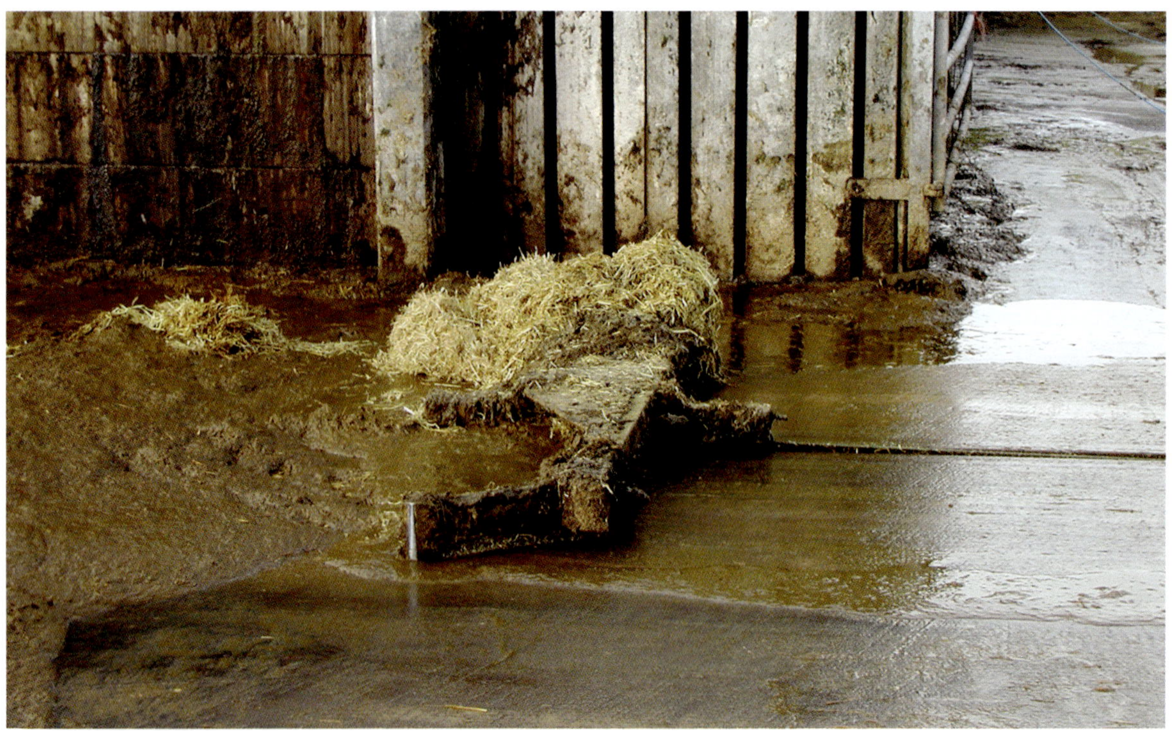

Automatic scrapers can cause problems if they produce lakes of slurry for the cows to walk through (digital dermatitis).

144

increasing wear on the feet and damaging the horn.

When using concrete as a housing surface take into consideration the following two factors:

1. The damaging effect it can have on the feet through abrasion or physical impact from too much standing.
2. The quality of the surface will dictate whether the floor is slippery and could cause damage to the cow's feet through shearing forces as they walk and turn on the surface. It could even damage the feet due to the cow's falling.

Newly laid concrete is very alkali when fresh and chemical attack on the horn will occur; excess wear can also be a problem if it is laid too rough. Worn surfaces due to deterioration caused by slurry and silage effluents can be damaging and wear the feet too readily. The advice once given for new concrete was to thoroughly wash it down to remove excess alkali before cows had access to it. Many farms now spread slurry on it, which is scraped off a few days before the cows have access. The type of aggregate used in the concrete could also play a role in exposing rough, sharp edges as it wears. Concrete made from rounded pebble gravel may be less abrasive than sharp, mined aggregate as it wears down. Many large dairy units in the USA actually grind off the new concrete surface to make sure it is flat and has no rough edges to damage the horn surfaces.

Slipping on concrete is damaging to both the legs and claw horn; it causes shearing forces as the cow walks, which are important in horn wear. Many units have concrete surfaces that are grooved to help with foothold. In the USA, long passages and feeding alleys, where the cow movement is in an almost straight line, are often grooved in longitudinal lines 75–150mm apart to allow a better grip when cows are being moved or are feeding. In areas where the cows cross between alleyways or rows of cubicles, the overall movement of the cattle is more random and a grooving pattern based on a diamond shape is more useful to give the cows grip in several directions.

Rubber mats or industrial belting has been used for passageways and feeding alleys, but the results are variable. Most scientific studies so far have shown little, if any, benefit from using rubber on cow surfaces. There is the real possibility that cows will actually stand in the alleys in preference to lying down if the cubicles are not of a good design. This has been observed in some dairies.

At grass, the way the cows move and the surface they move on to and from the grazing paddocks can have a huge effect on the incidence of lameness.

The surface is often poor because it is exposed to the weather, and it is usually not of a permanent structure but a combination of stones and mud. The Liverpool University team, in the early 1990s, showed that constructing special cow tracks was both simple and worthwhile.[24] The first principle is that machinery and cattle are incompatible both on tracks and gateways and they should ideally have separate access routes. The cow track can be constructed specifically to give good drainage and, with special road membranes, the top surface is protected from the lower stones coming through. The top surface can be made of bark peelings or 'cundy' peel, as it is known. This surface will usually last for a complete grazing season and, because the track is so comfortable to walk on, it need only be a metre wide to get good flow rates of cattle along its length; the same care of surfaces should be used for gateways through into the grazing area. Any collection of mud in gateways, especially in warm weather, can be associated with outbreaks of lameness due to 'foul' infection as the organism thrives in mud and faeces.

The way cows are moved along tracks is also an important environmental issue. Again, Liverpool University showed that cows like to walk along a track using the front feet to test the ground for the hind feet;[25] the cow will, if left to move under its own volition, place

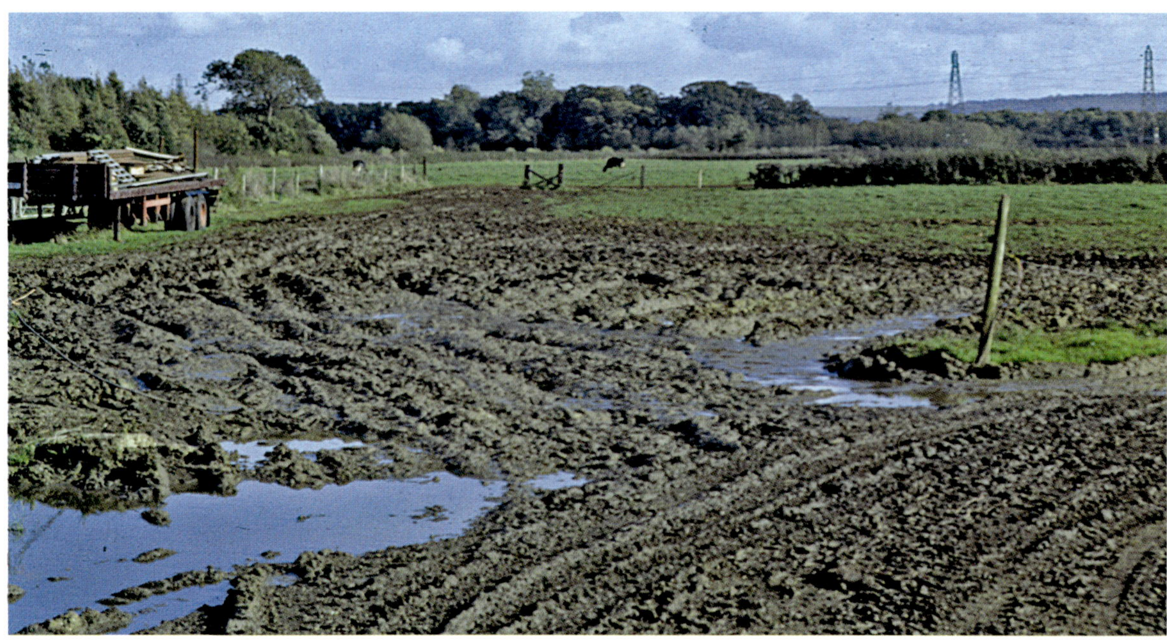

Machinery and cattle do not mix when it comes to sharing tracks at grazing.

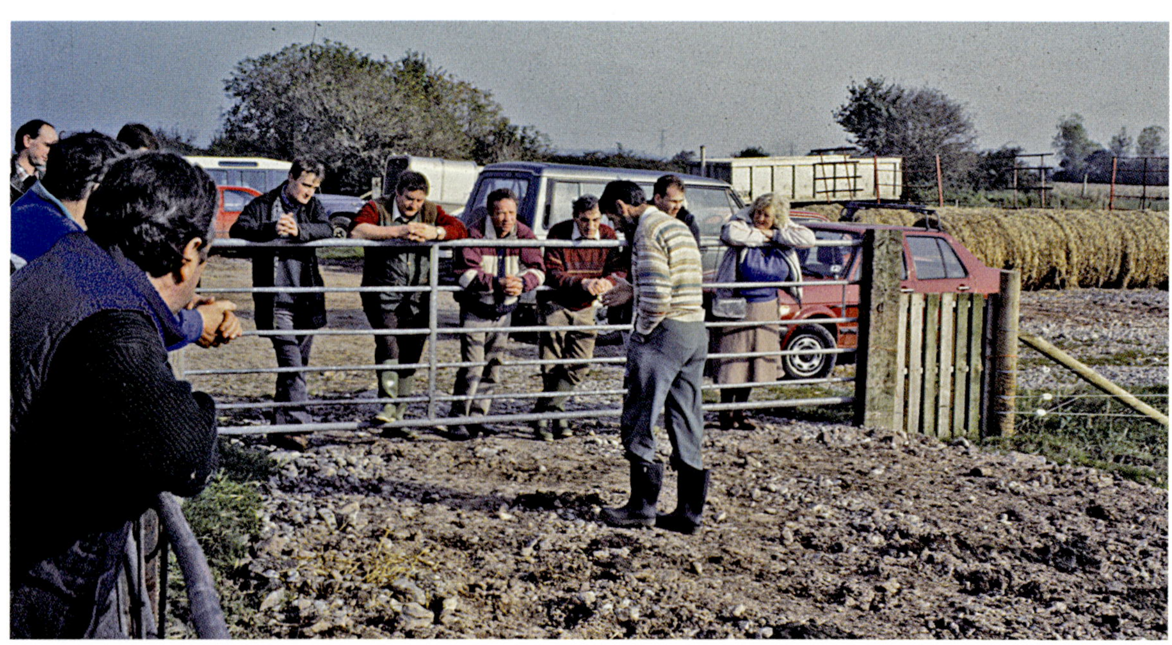

Gateways are pressure points when large numbers of cattle funnel through them. The drainage and construction needs to be right.

the hind foot in the same spot that the front foot has just vacated. This testing and adaptation of the cow's gait to the surface is for self-preservation and helps to prevent lameness. Problems can arise if cows are moved too rapidly and with coercion, such as using a dog or motorbike at the rear. Studies have shown that the cow then has to abandon the self-preservation gait to move more quickly. It is thus not surprising that this creates more lameness.

New Zealand studies also showed that if cows are left to walk at their own speed they follow the cow in front, walking roughly in order of social ranking in the herd.[26] They walk headdown to check the ground, and place their feet accurately, as described by the Liverpool team. If the dominant cow stops, all the rest behind will stop; when she moves on, so do the followers. If the cows are rushed in any way their heads will come up and they cannot use the same choice as to where they place their feet. They are more likely to step on a rough surface or a stone, which may cause lameness. The same sequence occurs when cows come into the collecting yard and the results can be the same. Do not use excessive force to get cows in from grazing or even into the collecting yard.

BEHAVIOURAL FACTORS

The role of cow behaviour in relation to cubicles and cow tracks has been mentioned above, and it is essential that we understand more about it. We can think that we have designed the best environment for the cow only to find that the cow's behaviour tells us differently.

Cows have distinct rankings within a pen and these rankings are related to the stability of the group. Moving cows from one pen to another results in a period of increased social interaction before they stabilize again and a hierarchy returns. These changes in social ranking have effects on the cow's nutrition, milk yield and the amount of time it spends lying down. In a recent study in the UK,

researchers looked at dairy herds over a 5-month period and recorded social rank, behaviour and lameness.[27] In all herds the stocking density was one cow per stall. Observation showed low-ranking cows spent less time lying, more time standing still and standing half in the cubicles, than middle- and high-rank cows. By 25 weeks into their lactations, more than 60 per cent of the low-rank cows had become lame compared with 18 per cent of the high-rank cows.

A typical cow, transferred at calving from the dry group to the main milking herd, is involved in about ten social interactions per hour immediately after the move. This is twice as many as occurs with other normal social interactions within the group. These interactions are bunting, pushing, fighting and non-physical, such as threatening and avoidance.

During the first 48 hours after changing groups all these interactions occurred, but they were mostly physical (65 per cent). After 48 hours the interactions became predominantly non-physical (65 per cent). These behavioural changes started to stabilize after about 7 days; however, there may be longer-term problems of social structure that have not been measured or detected, which may affect the cow's ability to lie in comfort.

When cows are mixed at housing, the following steps can be taken to minimize the effects to social structure:

- Use vinegar. Putting vinegar along the back of a new cow entering the herd will encourage the other cows to avoid it. This gives the cow a social advantage for a period of time whilst it adapts to the environment and the other cows in the group. This system works well with any cow, but it is particularly useful for heifers, who are usually subordinate to the older cows in the herd.
- Reduce the number of group changes. Using complicated groups during the transition and early-calved period can exacerbate the social disruption of the cows in a group, especially for the lower-ranking

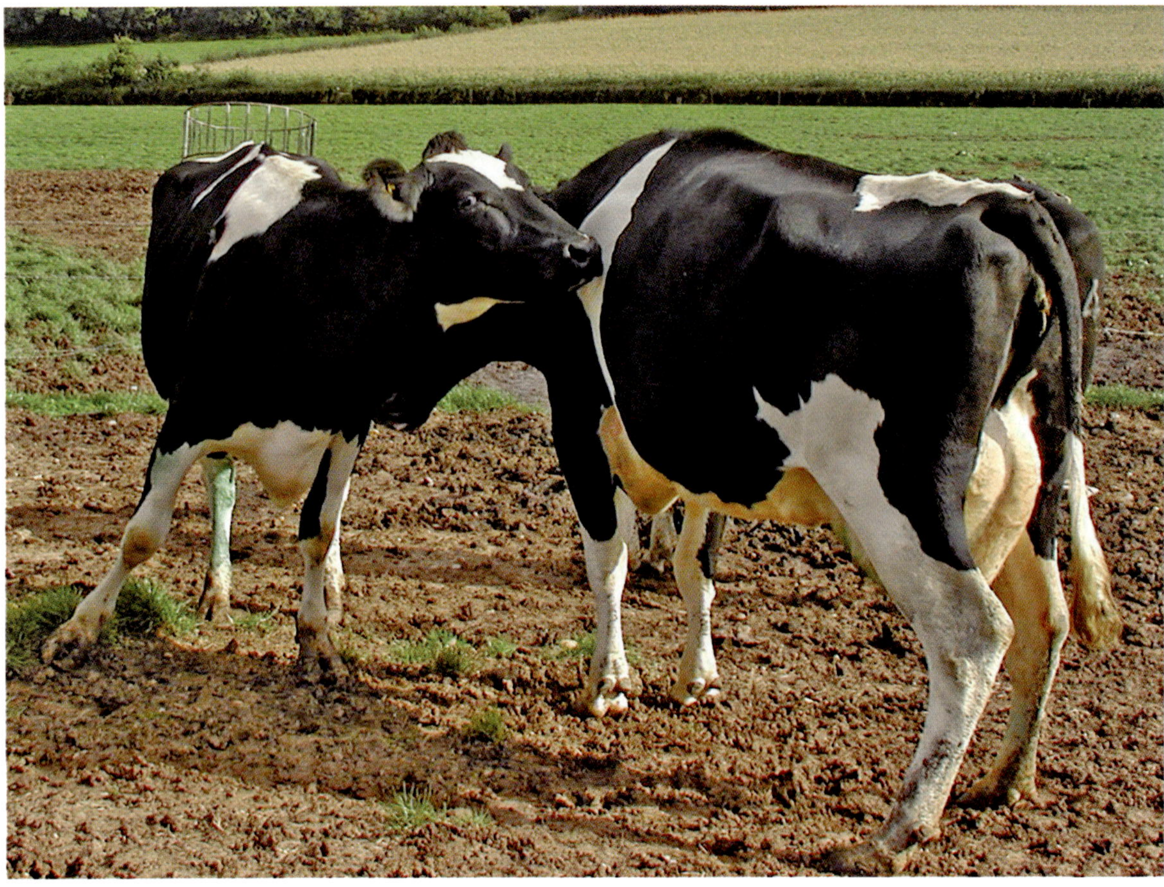

Physical interactions are common after changing groups.

animals such as the heifers. Constantly adding and removing cows is likely to set up fresh interactions and changes in dominance, particularly for the newly introduced animals. Simplify the number of group changes during transition and at calving to minimize this effect. Moving groups of animals is preferable because the social bond between a group of animals that are accustomed to each other reduces the stress of moving the animals into a new group. Work at ADAS Bridget's showed that introducing fresh-calved cows into the herd at night had advantages as the group was settled and there were few immediate social interactions with the newcomer.

- Use single size/age groups. Groups of cows that are of the same age or parity tend to have fewer social interactions, with less disruption to feeding or, more importantly, lying periods in the herd. Having a heifer group in the herd may be a problem in the milking parlour, but it can be an advantage for improving overall production through better feeding times, and may reduce lameness by reducing the standing time and increasing the lying periods.

- Excess cubicles. Many systems in the USA revolve round having more cows in the housing than there are cubicles. There is no evidence from the USA that increasing the stocking rate to 133 per cent (i.e. 133 cows per 100 cubicles) had any effect on resting time for the cows. This work, however, did not take account of the lower-ranking cows, who became affected by overstocking at quite low rates because they were the first animals to be dominated in the herd and pushed to lying in cubicles at different times to the main herd. This has always been a questionable principle in the UK. Cattle are described as showing allelomimetic behaviour. This means they prefer to perform the same activity at the same time, for example resting, feeding and other activities. Overstocking cows in a cubicle shed will frustrate this normal behaviour pattern. Lower-ranking animals spend more time on their feet and lying outside the cubicles when overstocking occurs.

- Adequate training. Introduction to the mysteries of a cubicle should occur at an early age, if possible. There are benefits in using cubicles of a proportional size for housing the maiden and in-calf heifers before they join the main herd; if a normal-sized cubicle is used, habits such as lying backwards in the cubicle may be learnt. Many heifers, if not used to cubicle designs before they join the main herd, can damage themselves by lying awkwardly in the stall area or trying to go through the front of the cubicle, especially on head-to-head rows.

Social interactions such as avoidance may be a problem in cubicles where there are head-to-head stalls or where the row is next to the feed passage. Social dominance may prevent a cow from using these cubicles or may affect the way it lies in the stall, for example diagonal lying may occur as discussed earlier in this chapter.

Heifers moving into the herd tend, on average, to be lower ranking and more prone to the effects of aggressive or dominant behaviour. These animals need special attention.

Behaviour of the lame cow is also different from that of a non-lame cow. The lame cow may become fearful of lying down in a cubicle and, once it gets down, may be afraid to get up. If it remains on its feet too long, healing will be delayed and it will be lame for longer. If it spends too long lying down in the cubicle,

its normal nutrition will suffer and pressure sores or hock damage will occur.

Lame cows may need to be removed from the normal housing environment to a straw yard or a set of sand cubicles that will give them more confidence to get up and lie down, and will prevent injuries or sores developing.

GENETICS

Genetics are involved in lameness, either through producing animals with poor conformation or through other factors that may affect claw horn quality. These effects are difficult to measure because there is such a large environmental component involved. For instance, we have shown in the section on nutrition that the feeding of the maiden heifer can markedly

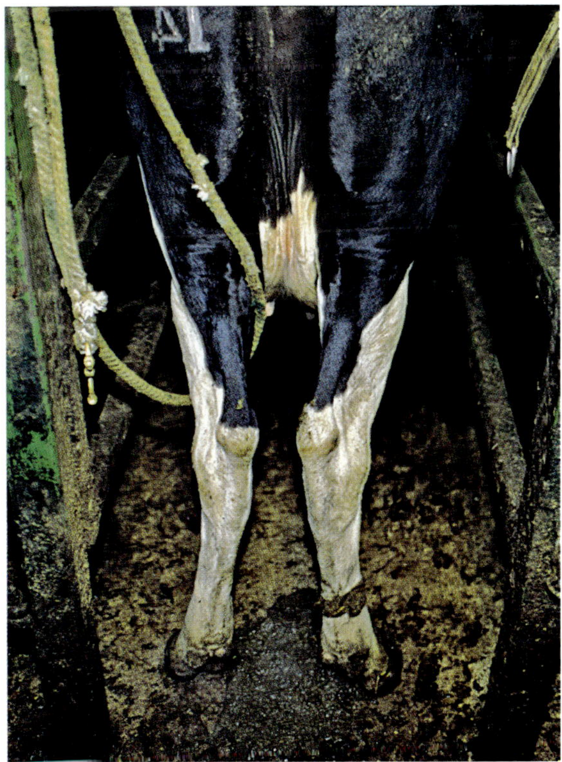

A cow with inward-pointing hocks; this will cause the hind feet to angle outwards and form overgrowths of horn on the sole. Is it due to bad breeding?

affect the incidence of lameness in subsequent lactations, without genetic involvement.

Breeding for improved 'soundness' characteristics is achievable, although difficult to do in practice because environmental influences have such an impact. The problem is recognizing what are good characteristics to choose and which are likely to have a strong genetic component that can be selected. Breeding from stock with high angles to the hoof and the legs may seem desirable, but it causes more 'shock' to be taken on the claws and joints, which is more likely to damage them.

Bull evaluations are now starting to address this problem by marking the bull's ability to pass on good scores for measures such as locomotion assessment. This will start to make some headway in producing less susceptible cattle.

The ideal would be to look for what are known as phenotypic markers. This means that, if the heritability of lameness is not good, we need to see if there are characteristics we can measure that will reflect the ability of parent stock to transfer improved characteristics for lameness incidence. These phenotypic markers could include such things as the angle of the hoof or the quality of the horn. Characteristics such as these can be measured at an early age to judge the potential of breeding stock, without waiting long periods for the outcome of lameness cases from several lactations.

There are reports of breed differences, sire differences and crossbreed differences, all of which indicate the possibility of genetic variation, which could be exploited to breed resistance to lameness. The problem with this approach is getting accurate records from farms and being sure about the diagnosis; skin lameness would be highly unlikely to show any genetic component, unlike horn disease. We need to be careful that the selection is not simply against milk yield, as there does appear to be a negative correlation.

CHAPTER TEN

Investigating a Herd Lameness Problem

This chapter attempts to bring together all the different facets of lameness that have been covered in previous chapters. The aim is to put them into an 'application' that we can use to investigate and improve lameness in cattle. We should now be in a position to use our skills with lameness recording, recognizing types of lameness, how they occur and how they can be prevented. Assembling these skills into a lameness health initiative will take the venture one step further – onto the farm to tackle lameness problems. The method described here is of an outside opinion, such as a veterinarian, dealing with a farm issue; but the farm itself could carry out the same approach to tackle lameness.

Any investigation of lameness in a herd needs to follow a series of carefully planned stages to look at relevant aspects of both the cow and its environment. We need to start by looking at the scale of the problem and specifically what types of lesions are involved. The next step usually involves a detailed investigation of the environment, specifically the cubicle and winter housing area or the tracks and gateways if outside grazing is used. The principles of this approach were laid down with the work of Liverpool University in the late 1980s and early 1990s, which defined some key parameters of cow housing. However, to take this approach further, we also need to ask some basic questions from the cow's point of view. This will indicate the impact of the housing on the animal. Can we 'weight' the various parameters of the housing to see which are more important? The issue is more difficult than it seems, because whatever we do or measure does not define what the cow thinks about it. We need to observe the cow in order to understand how it is interacting with its environment and how this could be affecting lameness. The most important part of understanding lameness is to try and appreciate things from the cow's point of view.

To make progress in preventing lameness, some form of active health initiative must be put in place to tackle the level of disease. The theory is simple. We need to set up a recording system to allow us to analyse lameness, undertake a herd investigation, and monitor any changes that are instituted to prevent lameness. In summary, the health initiative should:

- Record the level of lameness.
- Record the type of lameness.
- Draw up a simple investigation plan.
- Recommend and put in place changes.
- Monitor the progress.

This 'closed circle' approach to health initiatives makes progress possible. If the proposals put in place are not producing the results required, we can go back and review the overall prevention plan. Is the plan being carried out correctly or do some changes need to be made?

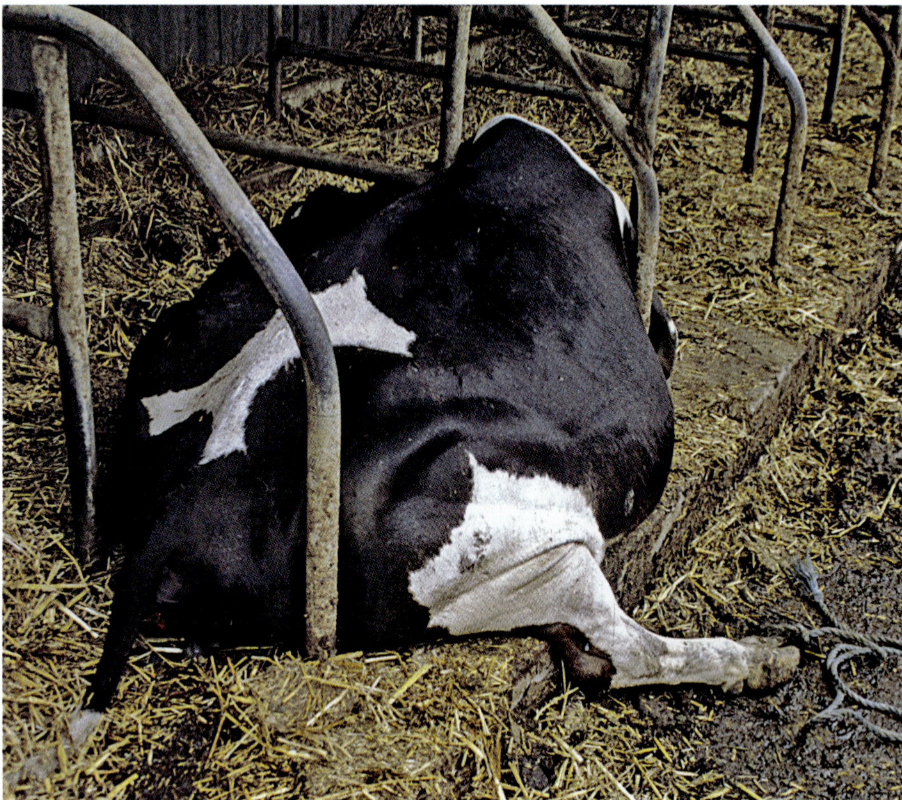

DEFINE THE PROBLEM

We need to be able to assess the lameness level both in terms of quantity and what type of lesion is occurring. In Chapter 3 we discussed in detail the recording of lameness and how this could be done. If we were to go out and look for lameness in the herd we would find much higher levels than if we relied on the farm's own records. The appreciation of when a cow is lame or not is very different for someone who is working with cows every day compared with a less frequent observer such as the veterinarian.

In most herds, lameness records are often non-existent or at best erratic. There is often considerable variation between what stock-persons describe as a lameness incident and their ability to diagnose and describe the lesions accurately and consistently. Therefore, when we look at lameness records we need to carefully define what they are based on – how the records were obtained, who diagnosed the lameness and who did the recording.

Record the Level of Lameness

The first step is to get any lameness records from the farm. Then assess how complete they are and if the information recorded is a reasonable reflection of the type of lesions found on that farm. It may be possible to get records from the foot trimmer if one is used.

One method of recording lameness is to use locomotion scores. In the 1990s the Liverpool team found that an accurate picture of the level of lameness in a herd could be found by doing a locomotion score on as little as two occasions, as long as one of them was during the winter housing period. Madison University (Wisconsin, USA) expanded this system to relate the prevalence of lameness seen at locomotion score visits to the actual

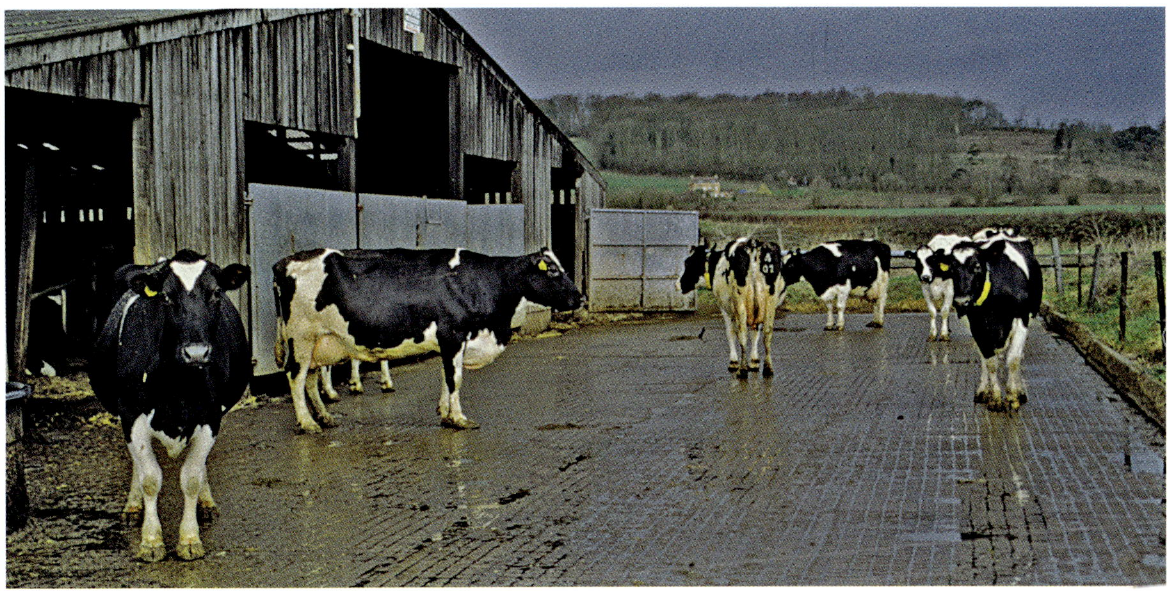

Can we get any information about lameness in the herd?

herd incidence. They found a relatively consistent relationship of three to one, in other words the actual incidence of lameness is about three times the prevalence based on an average of herd locomotion score visits. This is a useful way to compensate for poor recording and estimate the level of lameness present in a herd. Madison's results for Wisconsin show a herd prevalence of about 25 per cent and an overall incidence of 69 per cent (limb cases per 100 cows), which is in line with the proportions suggested by the Liverpool team.

Further analysis of these records may indicate seasonal trends or age group differences, for example if the heifers have a high level of solar ulceration.

Recording the Type of Lesion

Recording the type of lesion producing the lameness is a key feature in determining what is going on in a herd, and is necessary before trying to implement improvements. If there are no records, visit the farm on a couple of occasions and look at a sample of lame cows; examine the lesions present and the approach of the farm in treating them.

SITE INVESTIGATION

The farm records or previous visits should provide some background information about lameness incidence and type. To follow this up and establish some causal factors we need to carry out a farm investigation and look at key areas that affect lameness.

It is more efficient if you have a rational system for a farm visit with definite points to achieve. A checklist and a recording sheet will ensure a logical system to record key basic factors that we know are related to lameness.

General Issues

Start the process of investigation by following the typical route taken by a cow as it moves through the various functions of the day. For instance, start in the collecting yard and then progress through the milking parlour to the dispersal yard, then the cubicles, loafing area and feed area, and back round in a full circle. This should give some structure to the site visit and lend itself to a standard set of questions and scores.

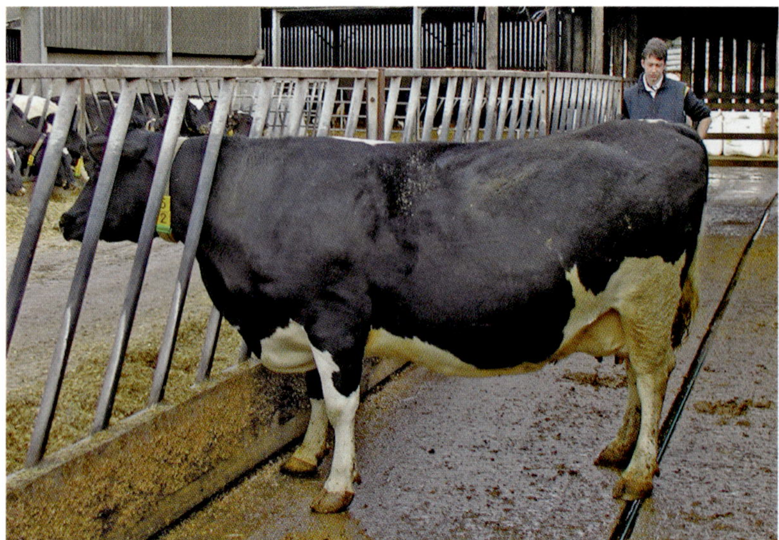

Start the investigation at a logical spot and follow the cow's daily routine.

There are a few items that will crop up at each stage of the route, such as surface condition. If possible, assess and score the surface for:

- Slip – feel it with your foot and watch cows moving over the surface. Do the cows ignore their basic 'one-foot-following-the-other' routine and go for a wide-based stance for safety, which may put uneven pressure on the foot and produce lameness lesions? Do the cows lose their footing, which, although not producing lameness of the foot, could indicate poor surface and abnormal posture?
- Physical damage – is the concrete such that it will physically wear the foot or produce damage?
- Hygiene – the amount of slurry present, any standing water, bedding being brought out onto the concrete surface (this may actually be an advantage if it softens the concrete surface). How often is it scraped, and so on?

Collecting yard. The size and capacity are basic measurements that can be assessed quickly against accepted standards. Does the collecting yard side load or rear load? The effect of dominance and aggression behaviour in cows is very significant with side-loading collecting yards. Dominant cows will push in and bully and stress the subordinates in the herd, forcing them to have longer standing times and possibly creating more aggression and slipping in the collecting yard. Rear-loading yards do not seem to have the same problems.

What is the exit like from the parlour? Is the turn very tight, producing a shearing motion on the foot? Is there a step up or down that could exacerbate this?

Dispersal yards and passageways. Many people think dispersal yards and passageways are unnecessary except to deliver the cows straight back to the feed or housing area. We have convinced ourselves that it is advantageous for a cow to stand for 30 minutes after being milked to allow for teat closure, but this may cause more difficulties than we are trying to avoid.

- Standing times are increased with no access to the bedding or cubicle.
- Slurry build up in this area can be very significant, which has implications for the hygiene of both the teat and the foot.

Housing. There are many issues related to the housing – its design, size, and how it is bedded.

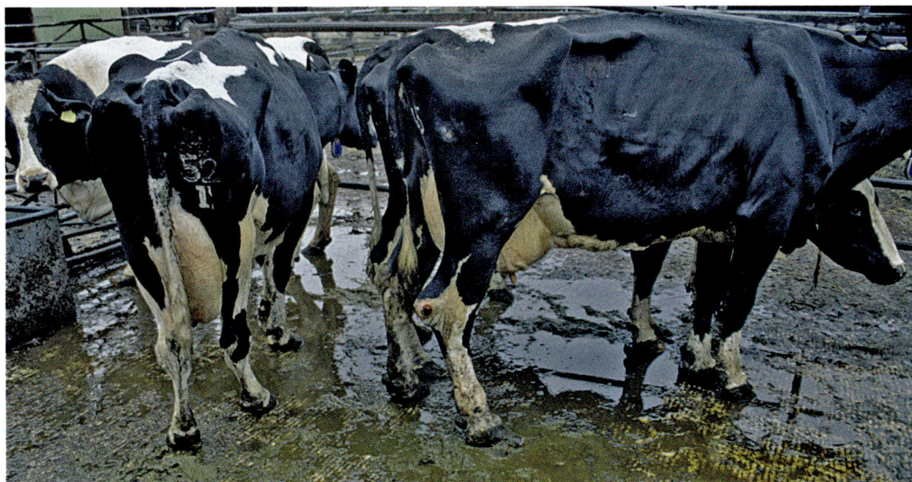

Check the cows for slurry contamination, and conditions underfoot.

However, first consider the type of housing – is it straw yard or cubicles?

Cubicles:
- The cubicle passages should be wide enough to prevent slurry becoming too deep and allow the cows to pass without aggression between them. Ideally they should be around 3m (10ft) wide and the feed passage 4.6m (15ft) wide.
- Is there an advantage in straw bedding coming out into the passage to allow a soft walking surface, especially when there are several cows that stand half-in cubicles? However, we have mentioned previously that passageways can be so comfortable that the cows will not lie in the cubicles.

Straw yard:
- Consider the overall layout, especially water troughs, bedding and loafing area.

Ventilation. Cows produce about 50ltr of water per day, from various sources. It must be got rid off to prevent it building up in the environment and having an impact on feet and other health issues. Ventilation can be specifically assessed using equipment such as hygrometers, but you can get a quick feel for the airflow through a building by looking for cobwebs and moisture streaking on the roof beams, which indicates high humidity and low air movement.

Stocking rates of the cubicles or loose housing can be assessed easily at this stage by

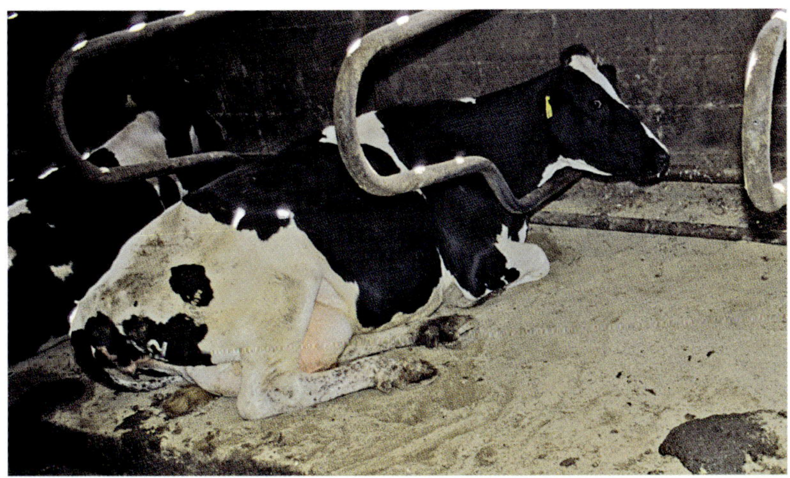

This cow is using the divider to 'borrow' space from the adjacent cubicle – the cubicle is too short.

checking yard size or cubicle numbers against the cow numbers.

Feed space at the barrier or manger. Competition will affect standing times. Agonistic behaviour will cause fighting and slipping, as cows jostle for access to the feed fence; any competition here will also reduce the subordinate animal's chance of getting enough food.

Loafing areas. These areas are essential for the expression of normal behaviour.

Tracks and gateways. These should be inspected if the cows are out at grazing.

Use a recording sheet, such as the one shown in Table 15 below, to fill in some detail whilst walking round. The 'size' column indicates stocking rate and area per cow for collecting yards and so on, so that it can be compared with accepted standards. The hygiene score can be used to assess slurry clearance in each area inspected and the surface score to assess the quality of the concrete underfoot in each site. The 'time' column records the proportion of the day the cows spend in each section of the farm and what they are doing

there, for example standing, feeding and so on. Knowing how long a cow is in each of the areas inspected will give a rough set of values for working out a 'time budget', which will be discussed in more detail in the section below on cow behaviour.

Specific Issues

The more specific issues will need a recording sheet of their own. Assess the cubicle using a specific checklist such as the one shown in Table 16.

Assess the straw yard as shown in Table 17.

Inspect the footbaths and check their construction and siting against what we listed as important features in Chapter 3. These are summarized in Table 18.

Nutrition is a difficult subject to cover fully at a single visit without a lot of extra work. Ask about specific consequences of feeding that might indicate a nutritional problem. Is there a high incidence of metabolic disease? Left displaced abomasum (LDA) and right displaced abomasum (RDA), and even endometritis, acetonaemia and milk drops, could

Area	Detail	'Size'	Hygiene score	Surface score	Time
Collecting yard					
Parlour	Width				
	Exits				
Passageways	Width				
	Turning				
Housing	Type				
	Passage width				
	Plan				
Feed fence	Width				
	Type				
Loafing areas					
Tracks at grass					
Gateways					

Table 15 General recording sheet

Detail required	**Notes**
Overall size	
Kerb height	
Surface material	
Bedding	
Divider	
Brisket rail	
Head rail	
Bob zone	
Space sharing	
Slurry scraping system	
Cleanliness score	

Table 16 Cubicle recording sheet

Detail required	**Notes**
Size	
Layout detail	
Water troughs	
Bedding depth	
Bedding management	

Table 17 Straw yard recording sheet

Detail required	**Notes**
Design	
Position	
Capacity	
Treatment agent	
Protocol for use	

Table 18 Footbath recording sheet

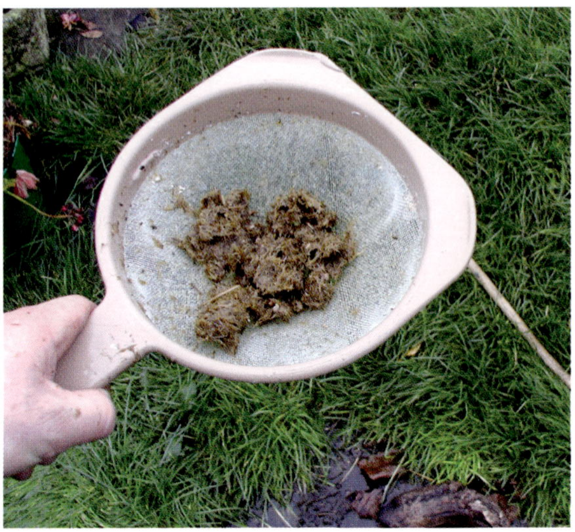

Sieving dung to look at the fibre content and check dietary fibre.

indicate that feeding is a limiting factor and could therefore be affecting feet. If there are indications of nutritional issues, it may be worth investigating further. Other quick indicators of overall herd nutrition are:

- Dung consistency in the housing area.
- Milk quality in terms of fat and protein.
- The fibre content of the dung. A quick method is to wash some through a sieve to check for fibre content.

Management of cattle movements within the herd, especially integration of cattle into the herd, is important and should be reviewed.

- Social integration. What is the policy for social integration? When introducing heifers, how are they mixed with the dry cows and what happens to them when they enter the main herd?
- Environmental integration. What is the policy of preconditioning the cows or heifers to life in the main herd? The best option may be 'concrete stimulation', which increases the sole thickness before calving, followed by a straw yard to buffer the effects of calving on the foot. This will help prevent pedal bone 'disruption' becoming lameness later in the lactation. Is there cubicle training for the heifers?
- Nutritional integration. What is the policy of introducing the production ration? There are various ideas about this at present. There may be an advantage in having short dry periods with very few diet changes so that the cow does not lose her adaptation to the last lactation diet before she again calves onto the new lactation diet. On the other hand, many dairy units are keeping the freshly calved cow on low-energy and high-fibre diets (e.g. the stale milker ration) until they have adapted to lactation and overcome the disruption of calving.

If the cows are at grazing, all aspects of track design and condition should be checked (Table 19).

Details required	Notes
Surface material	
Stones present	
Inclines and drainage	
Gateways	
Method of moving	
Shared with machinery	

Table 19 Grazing checklist

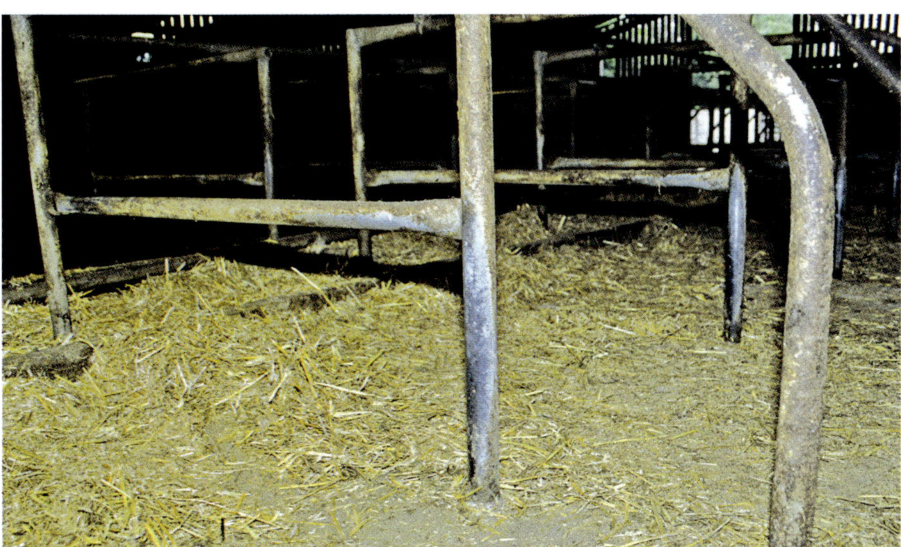

Look at the cubicles to check for smooth rub marks, which indicate where the cow 'does not fit'.

Conclusions

We can devise standards and recommendations for all the information gathered on a farm visit, but what does the cow think of the ideals we have set? Previous work has highlighted some basic minimums along with what might be the important issues, but what does the cow think of these minimums? Cow behaviour is the next step to address when investigating lameness.

COW COMFORT – WHAT ARE THE COWS TELLING US?

Most cows are winter housed in a cubicle environment. We need to examine the relationship between the cow and the cubicle because this is where understanding of most of the lameness issue lies.

The difficulty with describing the environment in detail is that it does not tell us how the cow is going to interact with it. We may have what we think is the best design and size for the cow cubicles, but are the cows using them? It would be disappointing to find that after using 'best knowledge' of cubicle design this has not resulted in the best results in terms of cow comfort. However, many parameters of housing design are still not absolutely specific. We often cannot 'gauge' the importance of any combination of design issues to find which factors are the most important when it comes to cow comfort; we need to look at the cow itself.

Investigating cow behaviour is very much an emerging science, but progress is being made and there are some very practical applications we can use in investigating a herd for lameness. Work in the USA and Canada has indicated that we should look at:

• Injuries and damage to the legs. This is a good indicator of how lying in the cubicle physically affects the cow.

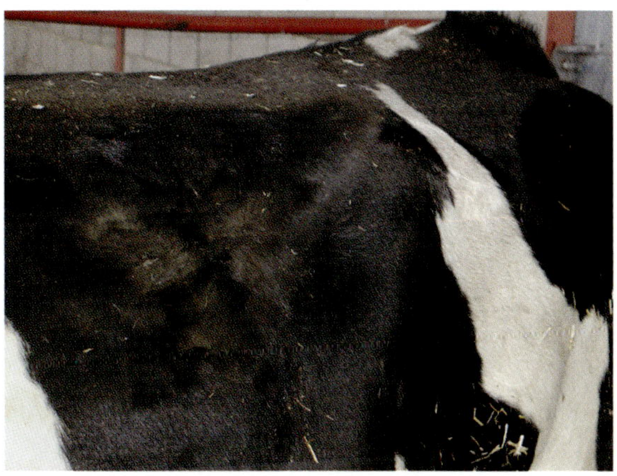

Check the cows to see if they are showing the same rub marks – the result of 'not fitting'.

- Cow hygiene. How is the way we keep the cow affecting how dirty it is?
- Time spent lying down as a proportion of the day. This is part of what are known as 'time budgets' and it allows us to see what areas of the cow's daily routine are limiting and interfering with cow comfort.
- Cow comfort by assessing the actual lying time in the housing.

Measuring Injuries and Damage to Cows' Legs

Cubicle design and the way it is managed affects the prevalence of hock lesions in cows. This can be used as a measure of how the cow is interacting with a cubicle design and bedding material. There are two main types of damage to look for:

- Lateral or medial hock damage. This involves the tarsal joint, and although it usually starts with simple hair loss it can proceed to skin necrosis or hygroma formation.
- Damage to the point of the hock. This is known as a 'capped hock' and involves the tip of the hock or tuber calcis as this bone is known. These lesions are described fully in Chapter 8.

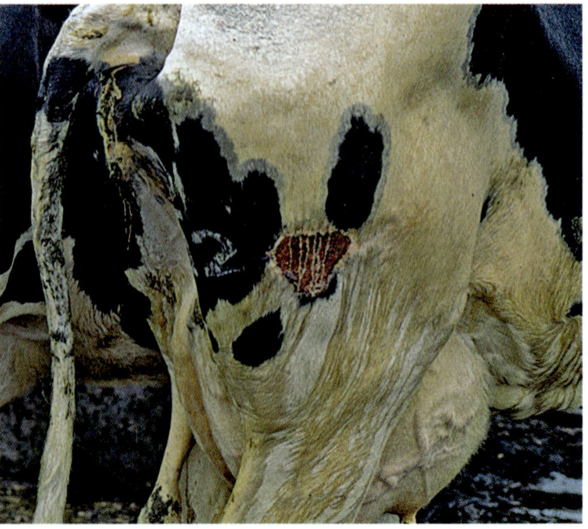

Pressure sores on the hindlimbs show that the cubicles are not soft enough or that the cow is lame and lying down for too long.

In the example shown below, what appears to be a good mattress construction in a reasonably proportioned cubicle is causing severe damage with pressure sores and hock lesions. There is a problem with the surface bedding material and this is producing superficial hock lesions in a lot of cows. The lame cows are spending too long lying in the cubicles and are showing pressure sores on the upper legs.

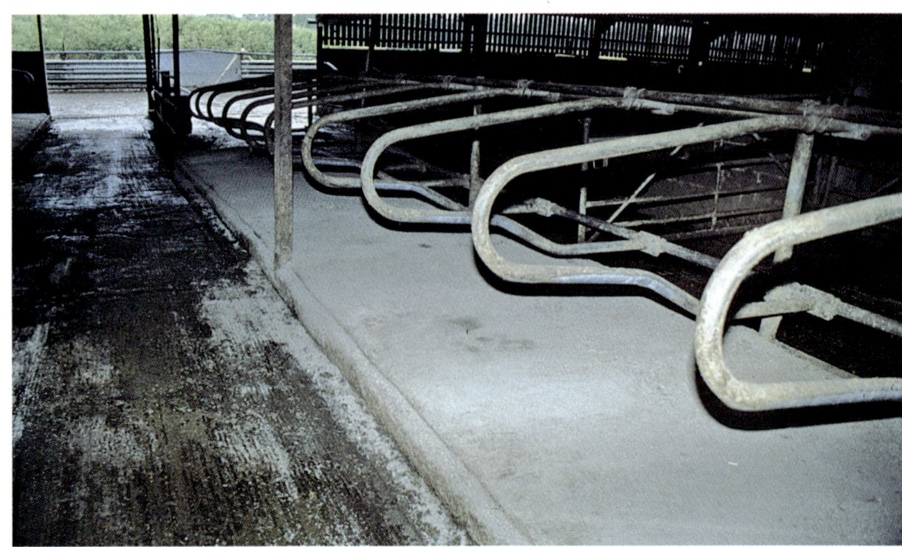

Example of mattress cubicles bedded with paper waste.

The dry cows in this herd are managed in cubicles on a deep sand bedding, which, when it is freshly bedded up, looks good. However, the retaining kerb is producing damage to the tuber calcis. The cow is telling us that what looks a good idea in theory is not working in practice and we must examine the cubicle surface, its bedding material and the way it is used.

Measuring Hygiene Score

The amount of manure staining on a cow is a good indicator of the hygiene conditions in which she is housed and managed. Look at the level of muck on the feet, udder and flanks and come up with a simple scoring system that is repeatable and can give a good assessment of farm hygiene. It has been shown that this sort of score is closely related to lameness, especially skin diseases such as digital dermatitis. It is also strongly associated with other health performance such as mastitis.

Time Budgets for Cows

Looking at the cows and how they spend their time in their environment are key steps in understanding the science of cow comfort. First determine a time budget for the cows; this is a 'time and motion' study to find out what they are doing and for how long they are doing it.

The key feature is lying time, which should be a minimum of 50 per cent of the cow's total time budget.

Comfort Measurements

There are more precise ways – that have a direct relevance to lameness – of defining what the cows are doing in relation to their housing environment. It is possible, with careful observation of cows in the cubicles, to put actual figures on comfort.

- Cow Comfort Index (CCI, the number of cows lying in a cubicle divided by the number of cows touching a cubicle surface) gives a numerical expression for the propor-

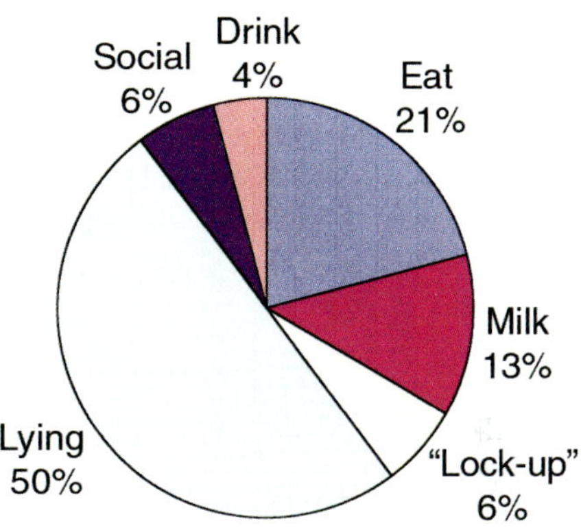

This pie chart shows a typical cow budget. 'Lock-up' equates to the time cows are penned away from the cubicles and feed fence for scraping out and other tasks.

tion of cows in cubicles that are actually lying down. Eighty five per cent or more of the cows should be lying in a cubicle 2 hours before morning milking.

- Proportion Eligible Lying (PEL, the number of cows lying in cubicles divided by the number of cows in the area not eating) shows how many of the cows in the housing that are eligible to lie down in the cubicles (i.e. they are not eating) are doing so. One hour after returning from morning milking 75 per cent or more of the cows should be lying in a cubicle.

- Stall Standing Index (SSI, the number of cows standing with two or four feet in a cubicle divided by the number of cows touching a cubicle surface) is the inverse of CCI and shows the proportion of cows in cubicles that are standing; so a lower percentage for SSI is desirable. Figures of 15 per cent or less for SSI at 2 hours before departure for morning milking are considered good.

These are not very user-friendly terms, but they can be defined and measured. We can simplify them to two straightforward measures:

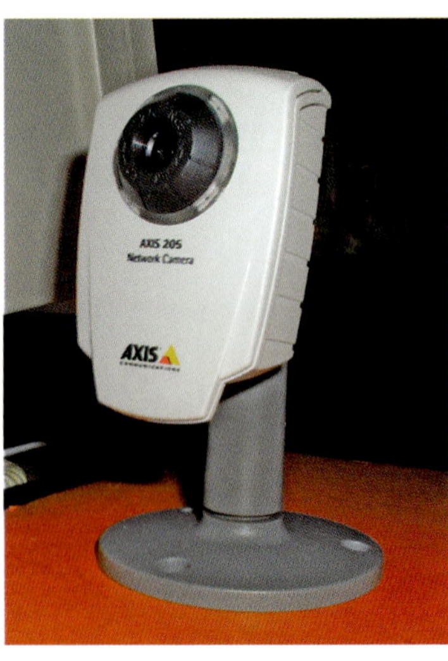

A web camera can make remote viewing of cow behaviour very simple.

the behaviour you are trying to measure is relatively short lived, for example standing in a cubicle amounts for only about 6 per cent of the cow's day and thus more frequent scanning is needed to be accurate with this measure. However, as lying down is a more prolonged behavioural expression, it can be assessed accurately from hourly snapshots. The graph below shows a typical scan for CCI based on two cubicle designs. The poorer result (lower line) comes from what appear to be the better cubicles, showing again the importance of the cow's point of view.

1. PEL describes cubicle acceptance by the herd.
2. CCI describes actual cow comfort.

Obtaining this information is not difficult as modern technology enables CCTV (closed circuit television) to be used on modern dairy herds. Even better, a web camera can be mounted to observe the cows and by using time-lapse images a good estimate of these behavioural characteristics can be derived from frames taken every hour. Be careful when

PRODUCING A HERD LAMENESS REPORT

It may be useful to work through an example of what a practical lameness investigation entails. In this section we will take a real farm and follow through a lameness consultation. We can use the items discussed above to produce a reasoned analysis of farm data and develop discussion points and recommendations from visiting the farm and carrying out a structured investigation. The skill is also to present this information for the farm so that it can be easily understood and hopefully form

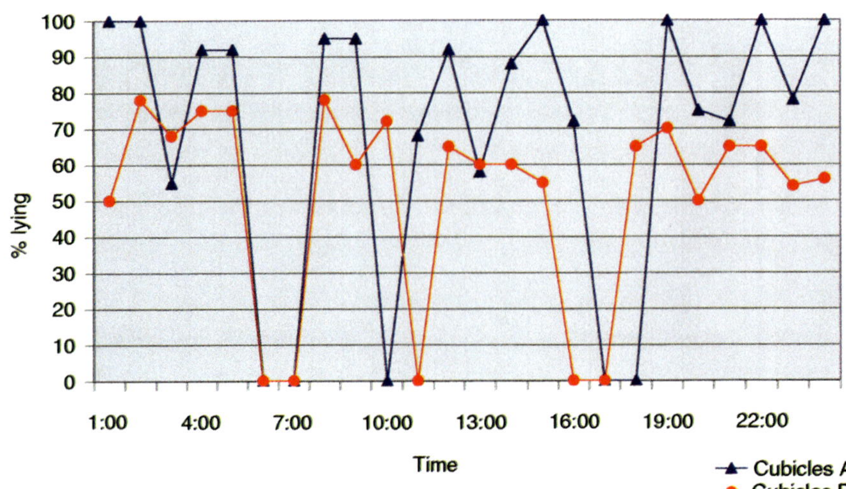

'Cow Comfort Index' measured over time for two sets of cubicles. The lower line shows that cubicles B are used less and could be less comfortable.

Lameness report for period ...

Herd data	**Results**	**Targets**
Herd size – average number of cows (A)	Cows incidence = B/A × 100	<20%
No. of cows recorded lame – cow cases (B)	Limb cases = C/A × 100	<25%
No. of limbs recorded lame – limb cases (C)	Repeat cases = D/B × 100	<10%
	(As a percentage of those affected)	
No. of cows affected more than once (D)	Cases per affected cow C/B	<1.2

Table 20 Lameness report summary

the basis of farm procedures for controlling lameness.

First choose a period of time for the report analysis. It would be best to look at a complete year because of seasonal variation and to be sure to get enough data in the period to reflect an overall level of lameness.

Use a table based on the outline shown in Table 20 to produce incidence figures for the herd.

The targets suggested here are for herds that are recording lameness accurately or if the records are based on locomotion scoring. If the records are poor and have no outside involvement (e.g. foot trimmers, veterinarians), the targets should be halved because the overall level of lameness will be half (we have covered the reasoning behind this in Chapter 2 on recording).

Herd Records for Incidence and Lesion Type

The example herd has computer-based records for lameness using the 'InterHerd' herd recording programme (NMR software). We can obtain an analysis of the lameness event

incidence from this system that will enable a more thorough look at the herd lameness records (Table 21).

We can also look at the spread of lesions in the herd from the list of lameness events recorded.

We can see the relative importance of the main lesions by quickly sorting them out from Table 21 and showing them as a percentage of the overall limb cases (*see* Table 22 on page 165).

The overall trend of lameness cases (limb cases) over the year is shown in the graph on the following page.

We can see from this example herd that the overall level of lameness in the 12-month period studied is very high at 59 per cent cow incidence or 59 cows per 100 cows in the herd. The limb cases incidence is 77 per cent or 77 limb cases of lameness per 100 cows in the herd. The seasonal distribution is what we would normally expect to see, with peaks in lameness during the winter and again at turnout in the spring. The two major lameness lesions on the farm are digital dermatitis and solar ulceration. We can make the site

Lameness report for period 1.1.2005 to 31.12.2005

Lameness records		**Herd parameters**	**Results**	**Targets**
Herd size	200	Cow incidence	59%	<20%
Cow cases	118	Limb case incidence	77%	<25%
Limb cases	154	Repeat cases	17%	<10%
Cows lame more than once	34	Cases per cow	1.3	<1.2

Table 21 Lameness record summary

Category	Overall	Jan	Feb	Mar	Apr	May	Jun	Jul	Aug	Sep	Oct	Nov	Dec
Overall	154	24	1	11	13	10	7	6	5	15	22	23	17
FR	19	2	0	1	1	1	3	0	2	0	3	3	3
BR	73	13	0	7	8	4	4	1	1	8	10	8	9
FL	21	2	0	0	1	1	1	1	1	5	3	4	2
BL	77	13	1	4	7	9	2	4	1	3	12	11	10
Sole Ulcer	76	10	0	9	8	8	6	2	2	7	8	7	9
Wtite Line Disease	16	1	0	0	2	1	1	1	0	3	2	4	1
DD Heel	40	7	0	1	2	2	0	2	1	2	7	10	6
DD Interdigital	17	4	0	0	2	0	0	2	0	3	3	3	0
DD Coronary band	0	0	0	0	0	0	0	0	0	0	0	0	0
DD Sole	1	0	0	0	0	0	0	0	0	0	1	0	0
Foul of the foot	6	0	0	0	0	0	0	0	2	0	2	2	0
FB Puncture	5	4	0	0	0	0	0	0	0	0	0	1	0
Septic Arthritis	2	1	0	0	0	0	0	0	0	0	0	0	1
Bruised Sole	0	0	0	0	0	0	0	0	0	0	0	0	0
Interdigital Hyperplasia	0	0	0	0	0	0	0	0	0	0	0	0	0
Under Run	2	0	0	0	1	0	0	0	0	0	0	0	1
Laminintis	0	0	0	0	0	0	0	0	0	0	0	0	0
No Diagnosis	0	0	0	0	0	0	0	0	0	0	0	0	0
O Claw	2	0	0	0	0	0	0	0	0	0	2	0	0
I Claw	3	0	0	0	0	0	0	0	0	0	3	0	0

The above analysis splits the lameness recorded into, first, the foot affected and then into the category of lameness that was recorded for each limb case entered.

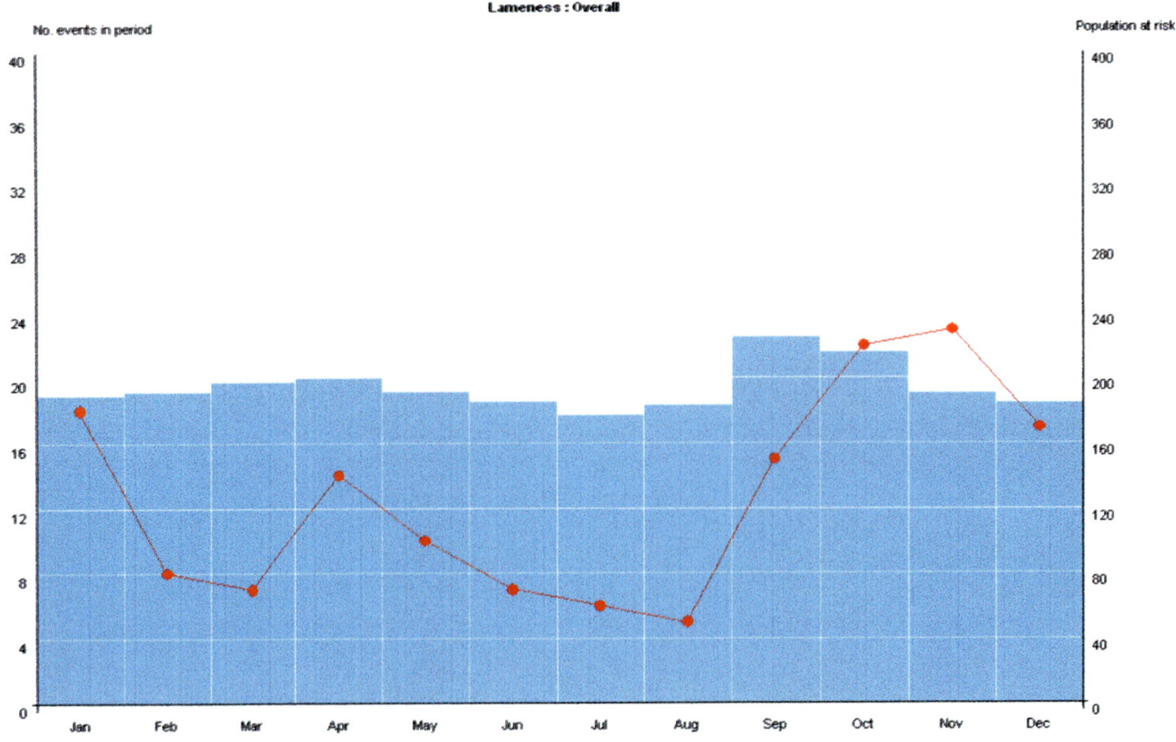

Cases of lameness shown over a 12-month period. The background bars show the herd size at the time of the lameness record. This keeps the lameness case incidence in proportion with the herd size if it was changing rapidly (buying new cows, heifers etc.).

Lesion	Number	Incidence as % of limb cases
Solar ulceration	73	47
White line	18	12
DD heel	44	29
DD interdigital	20	13
DD total lesions	64	42
Foul	6	4

***Table 22   Distribution of lesions
DD = digital dermatitis***

visit more targeted to issues that are likely to involve these two lameness diseases.

Farm Site Visit Report

Using the system outlined earlier in this chapter, we start the farm visit in the dispersal yard and work round following the same route that the cows take. Notes are filled in and rough time measurements are taken to allocate the cow's time spent in each area. The time budget is shown below in a graph.

A quarter of the total time budget is spent in the collecting yard at milking; this is partly because of three-times-a-day milking and also because the collecting yard is side loading and

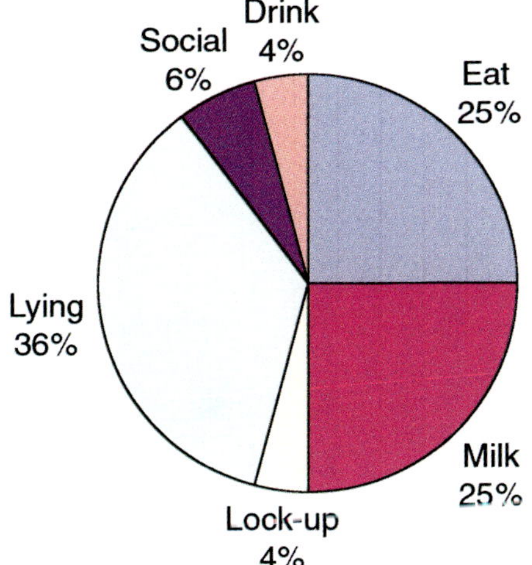

A time budget from the farm investigation

many cows are kept at the back whilst more dominant cows push through to the front. There is also increased feeding time because the feed fence is too short for the number of cows. Therefore, the amount of time for lying is reduced.

The cubicle score was also low, with a mattress surface covered thinly with a paper mulch bedding and obstruction in the 'bob zone' making it difficult for cows to get up and down. Hock lesions were evident on many of the cows, with areas of hair loss and reddening present as well as several large hygromas.

The footbath routine was not being carried out with enough attention to detail. The cows were not being cleaned off well enough before using an antibiotic footbath and the use of formalin was erratic; some weeks it would be every day and some weeks it was not done at all. Most importantly the dry cows were not receiving any treatment and there was a high level of infection of digital dermatitis in newly calved cows. Of the 30 per cent of cases of lameness occurring before 100 days after calving the majority of these were due to digital dermatitis.

Advice

Some points for the farm to address:

Short Term

- Better digital dermatitis control protocol; to include a consistent treatment approach and to include the dry cows.
- Improve the flow of cows at milking to reduce the length of time in the collecting yard. Use groups brought up in turn rather than the whole herd at once.
- Change the cubicle bedding material and use more of it to improve the surface quality.

Long Term

- Improve cubicle design.
- Increase the feed fence and trough area.

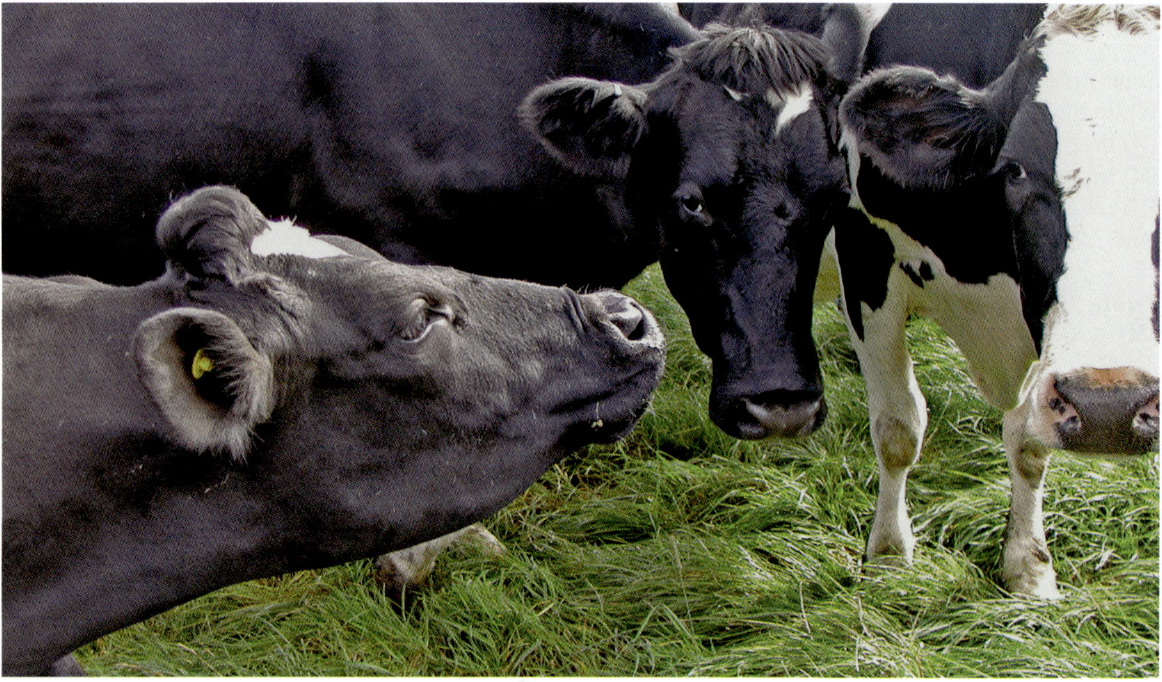

Watch the cows and they will tell you what they think of their environment.

SUMMARY

Collecting information from the farm will give the background to enable a lameness situation to be assessed. Using a well-rehearsed approach to review the farm layout, design, farm management, and cow behaviour patterns you can then undertake a thorough and constructive investigation of a herd lameness problem.

To achieve true benefits for the cow, look carefully at the impact of the environment on the animal through its behaviour.

- Investigate herd records or …
- Locomotion score the herd – preferably on two occasions, at least one of which is in the winter housing period, to determine the average lameness prevalence; the lameness incidence is calculated as three times the prevalence recorded.
- Try and obtain good records of the type of lameness.
- Investigate the herd in a logical fashion.
- Look at simple cow interactions – injuries, hygiene and cow behaviour.
- Formulate a health initiative.
- Monitor progress.

A logical approach based on understanding lameness will enable us to make progress and develop achievable herd initiatives that can deliver results.

Further Reading

Blowey, R.W., *Cattle Lameness and Hoofcare* (Farming Press, Ipswich, 2002).

Cook, N., Oetzel, G. and Nordlund, K., University of Wisconsin–Madison. www.vetmed. wisc.edu, www.cals.wisc.edu and www.cias. wisc.edu (accessed 2 August 2006).

Esslemont, R.J. and Kossaibati, M.A., *The Costs of Poor Fertility and Disease in UK Dairy Herds* (Intervet UK, Milton Keynes, 2003).

Greenough, P.R. (ed.), *Lameness in Cattle*, 3rd edition (W.B. Saunders, Toronto, 1997).

Kossaibati, M.A., Esslemont, R.J. and Watson, C., *Understanding and Tackling Lameness in Dairy Herds* (NMR and The University of Reading, 1999), 40pp.

Tucker, Cassandra and Weary, Dan from The University of British Columbia, Canada www.agsci.ubc.ca/animalwelfare

The Milk Development Council. www.mdc.org. uk

Notes

1. Whitaker, D.A., Kelly, J.M. and Smith, E.J., 'Incidence of lameness in dairy cows', *Vet. Rec.* **113**: 60–62, 1993.
2. Clarkson *et al.*, 'Incidence and prevalence of lameness in dairy cattle', *Vet. Rec.* **138**: 563–567, 1996.
3. Kossaibati, M.A., Esslemont, R.J. and Watson, C., 'The Costs of Lameness in Dairy Herds'. A paper presented to the National Cattle Lameness Conference, Stoneleigh, Warwickshire, 1999.
4. Weaver, D., 'Analysis of some epidemiological factors in lameness on 55 Somerset dairy herds'. Proceedings of the 10th International Symposium on Lameness in Ruminants, September 1998 (Lucerne, Switzerland, 1998), pp. 65–69.
5. Hedges, J., *et al.*, 'A longitudinal field trial of the effect of biotin on lameness in cows', *J. Dairy Sci.* **84**: 1969–75, 2001.
6. Cook, N.B., 'An update on dairy cow free stall design', *The Bovine Practitioner* (*Journal of the American Association of Bovine Practitioners*) **39**: 29–23, 2005.
7. National Animal Disease Information Service (NADIS), *UK Vet* (Blackwell Press, Oxford).
8. Cook, N.B., 'The prevalence of lameness in a selection of Wisconsin dairy herds', *JAVMA* **223**: 1324–1328, 2003.
9. Laven, R., 'Determination of the factors affecting the cause, prevalence, and severity of digital dermatitis as a major cause of lameness in dairy cows' (Milk Development, Cirencester, 2000), Study 95/R1/11.
10. Rodriguez-Lainz, A. *et al.*, 'Case control study of papillomatous dermatitis in southern California dairy farms', *Prev. Vet. Med.* **28**: 117–131, 1996.
11. Wells, S.J. *et al.*, 'Papillomatous digital dermatitis and associated risk factors in US dairy herds', *Prev. Vet. Med.* **38**: 11–24, 1999.
12. Bargai, U., 'Digital dermatitis, interdigital dermatitis and heel erosion associated with nutritional aetiology', *Israel J. Vet. Med.* **61**: 23–34, 2006.
13. Piromalli, G. *et al.*, 'Therapy of interdigital phlegmon in the cow, a novel protocol'. Proceedings of the XVIII World Buiatrics Congress (Bologna, Italy, 1994), pp. 587–591.
14. Baker, I.D., 'Amputation of the bovine digit as a treatment for septic arthritis', *Bovine Practice* (Bailliere Tindall, 1991), p. 123.
15. Watson, C.L. and Penny, C., 'Crushed tail head syndrome in cattle', *Vet. Rec.* **152**: 542–543, 2003.
16. Shaw, J., 'Acute tailhead trauma in Friesian Holstein cows', *Vet. Rec.* **140**: 612, 1997.
17. Nordlund, K.V. and Garrett, E.F., 'Rumenocentesis: a technique for the diagnosis of subacute rumen acidosis in dairy herds', *The Bovine Practitioner* (*Journal of the American Association of Bovine Practitioners*) **28**: 104, 1994.

18. Gummer, R., University of Wisconsin Department of Agriculture. www.cals.wisc.edu (accessed 1 September 2006).

19. Manson, F.J. and Leaver, J.D., 'The effect of dietary protein on lameness in cattle', *Anim. Prod.* **47**: 185–190, 1988.

20. MDC project 97/R4/14 (Milk Development Council, Cirencester, 2001).

21. Webster, A.J.F., 'Effects of housing practices on the development of foot lesions in dairy heifers in early lactation', *Vet. Rec.* **151**: 9–12, 2002.

22. Cook, N.B. *et al.*, 'A comparison of dairy cow behaviour in sand and mattress free stall barns in relation to lameness'. Proceedings of the 13th International Ruminant Lameness Symposium (Maribor, Slovenia, 2004).

23. Hughes, J.W, 'Environmental control of bovine lameness', *BCVA*, vol. 5, part 3: 235–246, 1997.

24. Clarkson, M.J. *et al.*, 'An epidemiological study to determine the risk factors of lameness in dairy cows', Liverpool University final report, ref CSA1379, 1993.

25. Clackson, D.A. and Ward, W.R., 'Farm tracks, stockman's herding and lameness in dairy cattle', *Vet. Rec.* **129**: 511–512, 1991.

26. Chesterton, R.N., 'Environmental and behavioural factors affecting the prevalence of foot lameness in New Zealand dairy herds – a case control study', *N.Z. Vet. J.* **37**: 135–142, 1989.

27. Galindo, F. and Broom, D.M., 'The relationships between social behaviour of dairy cows and the occurrence of lameness in three herds', *Res. Vet. Sci.* **69**: 75–79, 2000.

Glossary

Abaxial The area of the foot towards the midline or interdigital space.
Acetabulum The cavity in the pelvis that is the cup for the articulation of the femur.
Agonistic behaviour Relating to, or being aggressive, or defensive social interaction (as fighting, fleeing, or submitting) between individuals.
Allelomimetic In a group of animals it is undergoing the same behaviour at the same time.
Ankylosis When a joint is damaged so that the bones fuse together and no longer articulate.
Anterior (or cranial) The area nearer to the head end – 'the front'.
Arthrodesis Surgically entering a joint through the joint capsule to produce a fusion of the joint.
Arthrotomy The surgical exploration of a joint.
Avulsion The forcible tearing away of a joint or ligaments from their attachment.
Axial The area of the foot that is away from the midline – to the outside.

Bacteraemia The presence of bacteria in the bloodstream.
Bulbs of the heel The area to the posterior aspect of the sole that joins up with the skin of the foot. It is like the periople softer horn and is waxy to feel.
Bursae Fluid-filled sacs over specific points of the body to produce lubrication of tendons and so on that pass over this area.
Bursitis Inflammation of the bursae.

Caudal This means the structure or area nearer to the hind end – 'the back'.
Collagen A component of connective tissue (the dermis or corium).
Coriosis Damage to the corium producing disruption of tissues and loosening of the connective tissue between the horn and the pedal bone.
Corium The area under the horn in the foot. It is equivalent to the dermis of the skin.
Coronary band The area of the hoof that produces the specialized horn structure that extends down the foot as the wall of the hoof.
Corticosteroid Anti-inflammatory drug.
Cranial The area nearer to the head end – 'the front'.

Dermis The underlying layer of the skin.
Digital cushion A sac of fat and connective tissues under the rear of the pedal bone to absorb impact on weight bearing.
Dislocation Displacement of a bone from a joint so that it no longer articulates.
Dorsal The lower aspect of the standing body, i.e. downwards.

Endotoxin Poisons released by bacteria, especially when they are destroyed.
Epidermis The outer layer of skin.
Exostoses Excess bone that is formed trying to stabilize a joint that is affected after dislocation, arthritis etc. It often restricts the movement of the joint.
Extensor tendons Move to straighten the leg – they are at the front of the limb.

Fibrous Made up of fibrous tissue, a component of connective tissue.
Flexor tendons Move the leg in flexion – they are at the rear of the leg.
Flexor tuberosity The point on the pedal bone to which the deep digital flexor tendon is attached. It is at the rear of the pedal bone.

Granulation tissue This is very vascular tissue formed from the dermis (or corium) when a wound is healing.
Granuloma Excess production of granulation tissue.
Greater trochanter A bony extension of the femoral head.

Haematoma A cavity of blood producing a 'blood blister' or bruise.
Hoof The keratinized area covering the foot that is composed of horn.
Hygroma A lump of fibrous tissue.
Hyperplasia Formation of excess tissue.
Hypertrophy Formation of a larger structure. Excess tissue produces an increased size to the whole structure.
Hypocalcaemia Milk fever.

Incidence An occurrence happening once. It needs to be defined by stating a period of time, e.g. annual incidence.
Interdigital space The cleft that is between the two claws.
Interdigitating horn Produced at the white line by the sole to join sole with wall horn.
Intertubular horn Produced by the papillae between the tubules.
Ischaemic Deprived of a blood supply, which tends to produce death of the tissue and necrosis.

Keratin Specialized protein to produce hardness in skin or the hoof.
Keratinize To lay down keratin in cells to form horn or skin.

Laminae The folds of the corium on the wall that attach and secure the horn and produce leaflet horn to lubricate its movement downwards.
Laminitis Inflammation of the laminae.
Lateral claw The outside claw furthest away from the midline.
Leaflet horn Lubricating horn produced by the corium of the wall (the laminae) to allow horn to slip down from the coronary band to the sole. It forms an integral part of the white line.
Luxation Moving out of its normal position. It can refer to structures other than joints.

Medial claw The claw that is nearest to the midline of the body – the inside claw.

NADIS National Animal Disease Information Service.
Navicular bone Found at the rear of the foot allowing the deep flexor tendon to move across the pedal joint.
Necrobacillosis Infection producing death of tissues and necrosis.
Necrosis Death of tissue.
NSAID Non-steroidal anti-inflammatory drug.

Papillae The specialized area of the corium that produces tubular horn at the coronary band and on the sole.
Patella Kneecap, a small mobile bone over the stifle joint.
Pedal bone or third phalangeal bone The last bone in the foot. Fully encased in the hoof.
Periople The softer horn structure that marks the boundary between skin and horn. It is much more pliable and produces a wax that coats the horn and helps regulate the loss of water from the horn affecting how soft or hard it is.
Phenotypic marker A trait that can be seen and measured and that accurately reflects the genetic component of the trait.
Posterior (or caudal) The structure or area nearer to the hind end – 'the back'.
Prevalence The level of a condition seen at a single point in time. It is a product of the

number of incidences and the length of time they last for.

Sacrum Section of the spinal column fused together to form a plate of bone forming the roof to the pelvis (sacral vertebrae).

SARA (subacute ruminal acidosis) A mild reduction in the pH of the rumen producing vague clinical signs in dairy cows.

Scabeous Thickened areas of skin forming plaques or hard areas.

Septic arthritis Inflammation of a joint that is due to a septic or infective process.

Serum The fluid left when blood cells are removed by clotting. It is also used to refer to the fluid products of inflammation.

Sinus An open tract draining a fluid-filled cavity.

Stratum corneum The outer layer of the epidermis in which keratin is laid down (cornification or keratinization).

Stratum germinativum The germinal layer producing cells for the epidermis.

Stratum granulosum The layer below the stratum corneum where cells are dying off.

Subluxation To move out of place only a small amount, e.g. a joint.

Synovial Pertaining to a joint.

Tendon sheaths Fluid-filled sacs around the tendons to lubricate them through other tissues.

Tuber coxae The front 'wings' of the hips.

Tuber ischii The back pins of the pelvis.

Tubular horn Tubes of horn produced by the papillae (corium) of the coronary band or the sole. This is either wall horn or solar horn.

Vegetative endocarditis An infection of the heart valve producing cauliflower-type abscesses on the valve, which are often shed into the bloodstream to produce infection elsewhere.

Ventral The upper side of the body, i.e. upwards.

White line The thin, paler horn that divides the horn of the sole from the horn of the hoof wall.

Index